HANDBOOK OF COMMUNITY CANCER CARE

HANDBOOK OF COMMUNITY CANCER CARE

Mark N. Gaze
MD, FRCP, FRCPEd, FRCR
The Meyerstein Institute of Oncology
The Middlesex Hospital
London

Isobel M. Wilson
BSc (Med Sci), MB ChB
General Practitioner
Edinburgh

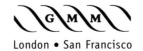
London • San Francisco

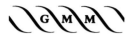

Greenwich Medical Media Limited
4th Floor, 137 Euston Road,
London
NW1 2AA

870 Market Street, Ste 720
San Francisco
CA 94109, USA

ISBN 1849 1 0001 3

First Published 2003

www.greenwich-medical.co.uk

Distributed by Plymbridge Distributors Ltd and in the USA by Jamco Distribution

Typeset by Charon Tec Pvt. Ltd, Chennai, India

Printed in the UK by the Alden Group Ltd, Oxford

Contents

Introduction

We realised some time ago that there is a void between the necessarily hospital based treatment of people with cancer, and care of these patients and their families in the community. Despite the fact that cancer comes second to cardiovascular disease as a cause of death, oncology is generally regarded as a "specialist" subject and therefore is seldom included in any depth in the undergraduate medical curriculum. Similarly, only a few vocational training schemes for general practice include an attachment in oncology or palliative medicine. The GP, therefore, often knows little detail about the specialist treatment of cancer, especially when new or experimental techniques are being used. Similarly, the consultant may be blissfully unaware of the difficulties faced by the GP in the diagnosis of cancer, and in the management of the side effects and the complications of treatment. In addition, communication between the hospital and the community – and also between the community and the hospital – all too frequently is suboptimal. Changes in the public perception of cancer and the internet have made patients and their families both better informed and also more enquiring. Accordingly, their expectation of their doctors is greater.

In recent years, various government initiatives have made the role of the GP in cancer management more important. The Calman-Hine report emphasised the need to deliver care as close to the patient's home as possible – in the community if practicable rather than the cancer unit or the cancer centre. Anxieties about poorer survival rates for some cancer types in Britain compared with abroad led to a focus on delays in the diagnosis and treatment pathway for cancer and the introduction of the two week rule and guidelines for early referral. The introduction of primary care trusts and their involvement in the commissioning of specialist services has also meant that GPs need to know more about cancer.

This volume is an attempt by the authors – one a consultant oncologist, the other a general practitioner with special experience of hospice care – to provide a practical guide to cancer and its management for GPs. We hope that others such as community nurses may also find it useful. Of course there are already many books about cancer, but these are often either far too basic to be of any real use or are texts aimed at specialists in one of the several hospital-based disciplines dedicated to cancer.

This book falls into several sections:

- The first is a general introduction to cancer, and deals with its incidence, causes and prevention. Although much is irrelevant to the actual treatment of someone who has developed cancer, it is surprising how often the first question a patient asks is "doctor, what caused this?"
- The second section relates to the diagnosis of cancer, not just in the patient who presents with symptoms, but also the screening of healthy individuals and those who for some reason are at increased risk.
- The third section is a series of chapters on treatment and rehabilitation, not just with orthodox medical techniques such as surgery and radiotherapy, but also considering complementary medicine and the role of paramedical carers such as speech therapists, dieticians, clinical nurse specialists involved in for example breast and stoma care, and community nurses.
- The next is a major section considering the different cancers by primary site. Collectively, the many rare types of cancer are not uncommon. Because of this, GPs are likely to encounter an unusual cancer from time to time, even though they may never have to look after a patient with most of the other rare cancer types. Rare cancers are therefore described in some detail here, as inevitably GPs will have less experience of these than, for example, breast or lung cancer. They may wish for a readily available source of at least some information on all varieties of cancer.
- There follows a brief section on the special needs of patients in particular age groups: children, adolescents and the elderly
- Section six is devoted to palliative care, death and bereavement. A symptom based chapter deals with the investigation and treatment of many of the more common and distressing symptoms, others with the practical aspects of coping with a death, and caring for the bereaved.
- The final section is a source of contact numbers and addresses of useful organisations such as patient support groups and charities dedicated to cancer research and the relief of cancer suffering, and pointers to sources of more detailed information.

There is inevitably some overlap and repetition between the different sections. This is not an oversight, but a deliberate attempt to make this book easier to use. It is not our intention that it should be read, like a novel, from cover to cover; rather that the reader should use it as a handbook consulting appropriate chapters when necessary.

MNG
IMW
2003

General introduction

SECTION CONTENTS

CHAPTER 1
What causes cancer? – aetiology

One of the most common questions patients ask when they first learn that they have cancer is "but what caused it, doctor?" The most honest answer in many cases is "I don't know". This response can be reassuring for people who seek comfort from knowing that they are not themselves to blame, but may be disturbing for those who like explanations, and who find the concept of "fate" or a random event frightening. In circumstances where the answer is well known, as in the case of the cigarette smoker with lung cancer, a very sensitive reply is required.

WHAT IS THE POINT OF KNOWING?

Is the knowledge of what did or what might have caused an individual patient's cancer ever particularly helpful for that person? Well, it might be. A smoker with early and potentially curable laryngeal cancer may be stimulated to kick the habit and thereby reduce the chances of developing a second and less curable malignancy, such as lung cancer. Similarly, the shock of dad getting cancer may lead other family members to realise the true dangers of smoking. This is a situation where the general practitioner (GP) is well positioned to be an advocate of public health and encourage a more healthy lifestyle.

If the cancer is an occupational illness, such as mesothelioma in a shipyard worker who has been exposed to asbestos, then financial compensation may be offered. If there is suspicion of a familial basis for the cancer, as in the case of a young woman with a strong family history of breast cancer, then appropriate genetic counselling can be offered and preventative measures undertaken if appropriate.

These are the principal reasons why knowledge of the causation of their cancer may benefit an individual patient. Society as a whole may be helped if the discovery of a cause enables avoidance of a risk. In these cases, it may be that government or institutions take on the responsibility for reducing risk, for example, in regulating exposure to hazardous substances in the workplace. Sometimes, individuals have to take responsibility for their own health, for example, by not smoking or by avoiding excessive sun exposure, perhaps encouraged by publicity campaigns which point out the risk.

Many cancers have no known cause, and it is always possible that a vigilant GP may be the first to recognise a possible relationship between an unusual cancer type and workers in a local industry who may be occupationally exposed to a new or unusual carcinogen. Of course, recognition of an association is not proof of cause, but it can be a starting point for further investigation. Remember, fortune favours the prepared mind!

SO WHAT DOES CAUSE CANCER?

Basically, all causes of cancer can be divided into two groups: environmental threats and inherited susceptibility. Sometimes there can be a relationship between these two factors, and it may not always be clear how they interact. For example, it has been noted that Japanese women have a lower incidence of breast cancer than women in the US. Does this have a genetic or environmental basis? The incidence in Japanese migrants living in the US is higher than in women who remain in Japan, but still less than that of American women as a whole. This suggests that there may be a combination of both a lower genetic risk in Japanese women, modified by adverse lifestyle or environmental factors.

> **CAUSES OF CANCER**
> * Environmental factors
> * Inherited susceptibility
> * Other factors

CANCER AND THE ENVIRONMENT

Many different environmental factors may predispose to, or directly cause, the development of cancer. These include occupational exposure to carcinogens, lifestyle factors such as diet, sexual practices and the use of tobacco and alcohol, viral infections such as hepatitis B virus (HBV) and Epstein–Barr virus (EBV) and immunodeficiency, and ionising and non-ionising radiation. These are considered in turn below.

Occupational exposure to carcinogens

Occupational cancers are a changing scene. This is because once a relationship between a cancer and a carcinogen in the workplace is recognised, occupational hygiene measures should be introduced which will, hopefully, make it of historic interest only. At the same time, many new substances are introduced into the working environment each year, and some of these may later be found to have risks which had not previously been appreciated. The eighteenth century surgeon Percivall Pott (after whom Pott's fracture is named) was the first to ascribe any type of cancer to an industrial cause. This was squamous cancer of the skin of the scrotum in London chimney sweeps, which he recognised was due to soot. More recently, shale oil has also been associated with scrotal cancer and there are measures in place to limit skin contact in workers who are exposed to mineral oils.

Exposure to aromatic amines and aniline dyes in the chemical rubber and dyestuffs industries is a definite cause of bladder cancer. This should no longer be encountered in advanced countries, but there may still be a considerable disease burden in countries which do not have effective occupational hygiene legislation.

> **INDUSTRIAL CARCINOGENS, PAST AND PRESENT**
>
> *Organic substances*
>
> | | |
> |---|---|
> | ◆ Polycyclic hydrocarbons in soot and oils | Skin cancers |
> | ◆ Wood or leather dust | Sino-nasal cancer |
> | ◆ Aromatic amines | Bladder cancer |
> | ◆ Aniline dyes | Bladder cancer |
> | ◆ Benzene | Leukaemia |
> | ◆ Vinyl chloride monomer | Hepatic angiosarcoma |
>
> *Inorganic substances*
>
> | | |
> |---|---|
> | ◆ Blue asbestos | Mesothelioma and lung cancer |
> | ◆ Nickel and chromium compounds | Sino-nasal and lung cancer |
>
> *Physical agents*
>
> | | |
> |---|---|
> | ◆ Sunlight | Cancer of the skin and lip |
> | ◆ Radon inhalation in miners | Lung cancer |
> | ◆ Radium ingestion | Bone sarcomas |

Unfortunately, not all industrial hazards can be escaped easily. The use of asbestos was widespread in shipbuilding and the construction industry before the association between blue asbestos (crocidolite) and mesothelioma of the pleura and peritoneum, and lung cancer was recognised. The latent interval between exposure and the development of cancer is measured in decades and is sometimes up to 50 years. Greatest exposure to asbestos dust comes not during construction (when it is known what materials are being used), but during demolition of older structures in which the presence of asbestos may not be expected. This means that although the hazards are recognised, and blue asbestos is no longer used in construction, we may expect to see new cases of mesothelioma for many years to come, as workers who were exposed many years ago develop the disease and current workers may be unwittingly exposed. Not only directly exposed workers may be at risk, cases of mesothelioma have been seen in women whose only exposure was to wash their husbands' work overalls.

An increased incidence of cancer of the nose and sinuses (particularly adenocarcinoma, a rarer type) has been reported amongst hardwood workers in the furniture industry in the Chilterns, and in boot and shoe workers in centres such as Northampton.

Similarly, sino-nasal and lung cancer is associated with workers in the industries which deal with the metals, namely nickel, chromium and arsenic where dusts get into the airways. Arsenic can also cause skin cancer, and one sometimes still sees patients who have repeated problems with Bowen's disease and squamous skin cancers having taken arsenic-containing medications many years ago.

Some workers have been occupationally exposed to radiation. These include the radium dial painters, usually young women, who worked in instrument factories around the time of the Second World War who painted clock faces and instrument dials with luminous paint-containing radium. They habitually moistened their brushes in their mouths, and so ingested radium which caused bone sarcomas. Miners who breathe air containing the radioactive gas radon underground are another occupationally exposed group of workers, at increased risk of lung cancer.

Almost all cancers are more common in industrialised or urban areas. The one type of cancer which is more common in rural workers is cancer of the lower lip in farmers and shepherds who spend long hours out of doors and whose skin is damaged by chronic sunlight exposure.

Lifestyle factors: tobacco and alcohol, diet, sexual practices

Smoking

Smoking has been recognised as an important cause of cancer for half a century. There is an increasing weight of evidence implicating cigarette smoking as the most important cause of lung cancer and also as being of significance in the aetiology of cancers of the oral cavity, larynx and pharynx, uterine cervix and bladder. Approximately, one-third of all cancers in the UK are directly attributable to tobacco use. In addition, smoking is, of course, related to coronary heart disease, stroke and chronic obstructive lung disease. Non-smokers who breathe other people's smoke are also at increased risk of illness. Smoking is hazardous for babies both *in utero* if the mother smokes in pregnancy, and postnatally when exposed to a smoker's atmosphere. More than 100,000 people die prematurely in the UK each year as a result of smoking – a Jumbo jet load every day.

SMOKING-RELATED CANCERS

- Cancer of the bronchus and lung (principally squamous and small cell types)
- Cancer of the oral cavity (also related to chewed or "smokeless" tobacco)
- Cancer of the oropharynx, hypopharynx, larynx and oesophagus
- Cancer of the pancreas
- Cancer of the kidney and urinary bladder
- Cancer of the uterine cervix

Despite widespread knowledge of all these, health warnings on cigarette packets and advertising, increasing taxation of tobacco products, a greater number of no-smoking environments and other measures, it is very disappointing that so many people continue to smoke. It is, perhaps, understandable that elderly life-long smokers may be addicted and are unable to give up, but the increasing popularity of smoking amongst young people, especially teenage girls and young women, is frightening. Another cause for concern is the spread of the smoking epidemic into parts of the world, such as India, Pakistan and China.

How great is the risk from smoking? Over 90% of lung cancer cases are thought to be due to smoking, and for an individual smoker risk increases with increasing number of cigarettes smoked, the number of years over which smoking has continued and smoking cigarettes with a higher tar yield. When a smoker stops, the risk of cancer gradually reduces over about 15 years to that of a non-smoker.

GPs and other health care professionals should be encouraged to be opportunistic in spreading the message about the dangers of smoking and other forms of tobacco use to their patients whenever a suitable moment arises. This could be in a well-woman clinic, or whenever a patient expresses an anxiety about a more trivial health risk, during a consultation for a chest infection (even in childhood) as well as in a cancer-orientated setting.

Alcohol

Alcohol is another widely used substance which can seriously endanger health. Again, other problems such as cirrhosis, malnutrition, dementia, trauma and accidents can be attributed to alcohol misuse as well as cancer. It has been estimated that about 3% of cancers are attributable to alcohol. It is sometimes difficult to separate out the risks of alcohol from those of tobacco as the two often go hand in hand and may be synergistic. Nonetheless, it is clear that alcohol is an independent risk factor for cancers of the mouth, throat and oesophagus. At these sites the combined risk from alcohol and tobacco may be greater than the sum of the individual risks for given level of consumption. Primary liver cancers are also related to alcohol use, and are more common in patients who have established cirrhosis. It is very difficult to separate out different types of alcoholic drinks as being associated with different levels of risk, and it seems likely that it is the alcohol itself rather than any congeners which are carcinogenic. It is probable that neat spirits may have a more damaging effect on oropharyngeal mucosa than the same quantity of alcohol well diluted. The discovery that resveratrol which is present in red wines may have a protective effect is probably not enough to compensate for the harm which alcohol may do. GPs are encouraged to promote moderation in alcohol consumption.

ALCOHOL-RELATED CANCERS

- Cancer of the oral cavity, oropharynx, larynx and hypopharynx
- Cancer of the oesophagus
- Hepatocellular carcinoma
- Cancer of the breast

Diet and nutrition

The effect of diet and nutrition in the aetiology of cancer has been under close scrutiny for decades, but its place is far less clear cut than the role of alcohol and tobacco. This is largely because of the complexity of measuring such a large number of variables in what people eat. Nonetheless, it is becoming increasingly clear that a healthy diet is of great importance. Part of the reason for this is that the main tumour sites for which diet is relevant are the breast, the stomach and the large bowel, which are common diseases.

There seems to be an association between increasing body mass index and breast cancer in post-menopausal women. This may be an endocrine effect as adrenal steroids are metabolised to oestrogens by the enzyme aromatase in fat. The theory that a diet high in saturated fats predisposes to breast cancer has only very limited evidence to support it. Some studies show that a diet rich in fresh vegetables may be protective, others show that deficiencies of dietary vitamin A may predispose to breast cancer.

Similar findings have been reported in relation to stomach cancer, that a diet rich in fresh fruit and vegetables containing anti-oxidants such as vitamin C and β-carotene may be protective. Possibly substances found in preserved food, such as salt and nitrates may predispose to stomach cancer. The high incidence of stomach cancer in Japan has been attributed to the high-dietary intake of smoked and preserved fish.

Saturated fats, particularly animal fats, may predispose individuals to cancer of the colon and rectum, and it is possible that the cooking of meat may produce carcinogens. People who are physically active have a lower risk of colorectal cancer, but obesity itself does not appear to be of importance in this regard. A high-fibre diet is thought to be protective, but whether this is a true effect of the fibre itself or whether it is just a proxy for a high-fruit and -vegetable diet with abundant vitamins and anti-oxidants is not clear.

Sexual lifestyle
Sexual lifestyle is important in relation to cancer risk. Carcinoma of the uterine cervix has many of the attributes of a sexually transmitted disease. It is more common in women who were young when they first had intercourse, and in women who have had many sexual partners. The association between cervical cancer and oral contraceptives may be a proxy either for the number of sexual partners, or correlate with non-use of barrier methods of contraception, such as caps and condoms. Many sexually transmitted viruses have been postulated as a cause for cervical cancer, but now all the evidence seems to implicate certain subtypes (16 and 18) of human papilloma virus (HPV). HPV is also thought to have a causative role in carcinoma of the penis and anus.

Human immunodeficiency virus (HIV) infection is predominantly a sexually transmitted disease, although of course there are other modes of transmission including the sharing of needles contaminated with blood by drug abusers, and the materno-foetal route. Patients with HIV infection are at risk of a number of cancers including Kaposi's sarcoma, squamous carcinomas of the cervix and anus, and non-Hodgkin's lymphomas (NHLs). Many of these cancers may not be due directly to HIV, but to coincidentally transmitted viruses which cause cancer in immunocompromised individuals.

Viral infections and immunodeficiency

That viruses may cause cancer, and that immunocompromised patients may be at greater risk has been alluded to above in relation to sexual lifestyle, but there are other examples of viruses which may cause cancer.

The Epstein Barr Virus (EBV) is widespread and almost everyone will have EBV infection, usually in the form of glandular fever, at some time in their lives. Cancers usually develop on a background of chronic infection, under the influence of other factors. For example, in the sub-Saharan region of Africa, children tend to acquire EBV infection earlier in their life than in the case in Europe or America. Chronic malaria and malnutrition are endemic and may result in some immunological compromise. It is this combination of factors which is thought to lead to the development of Burkitt's lymphoma in this area.

VIRUSES ASSOCIATED WITH CANCER	
◆ EBV	Nasopharyngeal cancer Burkitt's lymphoma Immunoblastic lymphoma Hodgkin's disease
◆ HPV-16, HPV-18	Cervical cancer Anal cancer HPV-5 Skin cancer
◆ HBV	Hepatocellular carcinoma
◆ Hepatitis C virus (HCV)	Hepatocellular carcinoma
◆ Human T-cell lymphotrophic virus (HTLV-1)	T-cell leukaemia
◆ HIV	Lymphoma
◆ Kaposi's sarcoma herpes virus (KSHV)	Kaposi's sarcoma

Nasopharyngeal carcinoma is uncommon in most of the world, but is one of the commonest types of cancer in south-east Asia, notably Hong Kong and certain provinces of China. Chinese communities in other parts of the world tend to have incidence rates intermediate between those of China and their adoptive country, whereas immigrant communities in China do not have increased risk. The cause is thought to be an interaction between EBV and dietary factors, such as salted and preserved fish with a high-nitrosamine content, in a genetically susceptible population.

Chronically immunosupressed patients, for example, those with congenital immunodeficiency syndromes, those who have had organ transplants and those with HIV infection are at risk of EBV-driven lymphoproliferative disorders. These may regress if immune competence can be restored, for example, by lowering the doses of immuno-suppressive drugs in transplant recipients if this can be done without causing rejection of the grafted organ.

However, it may progress to become a true malignant lymphoma. EBV infection is thought to be causally related to some other lymphoid cancers, including Hodgkin's disease and immunoblastic NHL, even in the absence of underlying immunosupression.

Immunosupressed patients are also at greater risk of squamous cancers, not just of the cervix and anus as described above in relation to sexual lifestyle and HPV types 16 and 18, but also of the skin. The epidemic Kaposi's sarcoma found in HIV-infected people is caused by another sexually transmitted virus, KSHV.

HTLV-1, found in the Japanese and Caribbean populations, causes adult T-cell leukaemia. This only arises many years after the original infection, and only in a small proportion of those infected. The other factors which promote carcinogenesis in this case are not known.

HBV is a widespread virus, transmitted sexually and by infected blood. It usually causes acute hepatitis, but sometime chronic liver disease develops leading to cirrhosis and hepatocellular carcinoma. The incidence of HBV-related liver cancer varies considerably worldwide. It is most prevalent in the Far East and in sub-Saharan Africa. Food stored in tropical regions is often contaminated by the mould *Aspergillus*, which produces a carcinogenic substance called aflatoxin. Aflatoxin and HBV are thought to work together in many cases to produce hepatocellular cancer. Chronic HCV infection, which was transmitted by blood transfusions before it could be detected, is now also linked with the development of liver cancer.

The possible role of as yet unidentified viruses causing childhood leukaemia in areas of population mixing is discussed in Chapter 46.

Taken together, all these viral causes of cancer account for a significant cancer burden worldwide. It is estimated that up to 20% of all human cancers may be caused by viruses, although the proportion in the UK is far less. Many are potentially preventable by screening, vaccination, improvement in the quality of food supplies and control of blood-borne infection.

Although most attention has been paid to viruses, other infections and infestations may play some part. *Helicobacter pylori* infection is now firmly associated with the development of stomach cancer as well as peptic ulceration. Both these diseases are now significantly less common than they used to be. In part this may be due to better food hygiene, but specific treatments of *H. pylori* may also play a part. Some bile duct cancers seen in Asia been attributed to liver fluke infestation.

Radiation

There is abundant evidence that ionising radiation is implicated in the causation of cancer. Studies of survivors of the two atom bombs detonated in Japan in 1945 showed a significant increase in both leukaemias

and other cancers. The incidence of cancer is greater in children whose mothers underwent X-ray pelvimetry antenatally. Use of radiological contrast media containing the radioactive element thorium had a higher risk of leukaemia and liver cancer than controls. Women undergoing repeated flouroscopic examinations in the era when artificial pneumothorax was a popular treatment for tuberculosis had a higher risk of developing breast cancer on the ipsilateral side. Patients treated with radiotherapy for benign conditions including ringworm of the scalp, ankylosing spondylitis, and presumed thymic enlargement in childhood had a significantly increased risk of developing a range of malignancies including leukaemia, basal and squamous skin cancers, and thyroid cancer. Second malignant neoplasms in survivors of cancer may in some cases be attributed to treatment of the original tumour with radiotherapy, although other factors such as smoking, chemotherapy and genetic susceptibility may also play a part.

The good thing about unnatural radiation exposure as a cause of cancer is that once the risk has been recognised it can to a very large extent be avoided, and so most of the problems referred to above are now only of historic interest. Natural radiation exposure may be more difficult to avoid. In some parts of the UK, the geological structure allows radon gas to leak from the ground. This can accumulate in houses and may result in lung cancer. The problem can be exacerbated by double glazing and the loss of natural ventilation, but can be prevented by sealing of the floors, although this is clearly an expensive investment. Cosmic radiation is unavoidable, and levels received are greater while flying in aeroplanes than at ground level. The full significance of this is not known, but there are some data to suggest that breast cancer may be more common in air stewardesses.

Skin cancer is the most common group of cancers worldwide. Sun exposure is probably the most important factor in the aetiology of all skin cancer types. Natural skin pigmentation is protective, and so non-melanoma skin cancer is rare in dark skinned races. Amongst "white" people, it is significantly more common in those with red hair and fair skins than in those who tan easily. Non-melanoma skin cancer is more common in men than women, and on the sun-exposed parts of the body, such as the face and the forearms and backs of the hands. In fact, more than half develop on the head and neck. In women, lower limb sites are more commonly seen. Chronic sun exposure may be more important for the development of squamous cancers whereas sunburn episodes may have a greater relevance for basal cell cancers and melanoma.

INHERITED SUSCEPTIBILITY

That some cancers are more common or less common in particular races or communities may be completely or in

Handbook of Community Cancer Care

part an inherited situation attributable to the genetic makeup. An example would be that black people are less likely to develop skin cancer. This fits in with Darwinian theories of evolution, in that over the millennia pigmentation clearly protects against carcinogenesis in sunny countries and confers a survival advantage. The epidemiology of nasopharyngeal cancer probably explained in part by genetics and in part by other factors. In other cases, such as the varying incidence of hepatocellular carcinoma throughout the world referred to above, the observation is probably an epiphenomenon related to lifestyle factors and infectious disease epidemiology rather than attributable to genetic differences between races.

Some cancers show a clear family history in a proportion of instances, but always sporadic cases outnumber familial ones. The classic example is retinoblastoma, discussed in more detail in Chapter 46.

Breast cancer is a common disease – the lifetime risk for a woman is about 1 : 12. So for, two women in the same family to have the disease purely by chance would not be uncommon. Familial breast cancer is in fact rare, accounting for only 5–10% of cases, overall, but a greater proportion of early onset disease. A familial form of the disease is more likely if there are at least three affected close family members, if it occurs in women under the age of 40, if there is bilateral disease, or if other family members have other cancer types, most notably ovarian or colon cancer. Several genes have now been identified in breast cancer families (see box). Of these, the *BRCA1* gene identified in 1994 and located on the long arm of chromosome 17, accounts for most familial cases. The prevalence of this gene in the community is only about 1 : 500, but in some populations, such as Ashkenazi Jews the prevalence may be as high as 1%. The individual risk of a *BRCA1* carrier developing breast cancer has been variously estimated as 60–85%.

FAMILIAL BREAST CANCER PREDISPOSITION SYNDROMES

- BRCA1
- BRCA2
- Li Fraumeni syndrome
- Cowden disease
- Hereditary non-polyposis colon cancer
- Ataxia telangiectasia

Bowel cancer is another common disease associated with a number of familial syndromes, the commonest being familial adenomatous polyposis, formerly known as hereditary polyposis coli. This is inherited as an autosomal dominant condition with a high degree of penetrance. Affected individuals have hundreds or thousands of benign colonic polyps, one or more of which will almost inevitably turn malignant given time. Patients are also at risk of developing other tumours including the rare connective tissue desmoid tumour. Other familial bowel cancer predisposition syndromes give rise to what is called hereditary non-polyposis colon cancer. Probably, only about 1% of colon cancer patients have a familial form. In all the familial forms, colon cancers tend to arise at an earlier age than usual, are more often multiple and arise with equal frequency in all parts of the colon, and so are more likely to be proximal than is the case for sporadic tumours.

FAMILIAL BOWEL CANCER PREDISPOSITION SYNDROMES

- Familial adenomatous polyposis
- Hereditary non-polyposis colon cancer
- Gardener's syndrome

The Li Fraumeni syndrome referred to above is another dominantly inherited susceptibility to cancer, due to a mutation of the tumour suppressor gene *p53*. The commonly seen tumour types are brain tumours, breast cancer, sarcomas and leukaemia. Characteristically, the age of onset of cancer is at a younger age in each succeeding generation of the pedigree.

Every cell in the body is at risk of sustaining DNA damage because of carcinogens, radiation or other factors. That so few people develop cancer as a result of these mutations, is because we are equipped with some very effective repair mechanisms to restore damaged DNA to normal. There are a number of rare diseases, inherited in an autosomal recessive manner, in which these repair mechanisms are defective. Affected individuals are, therefore, predisposed to cancer. These include xeroderma pigmentosum, in which multiple skin cancers of all types develop in sun-exposed skin. Most patients die before the age of 20, and before internal cancers develop. In Blooms syndrome, there is also a predisposition to leukaemia as well as skin cancer. In ataxia telangiectasia, homozygous individuals develop cerebellar ataxia and telangiectasia, usually first apparent on the conjunctiva. They are more at risk of leukaemia and brain tumours, such as medulloblastoma. Ataxia telangiectasia heterozygotes also have an increased susceptibility to breast cancer, and can be more sensitive to the side-effects of DNA-damaging treatments, such as radiotherapy and chemotherapy.

The management of families who might be at risk of having a familial predisposition to cancer is discussed further in Chapter 4.

OTHER FACTORS

Several other factors have been implicated in the development of cancer. The most important of these are endocrine in nature. Although breast cancer can occur in both sexes, female breast cancer is numerically by far the most important. Breast development is a secondary sexual characteristic under hormonal control. Breast cancer is more likely in women who have an early menarche and a late menopause, their breast tissue has been subject to the influence of a larger number of menstrual cycles. Early pregnancy is protective, especially if the baby was breast-fed. Nulliparity, or pregnancy late in the reproductive life-time is associated with a greater than average risk. There is some evidence that users of the oral contraceptive pill may be at somewhat higher risk. As it takes many years to get epidemiological data, it may be that the types of pill used decades ago, which had a higher oestrogen content, may be associated with more risk than more modern formulations, or that the risk relates more to effective contraception and delayed childbearing than it does to the actual contraceptive itself. For the majority of women, the pill has no effect on their chances of getting breast cancer, and any risk has, of course, to be offset against the risks associated with unwanted pregnancies. Taking hormone-replacement therapy (HRT), especially for very long periods such as for 10 or more years, may also be associated with a slightly increased risk of breast cancer. Again, such risks need to be considered in relation to the good which HRT may do. More modern forms of HRT, such as raloxifene (which is related to tamoxifen), may possibly be protective against the development of breast cancer.

Endometrial cancer is another hormonally dependent neoplasm. It is more common in obese women, as aromatase enzymes in fat cause peripheral conversion of adrenal precursors to oestrogen. Oestrogen-only forms of HRT, should not be used in women with an intact uterus as unopposed stimulation of the endometrium will occur which can lead to malignancy. Progesterone-containing preparations which are associated with a regular withdrawal bleed like a period should be used in non-hysterectomised patients.

The thyroid gland is another endocrine organ, and well-differentiated papillary cancers are more common if untreated hypothyroidism causes prolonged thyroid-stimulating hormone (TSH) stimulation.

CONCLUSIONS

At first sight, an understanding of the causes of cancer may be of little relevance to the GP, apart from enabling a reply to a question from a patient about causation in some instances. On the other hand, knowledge of potential causes may enable a GP to be proactive in both primary and secondary prevention, and these aspects are discussed further in Chapter 2.

Healthy lifestyle and the avoidance of cancer

General practitioners (GPs) are already playing an important part in preventive medicine and health promotion. Routine assessment of child development, immunisation programmes, family planning and antenatal care are all aimed at keeping people healthy and at picking up problems early at a stage when remedial action can be taken, hopefully preventing long-term harm.

The GP has many opportunities, some structured, some opportunistic, for intervention to reduce the incidence and effects of cancer. Some of this is truly preventive in intention, aimed at helping patients to avoid some of the risk factors described in Chapter 1. Others relate more to the early investigation of symptomatic cancer, and screening for asymptomatic disease with the aim of treating cancers at their earliest stages when they are hopefully more easily curable.

OPPORTUNITIES FOR PREVENTION

For the most part, the GP's greatest opportunity for preventative intervention must be in regard to lifestyle factors, smoking and drinking, diet and sexual health. Fortunately, a lifestyle which is healthy in regard to cancer is also healthy in regard to other major causes of illness and death, such as heart disease, stroke and peripheral vascular disease, and chronic obstructive lung disease. The GP is not in a good position to reduce occupational cancer risks; this is essentially in the remit of occupational health medicine and public health medicine doctors, and also a governmental responsibility in framing appropriate health and safety legislation and in ensuring that it is policed. Nonetheless, a GP can certainly reinforce good practice when talking to patients, such as in encouraging workers to use protective clothing when appropriate, and to reassure them that safety regulations in the workplace exist to protect them and should be adhered to.

Smoking is the single lifestyle factor of greatest importance in cancer causation. Most patients who smoke know that already, and many wish to give up but are addicted. Others, particularly teenage girls, feel that the immediate benefits of smoking in terms of social status, keeping their weight at what they perceive to be "correct" and appearing to be "grown up", outweigh any risks which may be decades away, and succumb to peer group pressure. Many teenagers consider themselves to be immortal.

GPs can reinforce in the patient's mind the benefits to health which will be gained; they can attempt to quantify the financial gain (let us face it, smoking is a pretty expensive hobby); and they can point out other reasons why it might be beneficial to stop or harmful to continue. Leaflets and posters in the waiting area and consulting room may be helpful. GPs who have any institutional role, perhaps as school doctors, can help to impart the message there. Evangelism alone, however, is not enough.

GPs need to be sympathetic to the difficulties faced by smokers who do wish to give up, but find it too difficult. More importantly, patients may value practical advice about how to stop, how to reduce that craving and how to respond in social situations where the temptation to light up again might be greatest. Nicotine patches, chewing gum and inhalers may be beneficial for those who wish to give up, but have a strong physical addiction to nicotine. Bupropion is a recently licensed oral therapy, designed to help adult smokers give up. It is said to be more effective than nicotine-replacement therapy. Advice about dietary modification and exercise may be helpful to those who fear weight gain as a consequence of smoking cessation. Nearly, everybody who stops smoking puts on weight, partly not only because of decreasing basal metabolic rate but also increased appetite. However, often about half of the initial weight gain disappears spontaneously. Patients who smoke more because of stress in their lives might benefit if they could be taught to reduce their stress levels, or to manage their stress more effectively. There are smokers' helplines, which can provide advice and support.

THE SMOKERS' HELPLINE

- England (Quitline): 0800 002200
- Scotland (Smokeline): 0800 848484
- Northern Ireland: 01232 663281
- Wales: 0345 697500

It is difficult for a person to stop smoking by himself, especially when others at home might continue to do so. How about encouraging a husband and wife to stop at the same time? How about promoting local self-help groups, perhaps tied in with well-publicised national events, such as the annual no-smoking day? Doctors who have an occupational health role can help by trying to get employers to institute a no smoking at work policy, or failing that to ensure that facilities, such as canteens and coffee rooms, are no-smoking environments. The GP as an employer can make the workplace a better environment. Is your practice a smoke-free zone?

As with smoking, the benefits from moderating excess drinking habits extend in the health field to more than cancer, and in society to more than just health. GPs can help to educate their patients about safe levels of alcohol consumption, and can keep an eye out for patients who may have a drinking problem as the underlying reason for an individual consultation. When patients with difficulties are identified, targeted help can be offered.

Of course, in many settings, heavy drinking and smoking may be too deeply entrenched habits personally or culturally for an individual GP to make any impact. Denial is commonplace, even in the face of unequivocal blood test results. Nonetheless, just because a problem often proves to be insoluble, it does not mean that a solution should not be sought. One may not win every battle, but each reformed character is a worthwhile achievement.

If it is difficult to influence people's behaviour with regard to tobacco and alcohol, it must be equally difficult to influence sexual practices. To advise fidelity within marriage, and sexual abstinence outside marriage in this era is an unrealistic counsel of perfection. Probably, the most sensible goal here is to encourage safer sexual practices, such as the use of condoms in casual sexual encounters, even if other contraceptive methods are also in use. People with high-risk patterns of behaviour should be immunised against hepatitis B, and sensitive consideration should be given to HIV testing with pre-test counselling in appropriate cases. Prompt treatment of sexually acquired infections should limit the spread of these and other infections. Cervical screening is considered in more detail below and in Chapter 6.

It may be somewhat easier to modify diet. Overall calorific intake should be reduced to treat obesity, and keep the body mass index at a healthy level. Greater benefit will be obtained by reducing the fat component to less than 30% of overall calories. It is, especially, important to limit saturated fat, which comes principally from animal sources. It may be helpful to limit red meat consumption, and, particularly, cured and preserved food, which contain salt and nitrates, such as salt beef and bacon. Fresh fruits, vegetables and fibre intake should be increased. This may help to offset the calorie reduction and will have independent benefits. Exercise should be encouraged as part of a healthy lifestyle. The principal benefits are cardiovascular, but it is also as important as dietary factors in limiting obesity, and it may have independent effects in reducing the risk from bowel cancer.

A further role for the GP as a lifestyle guru comes in advising about safe sun exposure and the risks of sunburn, especially in children and babies. Even children who go outside at school during break time and lunchtime in summer should use sunscreens, preferably under supervision. Modern sunscreens provide protection against both UVA rays, which cause malignant melanoma, and UVB rays, which cause non-melanoma skin cancer and sunburn. Use of broad spectrum (four star) and high-factor (e.g. 20) sunscreens is recommended. A good time to be opportunistic in respect of sun exposure is when families come for their immunisations prior to holidays in exotic overseas resorts. As the Australians say, "slip, slop, slap": wear a hat, cover bare skin and use sunscreen.

EARLY DETECTION OF SYMPTOMATIC DISEASE

The GP will be well aware that for most cancers, earlier diagnosis may increase the chances of cure. Similarly, it is well known that most of the classic symptoms of cancer are those of advanced disease, when the value of intervention may be significantly less. The trick, therefore, is to be aware that many vague and non-specific symptoms could herald the arrival of an early cancer, particularly, in higher-risk groups.

WHAT EVERY SMOKER SHOULD KNOW

What to look out for
If you have any of the following symptoms – especially if you smoke or have smoked in the past, you should go to your doctor for advice. But remember that often there is a simple explanation for such symptoms, so do not worry unnecessarily:

- A chest infection that does not get better
- Coughing up blood
- A cough that is changing or has been troubling you more
- Feeling more breathless than usual
- Chest pain
- Voice changes that last for more than 3 weeks, for example hoarseness
- Problems with swallowing
- Feeling generally unwell and tired

(from the Macmillan Cancer Relief leaflet *No time to draw breath?*)

Investigation of these patients will inevitably turn up a lot of negative results, but it might save a life or two. The government is at last beginning to take the cancer problem seriously, and one of its measures has been to introduce the 2-week rule. This means that patients with a suspected cancer should not have to wait for more than 2 weeks for hospital investigation after referral by their GP.

"One stop clinics" are being introduced for the investigation of women with breast lumps or other breast symptoms, such as non-menstrual pain, nipple discharge and breast deformity, which could be due to cancer. At these clinics, women will undergo triple assessment with clinical examination, imaging, usually with mammography and/or ultrasound, and fine needle aspiration for cytology in one session. Most of them will be found to have benign disease and be reassured or treated as necessary. It was used to be said that 1 in 10 women with a breast lump had cancer, nowadays because of increasing numbers of referrals to breast clinics, both GP initiated and on patients' own request, only 1 in 20 will have. Similarly, one stop clinics or "quick, early diagnosis clinics" are being introduced by appropriate hospital specialities for the investigation of, for example, persistent hoarseness, which could be due to laryngeal cancer; haematuria, which could be due to a variety of urinary tract cancers; and rectal bleeding and change in bowel habit.

Late diagnosis can often be attributed to patients' late presentation to GPs. Patients may fear that a lump in the breast is cancer, and go into a state of denial. Sometimes, having noticed a breast lump, a patient will arrange to visit their GP on a spurious pretext, being too embarrassed or frightened to mention the real reason. On other occasions, patients may notice, for example, a mole, and imagine that it is more likely to be benign than not. Although they wish for reassurance, they may fail to seek attention because they feel the doctor will be too busy, or worry that they may be ridiculed for presenting with something, which turns out to be trivial.

GPs can help this sort of anxiety by trying to encourage a climate of openness in their practice. They should be aware that the ostensible reason given for a consultation may not be the real one. They can promote, verbally or with posters or leaflets, a positive attitude about what can be done for cancer. Leaflets, which may be valuable may be obtained from various organisations, such as CancerBACUP and Macmillan Cancer Relief (see Chapter 57). GPs should encourage patients to seek advice about any symptom, which could herald a cancer, such as a lump, swelling or ulcer, any abnormal bleeding, any persistent unexplained fatigue, indigestion or abdominal pain, weight loss or change in bowel habit.

SCREENING FOR ASYMPTOMATIC CANCER

All GPs are involved in screening for cancer. The national programmes for cervical-cancer screening and breast-cancer screening are now well established and, generally, believed to be effective, although some issues remain controversial, and there have been well-publicised instances where the quality of the service has fallen short. Screening programmes for other cancers, such as colorectal cancer, prostate cancer, ovarian cancer and lung cancer are still experimental. Screening is considered fully in Chapter 6.

CONCLUSIONS

Much of this chapter can usefully be summarised by The European Union's guidelines aimed at reducing cancer risk and encouraging earlier diagnosis, called the European code against cancer.

THE EUROPEAN CODE AGAINST CANCER

- Do not smoke. Smokers, stop as quickly as possible and do not smoke in the presence of others
- Moderate your consumption of alcoholic drinks – beers, wines and spirits
- Avoid excessive exposure to the sun
- Follow health and safety instructions at work concerning production, handling or use of any substance, which may cause cancer
- Eat fresh fruits and vegetables frequently, and cereals with a high-fibre content
- Avoid becoming overweight and limit your intake of fatty foods
- See a doctor if you notice a lump or observe a change in a mole or experience abnormal bleeding
- See a doctor if you have persistent problems, such as a persistent cough, persistent hoarseness, change in bowel habit or unexplained weight loss
- Women: have a cervical smear regularly
- Women: check your breasts regularly, and if possible undergo mammography at regular intervals over the age of 50

CHAPTER 3

Patterns of cancer occurrence – epidemiology

Cancer is a very unevenly spread disease, or group of diseases. Incidence figures for different types vary not just between different countries, but also within countries. A particular cancer type may show varying incidence according to age, sex, race and social class. Over time, some cancers become more common, while the incidence of others decline.

> **VARIATIONS IN CANCER INCIDENCE**
>
> ◆ By country
> ◆ By age group
> ◆ By sex
> ◆ By social class
> ◆ By race
> ◆ Changes over the course of time

A knowledge of these patterns is necessary for those responsible for commissioning cancer services, and may also give some insight into the cause (Chapter 1). It can also be helpful for a GP in gauging how likely an individual patient in his practice presenting with a particular symptom is to have developed a certain cancer.

INTERNATIONAL VARIATIONS IN CANCER INCIDENCE

Globally, carcinoma of the breast is the most frequent cancer encountered in women; however, its incidence does vary geographically. It is most common in the US, from where incidence rates of from about 90 to over 100 per 100,000 are reported. Intermediate rates of 50–70 are seen in Europe, with the lowest rates of about 5–20 occurring in the Middle and Far East and in some African countries.

Lung cancer is the most common cancer reported in men worldwide. The highest incidence rates, often exceeding 100 per 100,000 are seen in the US, especially in the black population, and in New Zealand Maoris. The rate in the west of Scotland is similar. At present, low rates of the order of 5–15 per 100,000 are found in India, Africa and South America, where the level of cigarette smoking has not been high. These rates are set to rise in years to come as international tobacco companies seek new markets to replace lost cigarette sales in North America and Europe.

Colon cancer is most common in North America, from where incidence rates of between 25 and 35 per 100,000

are reported. By contrast, rates in India, Africa and the Far East are much lower at less than 5 per 100,000.

There is more than 10-fold variation in the incidence of stomach cancer across the world. It is commonest in Japan, where rates of 70 to over 90 are seen in men, contrasting with rates of about 5 per 100,000 in most of the US.

Oesophageal cancer has probably the biggest variability of any cancer throughout the world. It is most common in a band of southern Asia called the oesophageal cancer belt, which extends from eastern China through the southern republics of the former Soviet Union to Iran. In places, the rates here approach 200 per 100,000. Moderately high rates of 15–25 occur in parts of Europe and South America, but in many parts of the world, the incidence rates are only 1–2 per 100,000. There can be quite marked local variations, for example the highest rates in men in Europe are found in north-east France, and the highest rates in women in Europe occur in Scotland and Ireland.

Nasopharyngeal cancer is, in general, rare. It is, particularly, common in parts of China and south-east Asia, and to a lesser extent in immigrant Chinese populations in other countries.

Hepatocellular cancer, although rare in Europe and North America (rates about 1–2 per 100,000) is very common in sub-Saharan Africa and the Far East, with rates between about 30 and 90 variously being reported in different countries, including what is a rare cancer from the British perspective into the top 10 of cancers worldwide.

Top 10 cancers worldwide

	Men	(%)	Women	(%)
1	Lung	17	Breast	19
2	Stomach	12	Cervix	12
3	Large bowel	9	Large bowel	9
4	Prostate	8	Stomach	7
5	Mouth and pharynx	7	Lung	6
6	Liver	6	Ovary	4
7	Oesophagus	5	Mouth and pharynx	4
8	Bladder	5	Lymphoma	4
9	Lymphoma	5	Oesophagus	3
10	Leukaemia	3	Liver	3
	Others	23	Others	29

Cancer of the uterine cervix, although becoming increasingly rare in many countries with well-developed health services as a result of cytological screening, is the second most common cause of cancer in women world-wide, and the leading female cancer in sub-Saharan Africa, Central and South America and south-east Asia, where rates are about 30–50 per 100,000. The lowest incidence rates, only 2–4 per 100,000 are found in Kuwait and Israel. Endometrial cancer is most common in the US, where rates are around 20, and least common in India and some African countries, where the incidence is only about 2 per 100,000.

Prostate cancer shows large geographical and racial variations. It is second only to lung cancer among black populations in the US, where incidence rates range from 60 to about 100 per 100,000. In low-risk populations, such as China, Thailand and India, rates are under 5 per 100,000. The true incidence of prostate cancer may well be under-estimated, as many cases are asymptomatic and post-mortem studies often reveal the presence of undiagnosed prostate cancers in the elderly. Screening programmes will lead to the condition being diagnosed more frequently.

The international variation in bladder cancer relates to the histological type. Transitional cell carcinoma accounts for the majority of cases in much of the world, but in the Middle East and parts of Africa, where the parasitic condition schistosomiasis is common, there are high rates of squamous carcinoma of the bladder. In Cairo, bladder cancer accounts for 29% of all cancer cases in men, and 11% of cases in women.

AGE VARIATIONS

The incidence rates for most cancer types rise gradually with age. Most of the common cancer types are rare in children and young adults, becoming more common in the fifth decade of life and being seen with increasing frequency in older age groups. Exceptions to this pattern are discussed here. The incidence of childhood cancers at different ages is discussed in Chapter 46.

Osteosarcoma is often wrongly thought of as being exclusively a disease of adolescents and young adults. It is rare before the age of 10 years, and the peak incidence in young people is at around 20 years. Between 30 and 60 years, the disease is uncommon, but the incidence rises rapidly in old age, due to an association with Paget's disease of bone in the elderly. The incidence in 80-year olds is in fact two to three times as great as in 20-year olds.

Malignant melanoma, despite increasing incidence, is still a rare cancer accounting for only about 1% of all cancers. It does, however, occur earlier in life than many of the more common cancers, and is the leading cause of cancer incidence in white males aged 35–44 years in the US.

The two major types of testicular cancer, seminoma and non-seminomatous germ cell tumours (testicular teratoma) occur principally in young men, but the patterns of incidence vary. Non-seminomatous tumours have a peak in men in their twenties and are much less common in older men. Seminomas are less common in the twenties, and the band of peak incidence is wider than for teratomas extending through the thirties and forties with a lower incidence in older men.

Cancers of the salivary glands, thyroid gland and nasopharynx are all relatively rare in the UK. They may all occur at virtually any age, and constitute a greater proportion of the cancer burden in young adults than they do in the elderly.

Hodgkin's disease is also another relatively uncommon cancer, which can occur at virtually any age. In the UK and most Western populations, there is a peak incidence in the twenties, and a gradual rise in incidence in later life. In developing countries, the initial peak occurs earlier, in children under the age of 10 years, perhaps due to age at exposure to a possible viral cause.

SEX VARIATIONS

Some cancers, such as prostate, testis and penis cancers in men, and ovarian, cervical and uterine cancers in women, can only occur in one sex. The breast is often thought of as being an exclusively female organ, but men have breast tissue too, and so can get breast cancer. Because of the strong hormonal influences in the aetiology of breast cancer, and the very much smaller volume of breast tissue in men, fewer than 1% of breast cancers occur in males.

For most other common cancer types, men are at greater risk than women. The male preponderance of lung cancer is easily explained by the differences in smoking habits, and the disparity is lessening due to an increase in the number of female smokers and a reduction in the number of men who smoke. The male preponderance of cancers of the stomach, oesophagus, nasopharynx, liver, pancreas, kidney, bladder and non-Hodgkin's lymphoma is less easily explicable, although exposure to tobacco smoke and other carcinogens must play a part.

The sex ratio in some cancers, such as colorectal cancer, malignant melanoma and Hodgkin's disease is nearer to unity. The only example of a cancer in a non-sex-related organ, which is significantly more common in women than men, is thyroid cancer, and in this regard the sex ratio, about 3 : 1, mirrors that of benign thyroid disease.

SOCIAL CLASS DIFFERENCES

In the UK, there are strong social class differences for some cancer types. These are principally those related to lifestyle factors such as smoking and drinking. The incidence of lung cancer, cervical cancer, stomach cancer and squamous cancers of the upper aerodigestive tract are all associated with deprivation and lower socio-economic class. In addition to the increased incidence rate of cervical cancer in deprived areas of the UK, the likelihood of mortality rates is greater in these patients than it is for patients with cervical cancer from a more affluent background. Interestingly, however, stage for stage outcomes show no difference related to social class. This is because a greater proportion of cases in lower socio-economic groups are advanced at diagnosis, reflecting a failure of the screening programme rather than poor provision or utilisation of treatment facilities for established disease.

Fewer cancers seem to be more common in more advantaged sections of the community, but ovarian cancer seems to fall into this category.

RACIAL DIFFERENCES IN CANCER INCIDENCE

At first sight, one might expect many of the geographical variations in cancer incidence referred to earlier in this chapter to be related to underlying differences in racial susceptibility. However, environmental factors are often a more plausible explanation for geographical variations. For example, the high incidence of stomach cancer seen in Japan falls within a generation among Japanese migrants to the US, and conversely the low risk of breast cancer in women in Japan has risen in the same migrant community. In both cases, failure of the levels in the immigrants to completely equalise with those of the native populations may suggest a genetic component, or indicate that some cultural lifestyle differences are retained.

In other cases, apparent racial differences in some countries may be due to social factors and levels of deprivation rather than to true racial differences. For example, black populations in the US have significantly greater levels of cancers of the lung, oesophagus and prostate than the corresponding white communities. The uniformly high incidence of colo-rectal cancers in both black and white people in the US contrasts with the low incidence in African countries, and again suggests that it is environmental factors rather than race, which is important.

On the other hand, the very low incidence of both malignant melanoma and non-melanoma skin cancer in black people compared with white people is without doubt a true racial difference in susceptibility due to the protective effect of skin pigmentation.

CHANGES IN CANCER INCIDENCE OVER TIME

The patterns of cancer incidence described above are not stable and are changing over time. In the case of cervical cancer, this is as a result of successful screening for pre-malignant changes, but most often the changes are due to alterations in exposure to lifestyle factors. In some cases, the reasons are not known.

Cancer of the stomach used to be the world's most commonly fatal cancer, but the incidence has reduced significantly in all communities over recent decades. This probably has a multifactorial basis and is not fully understood.

Both the incidence and the mortality of cervical carcinoma are decreasing in the UK, despite lifestyle changes over the last 40 years, which could have been expected to have increased the incidence. This is largely due to the result of the efficacy of screening programmes based on exfoliative cytology. GPs are in a key position to ensure that women accept their invitations to attend for cervical smear tests. This remains true even if the invitations come from a well-woman clinic and not directly from the practice. Often, it is inertia which prevents women attending for their smear. If a GP directly contacts non-attenders by phone, a suitable appointment can often be arranged.

There is evidence for a reduction in the risk of ovarian cancer in the UK for women born later in the twentieth century, which may in part be due to the protective effect of the oral contraceptive pill.

As a result of the international smoking epidemic of the twentieth century, the incidence of lung cancer rose dramatically in the UK from the 1950s onwards. The levels in men peaked and have been gradually declining over the last 20 years. The rise in rates in women was later to start, but unfortunately is still continuing as an upward trend, reducing the difference between the sexes. Mortality from lung cancer in women now exceeds that from breast cancer in some parts of the UK.

Both malignant melanoma and testicular tumours are on the increase in the UK. The former relates to increased sun exposure, but the reasons for the latter have not yet been satisfactorily explained. Fortunately, the mortality from both these conditions is now declining, as a result of earlier diagnosis for melanoma, and because of the development of effective chemotherapy for germ cell tumours.

Prostate cancer is becoming more common. In part, the rise in incidence is due to the increasing discovery of early, so-called "latent" carcinomas, which might never have become clinically apparent. There is also a genuine underlying rise in incidence.

CONCLUSIONS

The variable patterns of the different cancer types in the community is a fascinating area of study. The association of various cancers with particular social and demographic factors has lead to a greater understanding of the causes of many cancer types. It is important for the future that trends are carefully monitored as these may give an early warning of new risks, and will prove or disprove the value of interventions designed to prevent or cure cancer.

Cancer in families – genetics

There is an inherited predisposition in about 5% of cancer patients (as mentioned in Chapter 1, along with a review of the various familial syndromes). In this chapter, we focus on the assessment of patients who may be at risk of one of the more common types involving breast, bowel or ovarian cancer, and the management of families in whom a genetic predisposition is identified. There is increasing public awareness of cancer genetics, but many people have an inaccurate perception of risk and unrealistic expectations of what a cancer genetics clinic might be able to do for them. The general practitioner (GP) may take the opportunity to explain, for example, to a young woman that her 20 cigarettes a day habit is a substantially greater health risk, both of lung cancer and of other smoking-related diseases, than the fact that her 85-year-old grandmother has just been found to have breast cancer.

RECOGNITION OF PREDISPOSITION

Usually, an unaffected individual, knowing that there is cancer in the family, will seek advice. Sometimes a patient with cancer will express anxiety to the GP or to another doctor that their own cancer may have a hereditary cause, and worry about the risk for others in the family. The family doctor, recognising a possible familial risk, may choose to raise the issue with the family directly.

The first step is to obtain a family history as comprehensively as possible and plot out the pedigree, noting the type of cancer and, particularly, the age at which each affected family member developed the disease.

Sometimes the level of knowledge of the first family member to be consulted is rather vague. The type of cancer may not be known, or primary and secondary sites may be confused. For example, "bone cancer" is more likely to have been metastatic disease in a woman with breast cancer than a primary osteosarcoma, and "liver cancer" is more often liver metastases from colon cancer than a primary hepatocellular carcinoma. Often, there are difficulties in accurately ascertaining the age at diagnosis in affected relatives. Old hospital records can be very useful. Most patients remember the full name, date of birth and date and place of treatment or death, and the GP can then write to the appropriate hospital and obtain full details of the case including the pathology.

Sometimes a particular pattern of cancers may immediately suggest a true familial condition. For example, a family with a grandmother with breast cancer in her forties, a mother with breast cancer in her thirties, and an aunt with leukaemia, an uncle with a glioma and a 3-year-old child with rhabdomyosarcoma seems very likely to have the Li Fraumeni syndrome described in Chapter 1. Sometimes an associated feature of a syndrome, such as the bowel polyps in familial adenomatous polyposis, may raise the suspicion in the absence of a cancer. Exceptionally rarely, the type of cancer by itself, for example retinoblastoma, indicates a high likelihood of a familial condition. Much more often, there are a few cases of common cancer types, such as breast or bowel cancer, which may well have arisen by chance. How then does one estimate the likelihood that that family does have an underlying genetic defect?

A number of authoritative bodies, for example, the British Association of Surgical Oncology (BASO), the American College of Medical Genetics and the Australian Cancer Society, have set out criteria by which individuals may be assigned to different risk groups, which can then be used to guide investigations, or as a basis for reassurance if the risk is low. The assigned level of risk can vary between different guidelines, however, and the recommended management plans differ. In the UK, there is not yet a national consensus on risk groups, advisable investigations or on management of those families shown to have a genetic condition. Most regional genetic clinics will have issued their own guidelines for referral. Alternative methods of estimating individual risk come from the use of one of a number of mathematical models, some of which are available as computer programs. Unfortunately, different models can assign significantly different risks using the same data, and their validity has been questioned. The following, however, illustrates the basic principles of risk group determination.

LOW-, MODERATE- AND HIGH-RISK GROUPS FOR BREAST CANCER

An individual can be considered to belong to a high-risk family, if any of the criteria below apply. Families at high risk should be referred to a cancer genetics clinic.

The number of high-risk families is small, only about 20–40 per million population, meaning that even a group practice with a list size of 10,000 may not even have one such family.

There is a greater number of families whose individual members are at moderate risk. Moderate risk defines a group of women with a likelihood of developing breast cancer before the age of 50 years, which is three times greater than the normal. The number of women at moderate risk aged between 35 and 49 in a group practice of 10,000 has been estimated to be about 50. These patients merit referral to a local breast unit for advice and screening. Individuals without any high- or moderate-risk criteria are in the low-risk group and can be reassured in the community without the need for specialist referral.

An alternative way to estimate the risk of a genetic basis for breast cancer is given in the two boxes below. These relate to the age at which breast cancer developed in an individual with no family history, and the mean age at the time breast cancer was diagnosed in two affected sisters.

GENETIC PREDISPOSITION IN AN INDIVIDUAL WITH BREAST CANCER BUT NO FAMILY HISTORY

◆ Age of onset (years)	25	35	45	55	65
◆ Genetic (%)	40	25	12	8	4
◆ Other factors (%)	60	75	88	92	96

GENETIC PREDISPOSITION IN TWO SISTERS WITH BREAST CANCER

◆ Mean age (years)	35	45	55	65
◆ Genetic (%)	90	62	38	13
◆ Other factors (%)	10	38	62	83

THE RISK OF FAMILIAL COLORECTAL CANCER

Familial adenomatous polyposis and hereditary non-polyposis coli are the principal familial conditions associated with the development of colorectal cancer and have been discussed in Chapter 1. The risk for an individual developing colorectal cancer based on the family history is shown below.

LIFETIME RISK OF DEVELOPING COLORECTAL CANCER

◆ Population risk	1:50
◆ One relative affected	1:17
◆ One first-degree and one second-degree relative affected	1:12
◆ One relative under the age of 45 years affected	1:10
◆ Two first-degree relatives affected	1:6
◆ Autosomal dominant family history	1:2

The Australian Cancer Society has recommended risk-based screening guidelines for individuals, depending on their family history. Those in the higher-risk group (Group B) should have colonoscopy 5 yearly and faecal occult blood testing annually from the age of 50 or from 5 years younger than the earliest diagnosis, whichever is the earlier. Those in the lower-risk group (Group A) should have flexible sigmoidoscopy or colonoscopy 5 yearly and annual occult bloods from the age of 50.

A diagnosis of hereditary non-polyposis colon cancer is made on the basis of the family history, according to the Amsterdam criteria (see box). Some genetic mutations have been identified, which are considered characteristic of hereditary non-polyposis colon cancer, but in about one-third of families meeting the Amsterdam criteria, no such mutation can be detected.

Screening for colorectal and other tumour types is recommended in those with a family history meeting the Amsterdam criteria, regardless of whether or not a mutation has been identified. There is no consensus about the best possible strategy for screening unaffected family members, but one reasonable system is described below.

THE RISK OF FAMILIAL OVARIAN CANCER

Ovarian cancer is, of course, much rarer than breast cancer with a population lifetime risk of only 1 in 70. Familial clustering of ovarian cancer cases is, therefore, much less likely to be due to chance than is the case with breast cancer. If an individual woman has a single affected first-degree relative of any age, then her own lifetime risk of developing ovarian cancer rises to 1 in 23. The most common familial syndromes involving ovarian cancer are the familial breast–ovarian cancer syndrome (described above and principally related to BRCA-1, where the lifetime risk of developing ovarian cancer reaches 60% by the age of 70 years, and to a lesser extent BRCA-2, where the cumulative risk by the age of 70 is only 25%) and hereditary non-polyposis colon cancer (described in Chapter 1).

REFERRAL FOR GENETIC COUNSELLING

Genetic counselling is the process by which patients or relatives at risk of a disorder that may be inherited are advised of the consequences of the disorder, the probability of developing or transmitting it and of ways in which this may be prevented, avoided or ameliorated. It is important to recognise that it is not a single event, but a process, which may well involve a number of stages, some of which may well involve the GP. The initial assessment by the GP of the level of risk an individual has may trigger either referral to a cancer genetics clinic, if such a service is provided locally and the risk seems to be high, or to a local breast, colorectal or gynaecological clinic, if the risk seems to be intermediate. Low-risk patients can usually be reassured without referral, and patients can be advised on measures to minimise their cancer risk (Chapter 2) and on the normal cancer screening programmes (Chapter 6).

THE BENEFITS AND DRAWBACKS OF MOLECULAR TESTING FOR INHERITED RISK

If a person is confirmed in a specialist cancer genetics clinic to be at high risk of a genetic mutation, such as BRCA-1 or BRCA-2, further counselling will follow, prior to a decision being made as to whether or not genetic testing should be undertaken. Testing may be diagnostic, that is, the detection of a genetic abnormality in a patient known to have cancer, or predictive, that is, the detection of a predisposing genetic abnormality in an unaffected individual with a family history.

Testing for genetic mutations is not a simple investigation like a full blood count, but is an individualised, very complex and time-consuming (and therefore expensive) procedure. Many different mutations can occur in the known inherited cancer predisposition genes, and these are usually constant within families. The first step, therefore, is to carry out diagnostic genetic testing in an affected family member. If a specific mutation is then found, other family members can then be offered predictive testing. Absence of a known specific mutation is a true negative. Initial assessment of an unaffected family member is not advisable as false negatives may occur due to failure of the test to detect a new and unknown mutation, and false positives may occur, if a rare but innocent genetic polymorphism is detected.

MANAGEMENT OF THE FAMILY WITH A PROVEN SYNDROME

Individuals with genetically proven family cancer syndromes (and perhaps also those with strongly suspected syndromes) should receive post-testing counselling including lifestyle advice to reduce risk, and discussion about early detection and screening and prophylactic measures. Patients may want advice about the risk that further children or grandchildren might inherit the cancer predisposition.

COUNSELLING OF THE PATIENT WITH A PROVEN FAMILY CANCER SYNDROME

- Lifestyle advice
- Early detection and screening
- Prophylactic surgery and medication
- Risks in other family members

Lifestyle advice is similar to that given in Chapter 2, concerning a healthy diet, avoidance of obesity, and probably (for patients at risk of breast cancer) avoidance of exogenous oestrogens, such as hormone-replacement therapy.

In breast-cancer families, breast awareness and regular breast self-examination should be encouraged. Different centres will have different policies regarding the age at which routine mammography should begin, and its frequency. Commencing annual mammography at the age of 35 or 5 years younger than the earliest familial case (with

a minimum age for mammography of 30 years), and less frequent mammography between the ages of 50 and 70 years is one reasonable policy. As there are anxieties about the possible carcinogenic effect of radiation on healthy breast tissue in younger women, alternative imaging techniques, such as magnetic resonance and ultrasound are sometimes used, but they have not yet been fully evaluated. A modern low-dose mammogram carries the same radiation exposure as a chest X-ray.

Patients at risk of colon cancer will usually be offered colonoscopy every 3–5 years. Sometimes regular testing for faecal occult blood is recommended. Women at risk of ovarian cancer can be screened with CA 125 measurements and transvaginal ultrasound, but the optimum frequency of screening has not been determined.

Prophylactic surgery, that is to say bilateral mastectomy or oophorectomy, seems a practical idea, but although it greatly reduces the cancer risk, it is still possible to get both breast and ovarian cancer after these operations. Mastectomy, especially the more cosmetically acceptable subcutaneous mastectomy with reconstruction does not remove all glandular epithelium, and ovarian cancer can arise from peritoneal cells after surgical oophorectomy. Similarly, although prophylactic restorative proctocolectomy is usually advised in patients with familial adenomatous polyposis, other gastro-intestinal cancers may arise in later life.

Chemoprevention of breast cancer in high-risk patients with either tamoxifen or its analogue, the selective oestrogen receptor modulator raloxifene, is an attractive alternative to mastectomy. A large US tamoxifen chemoprevention trial was halted in 1998 because a significant reduction of about 45% in the incidence of breast cancer was observed. No benefit has yet been demonstrated in terms of mortality. Similar European studies are continuing as significant benefit has not yet been demonstrated. Tamoxifen in healthy women is not without risk. There is an increase in the incidence of thromboembolic events and endometrial cancer, both of which may be fatal. Patients need to be counselled very carefully before commencing chemoprevention.

CONCLUSIONS

Family cancer syndromes account for only a small proportion of the cancer burden. An accurate and comprehensive family history can be used to estimate whether a patient is at significant risk of having a genetic predisposition to cancer, and this can be used to decide whether or not referral to a specialist cancer genetics clinic is indicated. In the rare instances, where a specific syndrome is identified, policies for advising on early detection and screening, and for prophylactic surgery or chemoprevention should be in place.

SECTION II

Diagnosis and assessment of cancer

SECTION CONTENTS

CHAPTER 5 — Presentation of symptomatic cancer

The overwhelming majority of cancers present with symptoms. Sometimes, as in the case of screen-detected breast cancer, they are purposefully sought in asymptomatic "well" individuals in an attempt to improve prognosis by early diagnosis. Only rarely are cancers discovered as unsuspected, incidental findings in asymptomatic patients being investigated for other conditions.

> **PRESENTATION OF PATIENTS WITH CANCER**
>
> ◆ With symptoms
> ◆ Through screening programmes
> ◆ Incidental finding

The symptoms may arise as a direct result of a primary tumour, such as haematuria in a patient with bladder cancer; from metastases, such as back pain in a woman with bone metastases from an occult breast cancer; or from the general effects of malignant disease such as fatigue or weight loss. One of the most important tasks of the general practitioner (GP) is to assess patients who present with symptoms which could be due to cancer and to decide whether any investigations are indicated, or whether immediate specialist referral is advisable. Sometimes it is appropriate to adopt a wait and see policy, only investigating or referring the patient if the symptom fails to resolve or worsens over the period of a few weeks. If this approach is adopted, the patient must be made aware of the necessity to return to the GP in say 2 or 3 weeks if the symptom has not fully resolved.

> **OPTIONS WHEN A PATIENT PRESENTS WITH A SYMPTOM WHICH MIGHT BE DUE TO CANCER**
>
> ◆ Keep under review to see, if the symptom settles
> ◆ Arrange further investigations
> ◆ Refer for specialist assessment

As the prognosis of cancer is better when it is diagnosed at the earliest possible stage, the UK Government had made the early diagnosis of cancer a priority in its 1997 White Paper *The New NHS – Modern, Dependable*. The plan is that all patients who are suspected by their GPs to have cancer should be seen by an appropriate specialist for assessment within 2 weeks. To facilitate the prompt referral of relevant patients, and also to prevent hospital diagnostic facilities being overwhelmed with patients unlikely to have cancer, guidelines have been published, which form the basis for this chapter. They can be found in full on the internet at www.doh.gov.uk/cancer.

Several factors have to be considered in addition to the symptom or symptoms themselves, which will enable better discrimination between those at high risk of having cancer, and those in whom there is little or no risk that the symptom might be due to cancer. These include socio-demographic characteristics, such as age and sex, tobacco and alcohol use, occupational and family history, and past medical history. In addition to the symptoms, findings on clinical examination and the results of investigations undertaken from the primary care setting need to be taken into account.

Incidence of selected cancers (England and Wales)

Type of cancer	Approximate number in (1,000s) per year	Approximate frequency in general practice
Lung	37	1–2 per year
Breast	32	1–2 per year
Colon	19	1 in every 1–2 years
Prostate	16	1 in every 1–2 years
Bladder, rectum	10–12	1 in every 2–3 years
Non-Hodgkin's lymphoma (NHL), pancreas, oesophagus, ovary	5–7	1 in every 3–4 years
Leukaemia, kidney	4.5	1 in every 5–6 years
Melanoma, endometrium	4	1 in every 6–7 years
Mouth/lip/pharynx, cervix, brain	3.5	1 in every 7–8 years
Myeloma	3	1 in every 9 years
Larynx	2	1 in every 12 years
Testis, soft tissue sarcoma, Hodgkin's disease	1.5	1 in every 20 years

While cancer is a major cause of morbidity and mortality, and therefore an important public health problem, it is important not to overestimate its frequency. The average GP with a list size of about 2,000 patients will see only eight or nine new cancer patients per year (see box).

Handbook of Community Cancer Care

Many symptoms which could be caused by cancer are very non-specific, and could well be due to benign causes. So while early referral for investigation and confirmation of cancer is important, it is also useful if the GP can give some estimate of the likelihood that the symptom for which they are being investigated is not, in fact caused by cancer. This may help to reduce unnecessary anxiety.

Among patients referred for investigation of a breast lump, or with symptoms suggestive of a possible gastro-intestinal cancer, the ratio of benign to malignant causes is likely to be of the order of 15 : 1. Among those investigated for post-menopausal bleeding, a testicular swelling or suspected lymphoma, the ratio of benign to malignant causes is likely to be about 10 : 1. Among those with suspected brain tumours or head and neck cancer the ratio may be only 5 : 1.

It is clearly important for all patients that they are seen and assessed quickly, to ensure that they can be reassured with confidence if the cause is trivial and insignificant, or to treat cancer or any other any serious pathology which may be present without delay. A hospital referral for a patient with symptoms suggestive of cancer is not a waste of resources if no cancer is found.

The age of the patient is a valuable guide to whether or not a symptom is likely to have a malignant cause. Ninety-nine per cent of patients with lung cancer are over the age of 40 years, and 96% are over 50 years of age. Similar figures pertain to both upper and lower gastro-intestinal tract cancers. Endometrial cancer is very rare in pre-menopausal women.

In some cancer types, younger people are more commonly affected. Although breast cancer is rare before the age of 35 years, 20% of cases occur in women under 50.

Younger people tend to be affected by rarer cancer types. Two-thirds of men with testicular cancer are under the age of 40. Nearly half of all patients with cervical cancer are under 50. One-third of patients with soft tissue sarcomas are under 50 and one-third of adults with bone sarcomas are under 40.

LUNG CANCER

The management of lung cancer is described in full in Chapter 22. Lung cancer is the commonest cancer and 85% of cases occur over the age of 60 years. About 90% are smokers or ex-smokers. More than 90% of patients are symptomatic at the time of diagnosis. The predominant symptoms are cough, dyspnoea, haemoptysis, weight loss, chest or shoulder pain and hoarseness. Often lung cancer will arise in someone with long-standing chronic obstructive airways disease, and the GP must be alert to a change in the nature of chronic symptoms, such as cough and breathlessness.

GUIDELINES FOR URGENT REFERRAL FOR A CHEST X-RAY

- ◆ Haemoptysis
- ◆ Unexplained or persistent (more than 3 weeks):
  - – Cough
  - – Chest or shoulder pain
  - – Dyspnoea
  - – Weight loss
  - – Chest signs
  - – Hoarseness
  - – Finger clubbing
  - – Features suggestive of metastasis from a lung cancer (e.g. brain, bone, liver or skin)
  - – Persistent cervical/supraclavicular lymphadenopathy

Chest X-ray findings are abnormal in the vast majority of symptomatic patients. However, a normal chest X-ray does not exclude a diagnosis of lung cancer. In most cases, it is appropriate for a GP to request a chest X-ray as an initial investigation, with referral to a chest physician if the chest X-ray is suggestive or suspicious of lung cancer.

GUIDELINES FOR URGENT REFERRAL TO A CHEST PHYSICIAN

Any of the following:

- ◆ Chest X-ray suggestive/suspicious of lung cancer (including pleural effusion and slowly resolving consolidation)
- ◆ Persistent haemoptysis in smokers/ex-smokers over 40 years of age
- ◆ Signs of superior vena cava obstruction (swelling of the face/neck with fixed elevation of the jugular venous pressure)
- ◆ Stridor (consider emergency referral)

Age at diagnosis for some adult cancers (values in %)

Site	Age (years)			
	<40	40–49	50–69	70+
Lung	<1	3	41	56
Breast	5	15	46	34
Colon	1	3	34	61
Stomach	1	3	32	64
Ovary	5	11	46	38
Cervix	28	19	29	24
Prostate	<1	<1	25	75
Hodgkin's	54	15	20	12
Testis	66	20	10	3
Thyroid	22	15	33	30
Soft tissue	19	14	35	33

In a limited number of circumstances, urgent referral to a chest physician is appropriate without requesting a chest X-ray. Sputum cytology is rarely indicated prior to referral for a specialist opinion.

After giving up smoking, the risk of someone developing lung cancer gradually lessens over a period of about 15–20 years, depending on the number of cigarettes smoked and the duration of the smoking history. The importance of referring ex-smokers as well as current smokers with persistent haemoptysis or other worrying symptoms is to be emphasised.

BREAST CANCER

Breast cancer is the commonest malignancy affecting women. Its management is described in Chapter 20. Five per cent of cases occur in women under the age of 40 years (i.e. over 1,250 patients each year in the UK), and only 2% (over 500 patients) in those under 35. An average GP may expect to see one or perhaps two new patients with breast cancer per year, but will see a considerably larger number of women with benign breast problems, from whom those at risk of cancer need to be distinguished.

COMMON BENIGN BREAST DISEASE

- *Diffuse nodularity*: common in all age groups up to the age of 50
- *Fibroadenoma*: peak age range 20–30 years
- *Cysts*: peak age range 40–60 years
- *Mastalgia*: breast pain *alone* is a very uncommon presentation of cancer

---

PRESENTING FEATURES OF SYMPTOMATIC CASES OF BREAST CANCER

- Lump   90%
- Painful lump   20%
- Nipple change   20%
- Nipple discharge   3%
- Skin contour change 5%

GUIDELINES FOR URGENT REFERRAL TO A BREAST ASSESSMENT CLINIC

- Patients over 30 with a discreet lump
- Patients with signs highly suggestive of cancer such as
  - Ulceration
  - Skin nodule
  - Skin distortion
  - Nipple eczema
  - Recent nipple retraction (present <3 months)

Patients under the age of 30 with a discreet breast lump, patients who have had a breast abscess, patients with breast pain and patients with nipple discharge are at low risk of having breast cancer. Nonetheless, non-urgent referral to a breast clinic may be advisable. It is important to be cautious in women who are breast-feeding, as it can be difficult to interpret changes in the lactating breast. If there are any suspicious symptoms or signs, referral is advised as there may be an increased incidence of breast cancer in recently delivered women.

UPPER GASTRO-INTESTINAL TRACT CANCER

The incidence of carcinoma of the stomach (Chapter 23), presently about 10,000 cases per year in England and Wales, appears to be decreasing, whereas that of oesophageal cancer (Chapter 24), presently about 6,000 cases per year, is increasing. Tumours at the gastro-oesophageal junction are increasing, particularly, rapidly. The incidence of pancreatic cancer (Chapter 25) is about 6,000 cases per year.

For all three tumour types, 99% occur over the age of 40 years, and for stomach cancer, 90% occur over the age of 55 years. The chance of a dyspeptic patient under the age of 55 having gastric cancer is only one in a million, and the age of 55 is taken as being a cost-effective age cut-off for investigation. Smoking and alcohol are both risk factors for upper gastro-intestinal cancer.

COMMON SYMPTOMS IN UPPER GASTRO-INTESTINAL TRACT CANCER PATIENTS

- Any upper gastro-intestinal cancer
  - Weight loss 60%
  - Anaemia   50%
  - Vomiting   25%
- Oesophagus
  - Heartburn   80%
  - Reflux   50%
  - Dysphagia   85%
- Stomach
  - Epigastric pain 90%
  - Dysphagia   40%
- Pancreas
  - Jaundice   80%

Dysphagia is a reasonably common symptom in the general practice setting. Patients with difficulty in swallowing food should always be referred for further investigation. Dyspepsia is an extremely common symptom in the community setting. The index of suspicion of cancer is considerably raised if dyspepsia is combined with an "alarm" symptom, such as weight loss, vomiting or anaemia. In patients aged over 55 years recent onset dyspepsia and/or continuous symptoms is associated with an increased risk of cancer.

COLORECTAL CANCER

The management of cancers of the large bowel is described in Chapter 21. There are about 19,000 cases of colon cancer and about 11,000 cases of rectal cancer occurring annually in England and Wales. Of these, 99% present over the age of 40, and 85% are over the age of 60 years. The principal symptoms include rectal bleeding and change in bowel habit. The latter is most commonly increased frequency and/or looser stools. Other symptoms include iron deficiency anaemia and signs of intestinal obstruction. On examination, there may be a definite rectal or abdominal mass.

It is recommended that the symptom and sign combinations listed above when occurring for the first time should be used to identify patients for urgent referral under the "2-week rule". The recommendation of age 60 years is considered to be the maximum age threshold.

Local Cancer Networks may elect to set a lower age threshold (e.g. 55 or 50 years).

GYNAECOLOGICAL CANCERS

Ovarian cancer (Chapter 32) is the commonest gynaecological malignancy. Only 5% of cases occur below the age of 40 years. The symptoms are often vague and non-specific, and most patients are diagnosed late. Women over 45 years with persistent abdominal pain or distension should have a pelvic examination performed as pelvic mass is present in 90% of cases of ovarian cancer.

Endometrial cancer (Chapter 33) is uncommon in premenopausal women. The overwhelming majority present with post-menopausal bleeding.

The incidence of cervical cancer (Chapter 31) is similar across all age groups over the age of 30 years. Typical symptoms are post-coital bleeding, persistent intermenstrual bleeding and post-menopausal bleeding. Usually 80% can be diagnosed on a speculum examination. The national screening programme aims to identify precursor lesions which can be treated, reducing the incidence of invasive cervical cancer, but up to 40% of cancers are detected on screening. Any clinical suspicion of cancer is an indication for referral, not for a cervical smear.

CLINICAL SUSPICION OF CERVICAL CANCER

- Refer to gynaecologist

Carcinoma of the vulva (Chapter 33) is rare. Most cases occur in women over the age of 65 years, and most have a visible tumour on clinical examination.

GUIDELINES FOR URGENT REFERRAL OF PATIENTS WITH SUSPECTED GYNAECOLOGICAL CANCER

- Lesion suspicious of cancer on cervix or vagina on speculum examination
- Lesion suspicious of cancer on clinical examination of the vulva
- Palpable pelvic mass not obviously fibroids
- Suspicious pelvic mass on pelvic ultrasound
- More than one or a single heavy episode of post-menopausal bleeding in women aged more than 55 years who are not on hormone-replacement therapy (HRT)
- Post-coital bleeding age more than 35 years that persists for more than 4 weeks
- Unexpected or prolonged bleeding persisting for more than 4 weeks after stopping HRT

Early but not "urgent" referral (i.e. to say within 4–6 weeks) is indicated for any other woman with post-menopausal bleeding not on HRT and to investigate persistent unexplained post-coital bleeding. Women on HRT can get gynaecological malignancy, and a change in the established pattern of bleeding while on HRT should be taken seriously.

UROLOGICAL CANCERS

Prostate cancer (Chapter 35) is the most common urological cancer. Only 1% of cases are diagnosed in men under the age of 50 years, and only 25% present in men under the age of 70 years when the life expectancy is greater than 10 years. Lower urinary tract symptoms are common in older men and are not, by themselves, a reason for suspecting prostate cancer. Presenting features include an abnormal rectal examination, bone pain and raised prostate-specific antigen (PSA) levels. Early, potentially curable prostate cancers are either impalpable or have only a small nodule and a PSA that is generally less than $15\,\mathrm{ng\,ml^{-1}}$. The age-specific upper limit of normal for PSA rises from 2.8 aged 50 up to 5.3 aged 70. Patients with a first-degree relative with prostate or breast cancer are at higher risk of developing prostate cancer, and black people probably have an increased risk. PSA testing of asymptomatic men or screening for prostate cancer is not national policy. It is recommended that PSA testing without a clinical suspicion of prostate cancer should only be performed after full counselling and provision of written information.

Urothelial cancer affects the bladder in 95% of cases, and the upper tracts in only 5% of cases. The management of bladder cancer is described in Chapter 36. The majority, 95%, present with macroscopic haematuria, microscopic haematuria is present in only 5–10%. Both macroscopic and microscopic haematuria, when caused by a urothelial cancer tend to be intermittent. A negative urine test for blood does not, therefore, exclude the possibility of malignancy. Microscopic haematuria is more likely to be due to malignancy if the individual is male, is over 50, or is a smoker. Microscopic haematuria in patients under the age of 40 years, especially if accompanied by proteinuria, hypertension or renal impairment, should be considered for referral to a nephrologist in the first instance.

GUIDELINES FOR URGENT REFERRAL OF SUSPECTED UROLOGICAL TUMOURS

- Macroscopic haematuria in adults
- Microscopic haematuria in adults over the age of 50 years
- Swellings in the body of the testis
- Palpable renal masses
- Solid renal masses found on imaging
- An elevated age-specific PSA in men with a 10-year life expectancy
- A high PSA ($>20\,\mathrm{ng\,ml^{-1}}$) in men with a clinically malignant prostate or bone pain
- Any suspected penile cancer

Macroscopic haematuria is the commonest presenting symptom of renal cancers (Chapter 37). Other features include loin pain, renal masses, microscopic haematuria, anaemia, weight loss and pyrexia. Renal cancers are increasingly found incidentally on abdominal imaging performed for other purposes.

Testis cancer (Chapter 38) is an uncommon urological malignancy, which occurs most often in younger men. Scrotal swellings occur relatively commonly in general practice. Solid swellings affecting the body of the testis are more likely than not due to cancer. Swellings outside the body of the testis are hardly ever due to cancer, and need not be referred urgently. Indeterminate swellings of the testicle have a low probability of being malignant, especially in men over the age of 55, and should be considered for ultrasound before urological referral.

Cancers of the penis (Chapter 45) are very rare. They usually present as swellings or ulcers under the foreskin in elderly men. They may be associated with enlargement of the inguinal lymph nodes.

HAEMATOLOGICAL MALIGNANCIES

Together, there are about 5,000 cases of all types of acute and chronic leukaemias each year in England and Wales (Chapter 40). Three-quarters of cases occur in patients over the age of 60, although people of any age can be affected. Risk factors include prior chemotherapy and radiotherapy, and non-therapeutic radiation exposure. Most cases are diagnosed following a blood count undertaken because of symptoms and/or signs of bone marrow failure, such as fatigue, pallor, bruising, bleeding and infections. Some leukaemias may present with lymphadenopathy and/or hepatosplenomegaly. Chronic lymphocytic anaemia (CLL) is an indolent disease normally diagnosed on a blood film, which does not usually require urgent referral.

NHL (Chapter 41) is slightly more common than leukaemia in adults. Again it can occur at any age, but two-thirds of cases occur over the age of 60 years. The presenting features include lymph node enlargement, hepatosplenomegaly, fatigue, weight loss and night sweats. Although the majority have lymph node enlargement, 40% present with a tumour outside lymph nodes.

Myeloma (Chapter 41) is rare; with only about 3,000 cases per year diagnosed in England and Wales an average GP might expect to see a new patient perhaps once in 10 years. It is a disease of the elderly, 95% of cases occur in the over 50s. Clinical features include bone pain and fractures, anaemia, hypercalcaemia and renal impairment.

The erythrocyte sedimentation rate (ESR) or plasma viscosity may be grossly elevated.

Hodgkin's disease (Chapter 41) is even rarer; the incidence rate is similar to that of soft tissue sarcoma and testis cancer, so an average GP might expect to see a new patient only once in 20 years. It occurs in individuals of any age, and half those affected are aged under 40 years. The clinical features are similar to those of NHL, but 95% present with lymph node enlargement.

HEAD AND NECK CANCER

The term head and neck cancer embraces different tumour types arising in a wide variety of primary sites. Those arising in the upper aerodigestive tract including the lips and oral cavity (Chapter 27), and larynx and pharynx (Chapter 26) are usually squamous cancer. They are often associated with smoking or other forms of tobacco use (e.g. chewing betel, gutkha and pan) and alcohol. They tend to occur in older, socially deprived people who often have a poor diet.

GUIDELINES FOR URGENT REFERRAL OF PATIENTS WITH SUSPECTED HAEMATOLOGICAL MALIGNANCIES

- Blood count/film reported as suggestive of acute leukaemia or chronic myeloid leukaemia
- Lymphadenopathy (>1 cm) persisting for 6 weeks
- Hepatosplenomegaly
- Bone pain associated with anaemia and raised ESR or plasma viscosity
- Bone X-rays reported as being suggestive of myeloma
- Constellation of three or more of the following symptoms:
  - Fatigue
  - Night sweats
  - Weight loss
  - Itching
  - Breathlessness
  - Bruising
  - Recurrent infections
  - Bone pain

COMMON SYMPTOMS OF SQUAMOUS HEAD AND NECK CANCER

◆ Larynx	Hoarseness	80–90%
	Pain on swallowing	30–40%
	Dysphagia	30%
◆ Nasopharynx	Lump in the neck	80–90%
	Nasal obstruction	60%
	Deafness	50%
	Post-nasal discharge	40–50%
◆ Oral cavity	Ulceration, visible lesion	80%
	Pain	60%
	Lump in the neck	20–40%
◆ Oropharynx	Persistent sore throat	90%
	Lump in the neck	80%
	Otalgia	80%
◆ Hypopharynx	Dysphagia	80%
	Otalgia	60–70%
	Hoarseness	50%
◆ Nasal cavity	Obstruction, congestion	80–90%
	Bleeding	70–80%

COMMON SYMPTOMS OF THYROID GLAND AND SALIVARY GLAND NEOPLASMS

◆ Thyroid gland	Thyroid lump	60%
	Discomfort in lower neck	80%
◆ Salivary glands	Lump in parotid or submandibular region	90%
	Pain	10–20%
	Lump in neck	10–20%

Salivary gland cancers (Chapter 28) and thyroid cancers (Chapter 29) are rarer and are not associated with the same risk factors. They occur more often in younger patients and thyroid cancer is more common in women than men.

> ### GUIDELINES FOR URGENT REFERRAL OF PATIENTS WITH SUSPECTED HEAD AND NECK CANCER
>
> ◆ Hoarseness persisting for more than 6 weeks
> ◆ Ulceration of the oral mucosa persisting for more than 3 weeks
> ◆ Oral swellings persisting for more than 3 weeks
> ◆ All red or white patches of the oral mucosa
> ◆ Dysphagia persisting for more than 3 weeks
> ◆ Unilateral nasal obstruction, particularly when associated with a purulent discharge
> ◆ Unexplained tooth mobility not associated with periodontal disease
> ◆ Unresolving neck masses for more than 3 weeks
> ◆ Cranial nerve palsies
> ◆ Orbital masses
>
> The level of suspicion is further increased, if the patient is a heavy smoker or heavy alcohol drinker and is aged 45 years or over and male. Other forms of tobacco use (chewing betel, gutkha, pan) should also arouse suspicion.

BRAIN TUMOURS

Brain tumours are not common. Their management is described in Chapter 39. With an incidence of 3,500 per year in England and Wales, the average GP may expect a case every 7 or 8 years. They are rare below the age of 30 years, but relatively evenly distributed thereafter, with a peak in the seventh decade of life. Patients with brain tumours typically present with one or more of the following: progressive neurological deficit, for example progressive weakness, sensory loss, dysphasia, ataxia, developing over days to weeks; seizure disorder; symptoms and signs of raised intracranial pressure such as headache, vomiting and papilloedema; and cognitive or personality (mental state) changes.

> ### PREVALENCE OF SYMPTOMS AMONG PATIENTS PRESENTING WITH BRAIN TUMOURS
>
> ◆ Focal neurological deficit   >50%
> ◆ Seizures   25–30%
> ◆ Headache   25–35%
> ◆ Papilloedema   25–50%
> ◆ Mental changes   15–20%

> ### PROBABILITY OF SYMPTOMS BEING CAUSED BY A BRAIN TUMOUR
>
> ◆ New onset seizure disorder (any type) in adults   2–6%
> ◆ New onset status epilepticus   10%
> ◆ Headache of non-migrainous type   <1%

> ### GUIDELINES FOR URGENT REFERRAL OF PATIENTS WITH SUSPECTED BRAIN TUMOURS
>
> ◆ Subacute progressive neurological deficit developing over days to weeks (e.g. weakness, sensory loss, dysphasia, ataxia)
> ◆ New onset seizures characterised by one or more of the following:
>   – Focal seizures
>   – Prolonged post-ictal focal deficit (longer than 1 hour)
>   – Status epilepticus
>   – Associated inter-ictal focal deficit
> ◆ Patients with headaches, vomiting and papilloedema
> ◆ Cranial nerve palsy (e.g. diplopia, visual failure including optician defined visual field loss, unilateral sensorineural deafness
>
> *Consider* urgent referral for
>
> ◆ Patients with non-migrainous headaches of recent onset, present for at least 1 month, when accompanied by features suggestive of raised intracranial pressure (e.g. woken by headache, vomiting, drowsiness)
>
> [This guideline is intended to provide the GP with the discretion to decline urgent referral if there are other known features (e.g. depression, somatisation disorder) making a diagnosis of brain tumour very unlikely.]

SKIN CANCERS

The management of skin cancers is described in Chapter 34. Malignant melanoma has an incidence which is rising by about 6% per year. It may affect all adult age groups. It is associated fair skin and a poor ability to tan, excessive ultraviolet light exposure (such as sun-beds), a large number of benign melanocytic naevi and a family history. Although they can occur anywhere on the body, half of melanomas in women occur on the lower leg, and one-third if melanomas in men occur on the back. Patients with suspected melanoma should not undergo biopsy in the general practice setting, but should be referred for specialist advice with the lesion intact.

Cutaneous squamous cell carcinoma is common, and the figure of about 10,000 new cases per year in England and Wales is, probably, an underestimate caused by incomplete registration as the mortality is so low. It is rare in patients under the age of 60 unless they are chronically immunosupressed, for example because of an organ transplant. Other risk factors include lifetime excessive sun exposure, especially in fair-skinned people with poor tanning ability and multiple small actinic keratoses. The commonest locations in both sexes include the face and the back of the hands. In men the scalp and ears are also at risk, and in women the lower legs. Cancers tend to be larger (>1 cm) than actinic keratoses and have a palpable component deep to the skin surface.

Basal cell carcinomas are very common, but as they grow so slowly and metastasise so rarely there is no need for urgent referral. Nonetheless, patients with a suspected basal cell carcinoma should be seen by a specialist within 3 months. The majority are on the face, particularly around the inner canthus and the nose. They appear initially as a slowly growing red or pearly nodule on the skin surface. Later they may break down with crusting to give the classic rodent ulcer.

SARCOMAS

Sarcomas are rare tumours. With an incidence of about 1,000 per year in the UK, the average GP may see only one patient with a soft tissue sarcoma in 20 years. Primary bone sarcomas are even rarer. With an incidence of only 400 per year in the UK, many GPs may never see a new case in a lifetime of practice.

Soft tissue sarcomas (Chapter 44) can occur at any age, but are more common in those over 30 years of age. Most soft tissue masses are benign, only 1 in 200 will prove to be malignant. Features of a soft tissue mass which are suggestive of malignancy include size greater than 5 cm, increasing size, pain, being situated deep to fascia and recurrence after previous excision. Lesions which are superficial, and painless, less than 5 cm and static in size are extremely unlikely to be malignant.

Primary bone tumours (Chapter 43) include osteosarcoma, chondrosarcoma and Ewing's sarcoma. They are most common in adolescents, but can occur in the elderly. About half occur in relation to the knee. Symptoms include pain which typically is non-mechanical, waking the patient at night. Bone swelling and limp are usually late features. Most are diagnosed on X-ray.

CHILDREN'S CANCERS

The management of cancer in children is described in Chapter 46. About 1,200 children aged less than 15 years in England and Wales are found to have cancer each year. This means that children's cancer as a whole is fortunately rare, having a similar sort of incidence to Hodgkin's disease, soft tissue sarcomas and testicular cancer. Put another way, one in between 550 and 600 children will be affected by cancer before the age of 15 years, which is a similar incidence rate for Down's syndrome, diabetes or meningitis in childhood.

There are, of course, many different types of cancer which present in childhood. Acute leukaemia is the most common, comprising about one-third of cases, and brain tumours comprise a quarter.

The incidence of commoner childhood cancers

Type	Cases per year (%)	Principal age group
Acute leukaemia		
ALL	310 (25%)	2–4 years
AML	60 (5%)	
Brain tumours	280 (23%)	
Lymphoma		
NHL	70 (6%)	
Hodgkin's	50 (4%)	10–14 years
Neuroblastoma	80 (7%)	<4 years
Soft tissue sarcoma	80 (7%)	
Wilms' tumour	70 (6%)	<5 years
Bone sarcoma	60 (5%)	10–14 years
Others	140 (12%)	

In most cases of childhood cancer no risk factors can be identified. However genetic susceptibility is apparent in some cases, and associated conditions or a family history may be important.

Children with leukaemia usually present with a relatively short history (weeks rather than months) with pallor, fatigue, irritability, fever, bone pain and bruising, and petechial haemorrhage. Two-thirds have hepatosplenomegaly and a half have lymphadenopathy. There is an association between childhood leukaemia and Down's syndrome. Neuroblastoma often presents with symptoms of metastatic disease including bone pain and bruising which may be indistinguishable clinically from acute leukaemia.

Brain tumours in childhood commonly present with symptoms and signs of raised intracranial pressure including headache and vomiting and, in infants, a rapidly increasing head circumference. Clear-cut neurological signs, such as squint and visual impairment, are less common. Vague and non-specific symptoms, such as changes in personality or mood, out of character behaviour and deterioration in school performance, are noted in the minority. Growth failure, due to hypothalamic/pituitary disturbance may lead to growth failure. There is an association between neurofibromatosis type I and brain tumours.

Lymphadenopathy may be a feature of Hodgkin's disease or NHL as well as leukaemia. In NHL, there is usually a rapid progression of symptoms. Hodgkin's disease, by contrast, usually presents with non-tender cervical or supraclavicular lymphadenopathy. The history tends to be measured in months and only a minority have classic systemic symptoms.

Abdominal swelling can be a presenting feature of NHL, and is the commonest presentation of Wilms' tumour. Children under 1 year may have localised abdominal swelling due to neuroblastoma. Very young infants may

---

GUIDELINES FOR URGENT REFERRAL OF CHILDREN WITH SUSPECTED MALIGNANCY

- *Abnormal blood count* if reported as requiring further urgent investigation
- *Petechiae* or *purpura* are always an indication for urgent investigation
- *Fatigue* in a previously healthy child when combined with
  - generalised lymphadenopathy
  - hepatosplenomegaly
- *Bone pain* especially if it is
  - diffuse or involves the back
  - persistently localised at any site
  - requiring analgesia
  - limiting activity
- *Lymphadenopathy* is more frequently benign in younger children but is suspicious in the absence of evidence of previous local infection if
  - non-tender, firm or hard and more than 3 cm diameter
  - progressively enlarging
  - associated with other signs of general ill health, fever and/or weight loss
  - involving axillary or supraclavicular nodes
  - seen as a mediastinal or hilar mass on chest X-ray
- *Headache* of recent origin which is either
  - increasing in severity or frequency
  - noted to be worse in the mornings or causing early awakening
  - associated with vomiting
  - associated with neurological signs (e.g. squint or ataxia)
  - associated with behavioural change or deterioration in school performance
- *Soft tissue mass* in an unusual location should be considered suspicious particularly if
  - it shows rapid or progressive growth
  - is greater than 3 cm in size
  - is fixed to or deep to fascia
  - is associated with regional lymph node enlargement

have rapidly progressive abdominal swelling due to liver metastases from neuroblastoma, or the primary liver tumour hepatoblastoma.

Soft tissue sarcomas can arise in many primary sites, and often present with a mass. Orbital masses will cause proptosis, and tumours in the nose or sinuses may present as polyps and cause nasal obstruction or discharge. Genito-urinary system tumours may cause urinary obstruction, vaginal bleeding or present as a mass within the scrotum.

In the process of carcinogenesis, there is in many cases a progressive change in tissues from normality, through the development of epithelial dysplasia, which becomes carcinoma *in situ,* to invasive cancer. Subsequently, there may be the development of lymph node spread and finally distant metastases.

Screening is the investigation of groups of asymptomatic people to identify pre-malignant lesions or established cancers. Appropriate treatment is then given. The aim of screening is to save lives. Eradication of pre-malignant lesions diminishes mortality by preventing the development of cancer. Screening-detected cancers have a better prognosis as they are usually found at an earlier stage than that at which symptomatic cancers present. The early diagnosis of established cancers is not truly preventive medicine, but nonetheless mortality should be reduced by early diagnosis.

THE AIM OF SCREENING FOR CANCER

To reduce cancer mortality by
- identification and treatment of pre-malignant lesions before cancer develops
- identification and treatment of early stage good prognosis cancers

---

Unfortunately, the aims of screening can only be met for certain cancer types at the present time. For most tumours, there is no effective system of screening.

CRITERIA FOR ESTABLISHING A POPULATION-SCREENING PROGRAMME FOR CANCER

Population screening can only be undertaken, when a number of prerequisites are in place, as given below.

Firstly, the disease must pose a significant public health problem. For example, there would be little value in establishing a national-screening programme for cutaneous basal cell carcinoma, when the overwhelming majority of cases already present at an early stage, when cure is a possible with simple treatment.

Secondly, the natural history of the disease should be understood, and there must be either a clearly defined pre-malignant phase, or a demonstrable progression from an early cancer with a good prognosis to more advanced disease with a worse outlook.

Thirdly, there must be a screening investigation with good sensitivity and specificity. By sensitivity, we mean that the test is good at picking up the majority of cases; in other words, there is a low false-negative rate. By specificity, we mean that the test picks out few people who on further investigation prove to be normal; in other words, there is a low false-positive rate.

- **Sensitivity** The proportion of patients with the disease being screened for who are actually detected, that is, the ratio of cases detected – true positives – to the total number of cases present (both detected – true positives – and missed – false negatives – by screening)
- **Specificity** The proportion of those with positive test results who actually have the disease, that is, the ratio of detected cases – true positives – to the total number of abnormal test results (both true positives and false positives)

The screening test must be acceptable to the general population. For a test to be acceptable, it must not be too uncomfortable, time consuming or embarrassing. If it is, then uptake of the test will be too low for any impact to be made on mortality. In addition, there should not be a significant possibility of it causing psychological or physical harm. There is no advantage when the mortality of the investigation exceeds the incidence of the cancer being sought.

Fourthly, there must be treatments which can eradicate pre-malignant lesions and are effective at controlling early stage established cancer. There is no advantage in identifying a cancer before it becomes symptomatic, if there is little chance of curing it.

It is of course helpful if groups of individuals at higher than average risk can be identified. This means that the incidence of the disease will be higher in the population which is screened. The simplest example of this is the limitation of breast-cancer screening to females aged between 50 and 64 years. In addition, younger women identified as being a high risk by virtue of family history can be screened.

Finally, in this era of evidence-based medicine, any new screening programme is only likely to be introduced, if there is unequivocal evidence from large scale, population-based, randomised trials that it is clinically effective and significantly diminishes cancer mortality and that it is also cost-effective, that is to say affordable, in comparison with other medical interventions. These factors are considered below in more detail.

ASSESSMENT OF THE EFFECTIVENESS OF SCREENING PROGRAMMES

How can we tell whether a screening intervention is truly effective? The only truly valid way is to demonstrate that mortality is lower in a screened population, compared with a comparison population. The best trials, in terms of the level of evidence they provide, are randomised controlled trials, but this is never easy and indeed not always possible in terms of screening programmes. One of the difficulties is that it takes many years to show a real reduction in mortality. There are a number of proxy outcomes, which may indicate that a reduction in mortality can reasonably be anticipated, but one must be cautious as these can be subject to bias.

When a screening test is applied to a population for the first time (the prevalence screen), more cases should be diagnosed than would have been expected to present with symptoms in the subsequent year. The implication of this increased yield is that cases have been diagnosed, which would otherwise have gone on to present later as more advanced disease with a worse prognosis. In subsequent rounds of screening in the same population (the incidence screen), the actual yield should be the same as the yield expected in the absence of screening. Nonetheless, the yield may well be higher as a result of finding tumours, which had been missed by the prevalence screen, and by the detection of non-progressive tumours, which may never present symptomatically.

If a screening programme is effective, the stage distribution of screen-detected cancers is expected to be skewed towards more favourable, early disease than would be the case in a control population of symptomatically presenting disease. For example, in one trial of screening for colorectal cancer by faecal occult blood testing, Dukes' A cancers accounted for 26% of screen detected versus only 11% of cancers occurring in controls.

If a screening programme is effective, one would anticipate that survival among patients with screen-detected cancers will be better than that of symptomatic patients. There are, however, several possible biases, which can make an intervention seem to prolong survival, when this is not in fact the case.

For those screening tests that aim to detect pre-malignant lesions, such as cervical cytology, which can pick up dysplastic changes in cervical epithelium, and faecal occult blood testing or flexible sigmoidoscopy, which can detect adenomatous colorectal polyps, a reduction in the incidence if invasive cancer in the screened population in comparison with unscreened control populations is a good marker of effectiveness.

If a cancer is diagnosed earlier as a result of screening than would otherwise have been the case, but no more effective treatment is possible as a result of this earlier diagnosis, then the survival period from the time of diagnosis to death lengthens, although the outcome has not in fact changed. This is called the lead-time bias. For example, several studies evaluating screening programmes for lung cancer have shown that some cases are detected at an asymptomatic stage. However, there is no reduction in mortality in the screened group, as results of treatment, even of relatively early disease, are so poor.

Because slow-growing tumours spend a longer time in the detectable, asymptomatic phase than more aggressive, poorer prognosis cancers, the case mix of screen-detected cancers includes a greater proportion of such slow-growing (good prognosis) cancers than the case mix of cancers which present with symptoms. This is called length bias.

As some cancers, which would never have progressed to a symptomatic stage will be screen detected, there may be an over-diagnosis bias. For example, post-mortem studies in older men show a significant incidence of early prostate cancer, which was both undiagnosed before death and unrelated to the cause of death.

Finally, selection bias results from the fact that health aware, well-motivated, socially advantaged individuals, who are likely to have a better prognosis anyway, are more likely to attend invitations for screening.

FACTORS AFFECTING THE EFFECTIVENESS OF SCREENING PROGRAMMES

THE EFFECTIVENESS OF SCREENING DEPENDS ON THE FOLLOWING

- Clear identification of the target population
- Acceptance by the target population
- Sensitivity of the screening test
- Interval between screening rounds
- Efficiency of follow-up of people with abnormal test results
- Effectiveness of treatment
- Audit and quality control

Several factors can affect the effectiveness of a screening intervention. Many of these can be manipulated to make a screening programme more effective. Conversely, neglect or complacency may mean that what should be an effective programme becomes ineffective. There have been several incidents involving cervical smear tests which have received much media attention, and have rightly been portrayed as scandals, where, for a variety of different reasons the quality of screening was suboptimal

and appropriate audit and quality control measures were not in place.

Clear identification of the target population depends not just on the definition of those to be screened, for example women aged between 50 and 64 years in the case of breast cancer, but also upon accurate-screening programme and community held records. In most cases, this will include the general practice age and sex register. Prior to a set of invitations for screening being issued, each GP will be contacted with a list of patients believed to be eligible for invitation. These are then cross-referenced to the general practice records. Any ineligible patients (e.g. women already treated for breast cancer and under hospital follow-up) can be removed from the list, and any additional patients who have been omitted can be added.

For a screening programme to produce the maximum possible reduction in mortality, there has to be a high level of uptake of the screening test by the target population. Older people, and those in lower socio-economic groups, are less likely to respond positively to invitations for screening. Education can be helpful here, and the GP is well placed to encourage people in the target population to attend for screening. Encouragement can be easily given opportunistically during consultations, and supported by posters and leaflets in the general practice waiting room.

A screening programme is clearly more effective if the test or tests used pick up the greatest proportion of true abnormalities possible. The sensitivity of a screening test depends on a number of factors. No test is absolutely perfect, and many tests are dependent on human observers. The sensitivity of mammography, for example, is increased when two views rather than one are used, and when each set of films is read independently by two observers. In colorectal cancer, screening by the use of both faecal occult blood testing and flexible sigmoidoscopy are better than either test alone. Meticulous staff training and careful audit and quality control measures are necessary to maintain maximum sensitivity.

Sometimes new cancers will present symptomatically between screening rounds. These so-called interval cancers comprise both cancers which were present at the time of the earlier screen, but missed due to the insensitivity of the test, and also new cancers that have arisen since the previous screen.

INCIDENCE OF INTERVAL CANCERS IN THE NHS BREAST SCREENING PROGRAMME

- First year after screening   15%
- Second year after screening   30%
- Third year after screening   45%

Clearly, if the interval between screening rounds is shortened, some of the new cancers will be picked up at an earlier, asymptomatic stage. In the breast-cancer-screening programme, with a 3-year interval between screens, about 15% of interval cancers manifest in the first year, 30% in the second year and 45% in the third year. Reduction in the screening interval to 2 years or 18 months might, therefore, lead to a worthwhile increase in yield, but an annual interval is likely to be too frequent. There is a balance to be struck between what is reasonable, affordable and practicable and what may be counter-productive. For example, if the interval is too short, some people invited for screening may perceive it as being inconvenient or less valuable, and the proportion attending might drop.

It is not enough for screening tests to identify abnormalities. There must be a streamlined and comprehensive assessment system, which can investigate abnormal-screening results and differentiate reliably and simply between true positives and false positives. Because of the anxiety created by a recall for further investigation by the multidisciplinary team, it is important that healthy people with false-positive results can be investigated and reassured quickly, and that patients with true-positive results can have the diagnosis confirmed without delay.

There must also be adequate facilities in place for the swift and effective treatment of patients with screen-detected cancer. The effectiveness of the treatment available impacts hugely on the benefits or otherwise of a screening programme. If the treatments available are inefficient or only sometimes helpful then it is probably not worthwhile screening for the cancer in the first place. Conversely, if treatments progress to a stage where they are highly effective even in advanced disease, then the benefit conferred by earlier detection and treatment are lost and it would become reasonable to abandon the screening programme and devote resources to the effective treatment of patients who present with symptoms.

Quality is at the heart of the new NHS. Clinical governance demands that audit, quality assurance and education programmes are in place. All screening programmes are, therefore, required to maintain meticulous records of, for example, the number of people invited for screening, the number who attend, the number recalled for assessment, the number of true positives, the number of false positives and number of interval cancers. Data relating to the sensitivity and a specificity of an individual centre can then be correlated with national standards. For example, following the initial screen in 10,000 women, 500–700 should be recalled for assessment. Following clinical, radiological and fine needle aspirate for cytology or core needle biopsy investigation, fewer than 100 should require an open surgical biopsy for diagnosis. Breast cancer should be detected in 50–60 women. When comparable data for an individual centre are known, it is possible to investigate the reasons behind any discrepancies and institute remedial action. For example, if the sensitivity or specificity are found to be a lower than the national average, there might be a need for additional staff training.

SCREENING FOR INDIVIDUAL CANCER TYPES

Cancers can be divided into four groups with regard to screening. Firstly, there are those types for which population-screening programmes are already in place, such as cervical cancer and breast cancer. Secondly, there are those cancers for which population screening is currently being evaluated and which in time may become the subject of national-screening programmes, if the evidence of benefit is substantial and funds are made available, for example colorectal and prostate cancer. Thirdly, there are those cancer types for which present evidence shows that screening is not justified, such as lung cancer, testicular cancer and neuroblastoma.

SCREENING FOR INDIVIDUAL CANCER TYPES

- Established population-screening programmes
  - Cervical cancer
  - Breast cancer
- Population-screening programmes under evaluation
  - Colorectal cancer
  - Prostate cancer
- Population screening not justified
  - Lung cancer
  - Testicular cancer
  - Neuroblastoma
- Screening of high-risk individual recommended
  - BRCA 1 and BRCA 2 families
  - FAP and HNPC families
  - Retinoblastoma families

Finally, there are those where screening is not justified for the population at large, but is advisable for carefully selected groups at high risk, for example ovarian and breast cancer in women from identified cancer families; colorectal cancer screening in people with known familial adenomatous polyposis or from families known to have hereditary non-polyposis colon cancer, and new babies in families with retinoblastoma.

CERVICAL CANCER

Cancer of the uterine cervix was the first type of cancer for which population screening became feasible. The hypothesis was that the detection of epithelial dysplasia and carcinoma *in situ* by examination of a Papanicolau stained cervical smear and its eradication would reduce the incidence of, and mortality from, invasive cervical cancer. However, cervical smear testing was introduced in a sporadic way in the mid-1960s without preliminary evaluation of its effectiveness and without specific funding or a uniform quality assurance programme. The lack of organisation of cervical cancer screening on a national basis and concurrent changes in sexual practices, which increased the incidence of pre-malignant cervical change meant that it took over 20 years before convincing evidence of benefit was obtained and before a uniform service was provided. There is now very good evidence from studies in Scandinavia that the mortality of cervical cancer reduced very substantially between the 1960s and 1980s in those countries (Denmark, Finland, Iceland and Sweden) with carefully co-ordinated national programmes compared with Norway, which did not introduce an organised programme at the same time. In the UK at this time, there was a failure of policy to introduce an equitable national system. This resulted in resources being wastefully deployed in the unnecessarily frequent screening of low-risk, educated women who demanded it, while at the same time the women most at risk were left out.

The NHS Cervical Screening Programme was set up in 1988, since which time there has been a national call and recall programme, clearly defined and audited quality standards, and there is now good colposcopy provision for the assessment of women with abnormal smears. All women between the ages of 20 and 64 are eligible for a free cervical smear test at least once every 5 years. Five-yearly screening between 20 and 64, assuming 100% coverage, can reduce cumulative incidence of invasive disease by 83.6%, 3-yearly screening by 91.2% and annual screening by 93.3%. Around 60% of health authorities invite women at 3 years and 15% have a mixed policy, inviting women every 3 or 5 years depending on their age. Health authorities inviting women are registered with a GP using a computerised call–recall system. This also keeps track of any follow-up investigation, and, if all is well, recalls the woman for screening in 3 or 5 years' time. It is, therefore, important that all women ensure their GP has the correct name and address details and inform them, if these change. Women who have not had a recent smear test may be offered one when they attend their GP or family planning clinic on another matter. Women should receive their first invitation for routine screening before their 25th birthday.

The priorities of the national office of the NHS Cancer Screening Programmes, set up in 1994, are to develop systems and guidelines which will ensure a high quality of a cervical screening throughout the country, to identify important policy issues and help resolve them, and to improve communications within the programme and with women. The system now seems to be efficient in ensuring uptake: of the 12.2 million women aged 25–64 eligible for cervical screening in 1998/99, 84% had been screened within the previous 5 years at an estimated cost of about £34 per woman screened.

> **REMIT FOR NATIONAL QUALITY ASSURANCE CO-ORDINATING GROUPS**
>
> ◆ Set quality assurance standards
> ◆ Monitor and review performance against these quality assurance standards
> ◆ Identify training needs and advise on how they should be met
> ◆ Identify research needs
> ◆ Advise the programme on professional matters

Quality is a key issue at both national and regional levels. National quality assurance co-ordinating groups are being set up for each of the four main areas of activity in the cervical-screening programme. Three groups have already been established to cover health authority activities, laboratories and colposcopy. A group for primary care is currently being established. Regional quality assurance co-ordinating groups have also been established.

The effectiveness of the present cervical cancer-screening strategy is shown by the fact that the death rate has fallen from 7.0 per 100,000 in 1979 to 4.1 per 100,000 in 1997, a reduction of 40%. Deaths are falling by about 7% per year. The incidence of invasive cervical cancer, at 2,740 cases in England and Wales, has fallen by more than a quarter over the preceding 5 years.

> **FEATURES OF THE REGIONAL SYSTEMS OF QUALITY ASSURANCE**
>
> ◆ A quality assurance director for cervical screening
> ◆ The identification of lead professionals to oversee co-ordination of audit in each area of professional activity in the cervical-screening programme
> ◆ The review of the performance of the screening programme against national quality standards
> ◆ Participation in external quality assessment schemes
> ◆ The development of an administrative structure including a quality assurance reference centre to co-ordinate professional activity, statistical returns, and liaison with national activities
> ◆ The development of training programmes within the region and support of training efforts in each laboratory and regional cytology training schools
> ◆ Liasing with the regional cancer registries to identify and audit cases of invasive cervical cancer and evaluate the effectiveness of the screening programme

BREAST CANCER

Randomised controlled trials have shown that screening by mammography can significantly reduce mortality from breast cancer by up to 40% in those who attend. The benefit is greatest in women aged 50–70 years. In contrast to the *ad hoc* introduction of cervical-cancer screening, the NHS Breast Cancer Screening Programme was introduced in a planned, co-ordinated way in 1988 after the publication of the Forrest report. Quality assurance and audit were structured into the programme, the first scheme of its kind in the world, from the beginning. Each NHS region has a quality assurance director supported by a multiprofessional team. There are quality assurance reference centres, which collect and collate process and outcome data to ensure that national standards are being met.

The programme routinely invites all women between the ages of 50 and 64 to attend for mammography on a 3-yearly basis. Invitations are sent out in batches corresponding to the GP practice, meaning that women may receive their first invitation anytime between their 50th and 53rd birthdays. All women will have been invited routinely five times before their 65th birthday. Women aged 65 and over are entitled to breast screening every 3 years. At present, they are not invited routinely, but are encouraged to make their own appointment, if they wish. There is no upper age limit on screening by request.

Women under the age of 50 are not offered routine screening. Research trials into breast screening by mammography have not so far shown a benefit in reducing deaths from breast cancer in pre-menopausal women. This may partly be because breast cancer is less common in younger women, and partly be because breast tissue is more dense in women who have not reached the menopause, which makes it more difficult to detect small cancers. As women go past the menopause, at an average age of 50, the glandular tissue in the breast atrophies and the breasts contains an increasingly high proportion of fat. This makes interpretation of mammograms more reliable. Research continues into ways of improving the effectiveness of breast-cancer screening in women aged 40–49 years. Of course, women who have breast symptoms (Chapter 5), should be referred directly to a breast assessment unit, and asymptomatic women at high risk (Chapter 4) may be considered for screening.

As a result of the breast-screening programme, more early and non-invasive cancers are being seen. In 1997/98 7,932 cancers were detected of which almost half (3,381) were less than 15 mm diameter and 1,718 were *in situ* disease. These cancers are associated with a better prognosis. Screen-detected cancers are also smaller and more likely to be node negative than cancers which present with symptoms. Data have recently been published covering the period from 1990 to 1998, the early years of the breast-cancer-screening programme, demonstrating that overall mortality has reduced by 21.3%. Of this, it is estimated that 6.1% is directly attributable to the screening programme and better treatment and earlier presentation outside the screening programme accounts for 14.9%. Because of the relatively long natural history of breast cancer, it is predicted that further substantial reductions in mortality will occur by 2010 directly as a result of the screening programme working at its present level of efficiency.

POSSIBLE WAYS OF MAXIMISING THE EFFICIENCY OF SCREENING

- Use two view mammography
- Decrease the screening interval
- Use double reading of films
- Encourage greater participation by women

When an abnormality is found on screening, patients will be recalled for assessment. Assessment is best carried out by dedicated assessment team consisting of an experienced radiologist, surgeon and pathologist supported by radiographers and breast care nurse. This will involve so-called triple assessment, a combination of clinical examination, further imaging with mammography and/or ultrasound and cytology from a fine needle aspirate or histology from a core needle biopsy. If the lesion is not palpable, cells or tissue can be obtained under imaging guidance at ultrasound or stereomammography.

TRIPLE ASSESSMENT

- Clinical examination
- Imaging (mammography, ultrasound)
- Tissue examination (FNA cytology, core needle biopsy for histology)

About two-thirds of patients can be reassured on the basis of imaging. Sometimes it is suggested that no further investigation is needed at the present time, but that the mammography should be repeated after an interval of, say, 6 months to ensure that the visible abnormality is not progressing. When the results of all the investigations are available, they should be considered by the multidisciplinary team and an appropriate action plan formulated. A definite diagnosis of malignancy can be made in the majority of cases, and then definitive surgery can be arranged. The screening programme minimum standard for preoperative diagnosis is 70%, but diagnosis may be possible in 95% or more.

If triple assessment has not confirmed the nature of a suspicious lesion, or if a confirmed impalpable cancer needs to be removed, then the radiologist will localise the position of the lesion using one of a variety of hooked wires under imaging guidance. The patient will then go to theatre for surgical excision biopsy of the area of tissue marked by the wire. A radiograph will be taken of the excised specimen to ensure that the abnormality, often an area of clustered microcalcification, has, in fact, been excised.

The NHS Breast Screening Programme is not set in tablets of stone, and research is underway looking at both the screening programme itself and the management of screen-detected early breast cancers. Some of these studies have completed recruitment and outcome data are maturing.

KEY ISSUES FOR RESEARCH IN BREAST-CANCER-SCREENING METHODOLOGY

- **The age trial** Annual screening for 7 years from age 40 is being assessed
- **Over 65s project** To assess the practical implications and resources required if routine screening was extended up to the age of 69
- **Frequency trial** Compares 3 yearly with annual screening
- **Genetics trial** Compares mammographic screening with magnetic resonance imaging in women at high risk of carrying one of the breast cancer predisposition genes

---

KEY ISSUES IN THE MANAGEMENT OF SCREEN-DETECTED CANCER

- **UK DCIS trial** To see whether surgery alone is enough for completely excised localised DCIS, or if radiotherapy and tamoxifen are required in addition
- **BASO II trial** To see whether surgery alone is enough for very small invasive cancers of special type, or if radiotherapy and tamoxifen are required in addition

---

COLORECTAL CANCER

Bowel cancer is a common condition, the second biggest cause of cancer death in the UK. Adenomatous polyps are a recognised pre-malignant lesion. About 10% of 1-cm-diameter adenomas become malignant after 10 years. The incidence of adenomatous polyps in the colon increases with age, and although adenomatous polyps can be identified in about 20% of the population, most of these are small and unlikely to undergo malignant change. The vast majority (90%) of adenomas can be removed at colonoscopy, obviating the need for surgery. Other types of polyps occurring in the colon – such as metaplastic (or hyperplastic) polyps – are usually small and are much less likely than adenomas to become malignant. As outcomes are markedly improved by early detection of adenomas and early cancers, the potential exists to reduce disease mortality through screening asymptomatic individuals for adenomas and early cancers. There is as yet no national-screening programme for cancers of the colon and rectum. At the moment, the effect that screening will have on the incidence of and mortality from colorectal cancer is uncertain, but various studies are underway evaluating different screening strategies.

SCREENING TESTS FOR COLORECTAL CANCER

- Flexible sigmoidoscopy
- Colonoscopy
- Barium enema
- Faecal occult blood testing

Although flexible sigmoidoscopy is more expensive than rigid sigmoidoscopy, it is generally more acceptable to patients (it is less uncomfortable) and has a much higher yield than the rigid instrument. Flexible sigmoidoscopy can detect 80% of colorectal cancers as it examines the whole of the left colon and rectum. Many nurses are now trained to perform flexible sigmoidoscopy, making potential-screening programmes using this technique more cost-effective.

A strategy of providing single flexible sigmoidoscopy for adults aged 55–65 years – with the aim of detecting adenomas – may be cost-effective. A multicentre trial of the flexible sigmoidoscopy for population screening is currently under evaluation. In a population-screening programme, uptake of the offer of the screening test is crucial. Uptake is likely to be around 45%, and, of these 6% will subsequently need full colonoscopy.

Colonoscopy is the gold standard technique for examination of the colon and rectum, but it is expensive, the need for full bowel preparation and sedation, and the small risk of perforation of the colon make it unacceptable for population screening. Colonoscopy is, however, the investigation of choice for screening high-risk patients (those at risk of hereditary non-polyposis colon cancer or with a long-standing ulcerative colitis).

Barium enema, like colonoscopy, examines the whole colon and rectum, and although it is cheaper and has a lower complication rate than colonoscopy, it is invasive and requires a full bowel preparation. Whereas polypectomy undertaken at colonoscopy may be therapeutic, barium enema does not allow removal or biopsy of lesions seen. There are no population-screening studies using barium enema.

"Virtual colonoscopy" or computed tomographic colography is a new investigational technique, which allows excellent imaging of the whole bowel. Although it is an expensive high-technology investigation, the quality of the data coupled with patient acceptability may make it a valuable adjunct to other techniques used in population screening.

Faecal occult blood tests are the most extensively studied screening tests for colorectal cancer. These tests detect partially digested blood in the stool. Their overall sensitivity for colorectal neoplasia is only 50–60%, though their specificity is high. In screening studies of faecal occult blood tests, individuals are invited to take two samples from each of three consecutive stools. Compliance is around 50–60%, but with population education this might be improved. Individuals with more than four out of six positive tests (about 2% of participants) need colonoscopy.

Randomised studies have shown that faecal occult blood testing is feasible. Screen-detected carcinomas are more likely to be Dukes' stage A than symptomatic cancers, and screening may reduce mortality from colorectal cancer. The disadvantage of faecal occult bloods is its relatively low sensitivity and specificity. Only about one-third of those with positive test results will have a lesion and a third to a half of cancers will be missed on each round of screening. Sensitivity and specificity could be increased by more frequent (perhaps annual) faecal occult blood testing combined with less frequent flexible sigmoidoscopy. This clearly deserves further investigation and an NHS commissioned pilot study is being conducted in England (Coventry and Warwickshire) and Scotland (Fife, Grampian and Tayside) to assess the outcome of population-based screening in those aged 50–69 using faecal occult blood testing.

In summary, current evidence on screening for colorectal cancer points towards benefit, but further reliable data about the efficacy and acceptability of different techniques are needed before an optimal-screening strategy can be defined. An economic assessment and identification of additional funding will also be required before a national programme can be implemented.

PROSTATE CANCER

Prostate cancer is common in older men, and the incidence is increasing. It has a very variable natural history. At one end of the spectrum, there is a high incidence of occult prostate cancer in older men, which is destined never to become symptomatic or life threatening. On the other hand, many patients present with locally advanced or metastatic disease, which can be rapidly progressive and is not usually curable.

> ## CAUSES OF ELEVATED PROSTATE-SPECIFIC ANTIGEN (PSA)
>
> - Prostate cancer
> - Benign prostatic hypertrophy
> - Prostatitis

Screening by, for example, digital rectal examination and measurement of serum PSA will undoubtedly detect asymptomatic cases. False-negative PSA results are common. Fifteen per cent of men over the age of 50 years are likely to have a PSA level greater than the upper limit of normal, which is 4 ng/ml, and will require further investigation including, possibly, a biopsy. Of these, 80% will have benign disease, such as benign prostatic hyperplasia or prostatitis. Only 3% of the total will have a cancer.

The treatment of prostate cancer is, however, associated with a certain morbidity (Chapter 35), and whether or not every patient who presents with symptomatic cancer merits treatment is controversial. Surveillance seems a good option for some categories of patient, and avoids the side-effects of treatment, at least until it becomes clear that the disease is progressing.

> ## DRAWBACKS TO SCREENING FOR PROSTATE CANCER
>
> - Initial-screening tests may yield false-positive results and cause unnecessary anxiety and expose patients to the hazards of additional investigation
> - Initial-screening tests may be falsely negative and provide false reassurance
> - Treatment of screen-detected cancers may fail to save lives because
>   - the disease may already be disseminated
>   - the disease may be so indolent that it does not pose a threat to life
> - Treatments are associated with morbidity

It would certainly be undesirable for an asymptomatic man to undergo a screening test and have a cancer detected, only to be told that he did not require treatment. It would similarly be undesirable for those with an early prostate cancer, which might never cause any trouble to be exposed unnecessarily to the risk of side-effects from surgery or radiotherapy. In the absence of evidence that treatment of screen-detected early prostate cancer results in any reduction in mortality, this cannot be recommended on a population basis.

Despite the lack of evidence that screening for prostate cancer leads to a reduction in mortality, it seems intuitively to many people to be a good idea. As acceptable, sensitive and specific-screening tests are available, it has become widely practised in some parts of the world, most noticeably in the US. Population-based trials, however, continue with the aim of identifying which groups of men, if any, will genuinely benefit from screening.

LUNG CANCER

Lung cancer causes more deaths in the UK than any other malignant disease, and anything which could reduce this mortality would be welcome. Smoking is, of course, known to be the cause of the majority of cases. Because primary prevention is, therefore, possible, there has been little enthusiasm for screening for what many people regard, rightly or wrongly, as a self-inflicted illness. Over the years, however, a number of trials have been performed to evaluate screening for lung cancer. Most of them have been based on chest radiography, stimulated by the success of the mass miniature radiography programmes of the 1950s, which screened for pulmonary tuberculosis. Some trials have also included sputum cytology. There is no evidence that screening for lung cancer in this way is of any significant value.

Computed tomography (CT) scanning is a more sensitive investigation for lung abnormalities than a standard chest X-ray, but the drawbacks include cost, availability and a relatively high-radiation exposure. A new type of CT scanning has recently been developed, which exposes the patient to a much smaller dose of radiation. The image quality of the lung parenchyma is good, although the technique does not allow proper assessment of the mediastinum and other thoracic structures. This low-dose CT scanning technique is currently being evaluated as a potentially better screening investigation for lung cancer in high-risk groups.

TESTICULAR CANCER

Testicular cancer (Chapter 38) is the most common malignancy of men in their twenties and thirties, and is becoming more common. As the testicles are amenable to direct physical examination or imaging by ultrasound, testicular cancer might seem to be a good candidate for screening. However, as there is no recognised pre-malignant phase, the process of screening would not reduce the incidence of cancer. In addition, the results of treatment for testicular cancer, even when it is disseminated, are excellent. Taken together, these factors mean that there would be no value in establishing a formal-screening programme, but of course it is wise to educate men to be aware of any changes in their own genitalia, and to encourage them to seek advice at an early stage.

NEUROBLASTOMA

Neuroblastoma (Chapter 46) is rare in absolute terms, although it is the commonest extracranial solid tumour of childhood. Early stage disease carries a good prognosis, but the outlook for children with advanced disease is very poor. The metabolites of catecholamines produced by neuroblastoma cells can be detected in urine, and this makes for a simple-screening test. It is, therefore, tempting to think that the early detection of asymptomatic children with neuroblastoma by screening would lead to an improvement in survival.

A number of population-based studies have been carried out, most notably in Japan, but also in Europe and America. Unfortunately, the process of screening leads to an increase in the incidence of neuroblastoma, while the mortality remains stubbornly unchanged. The reason for the increased incidence is that asymptomatic, essentially benign, tumours which were never destined to progress and present clinically are detected. Children with these tumours are then needlessly exposed to the risks of surgery and other treatment. The reason for the stable mortality rate is that those tumours which have the potential to kill have unfavourable biological characteristics, which determine outcome. They are rapidly progressive and are not likely to be detected at an early stage. Screening for neuroblastoma is, therefore, not recommended.

The tissue diagnosis

It is necessary to confirm a suspected diagnosis of cancer by pathological examination of tumour tissue in almost every case. Benign processes can mimic malignancy clinically and radiologically; for example, a small fibroadenoma may be indistinguishable from an early cancer of the breast and an area of fat necrosis can resemble a more advanced breast cancer. It is clearly important to distinguish benign from malignant disease reliably for two reasons. Firstly, to ensure that the signs of an early cancer are not wrongly attributed to an innocent process, thereby delaying its treatment while it is still potentially curable. Secondly, it could be disastrous to treat a benign lesion as cancer because of the possibly mutilating surgery or toxicity of the treatments used and because of the psychological consequences of wrongly labelling someone as having cancer.

> **WHY OBTAIN PATHOLOGICAL CONFIRMATION OF SUSPECTED CANCER?**
>
> ◆ To distinguish benign from malignant conditions
> ◆ To identify and fully characterise the tumour type
> ◆ To guide treatment choices
> ◆ To give information about prognosis

Pathology is an indispensable guide to treatment and prognosis. The amount of information depends on the quantity of tissue which is available for examination. Fine needle aspiration cytology, or exfoliative cytology, may enable a confident diagnosis of malignancy to be made, and it is sometimes possible to determine the type of cancer. Accurate recognition of the cancer type is important, for example small cell and squamous cell lung cancer can present a similar clinical picture, but they are treated in different ways, and the prognosis is different. Different tumour types cannot always be reliably distinguished by cytology, for example, it may not be possible to distinguish ductal carcinoma *in situ* of the breast from invasive ductal cancer, and so a biopsy is needed for histological examination.

In addition, a biopsy may reveal features indicating the degree of biological aggressiveness of the tumour, such as tumour grade and the presence of invasion of lymphatic and vascular channels, and nerves. However, absence of these features on a small biopsy can be due to sampling

error, and they may be apparent when the larger samples are sectioned.

The definitive histology report follows from examination of a surgical resection specimen. This will give much more information than is possible from a biopsy alone. The size and degree of extension of the tumour through the organ will enable a pathological T-stage to be assigned. Completeness of excision can be assessed by examination of the margins of the resection specimen, and the presence and extent of nodal involvement (the N-stage) can be determined. The principles of staging are fully considered in Chapter 8.

CYTOLOGY

Cytological examinations can broadly be divided into groups according to how the cells are obtained. Exfoliative cytology refers to examination of cells scraped from the surface of an organ or lesion or shed into a fluid, such as sputum or urine. Cells can also be obtained from solid lesions by fine needle aspiration. If an open or needle biopsy is taken for histological processing, a slide can be pressed against the surface of the tissue, and cells from this imprint can be examined cytologically.

> **CYTOLOGY**
>
> ◆ Exfoliative cytology
> ◆ Fine needle aspirate cytology
> ◆ Imprint cytology

The most common example of the use of cytology in general practice is the cervical smear, used for screening for dysplasia, cervical intra-epithelial neoplasia (CIN) and invasive cancer. An Ayres spatula or cervical brush is used to exfoliate cells from the cervix. The cervix should be fully visualised using a speculum and the end of the spatula inserted into the os. The spatula is then rotated through a full circle to ensure that cells are obtained from the whole transition zone where the squamous epithelium of the ectocervix meets the cuboidal epithelium of the endocervix. The cells are then spread onto glass microscopic slides, fixed to preserve cytological detail and then dried, labelled and sent to the laboratory. There they are stained, usually with the Papanicolau (Pap) stain and examined under the microscope. The first question to be asked should be whether or not the sample is adequate and of good quality. If not, no opinion can be given and the procedure should be repeated. For a cervical smear to be considered to be "well taken", transition zone cells must be present. It is possible to audit the quality of cervical smears with an assessment of the percentage of smears which have transition zone cells present.

The cells may be seen to be normal, or they may show various degrees of dysplasia, progressing towards definite malignancy. These changes are usually graded as CIN I, II or III. CIN III used to be referred to as carcinoma *in situ* of the cervix. The presence of infection and other changes may also be noted. If the report says "cells obscured by purulent exudate suggest treat infection and repeat" and a high vaginal swab is negative, one should be cautious as there could be an underlying problem obscuring cells.

Other types of commonly used exfoliative cytology are used in patients with suspected cancer. These include sputum cytology to look for evidence of lung cancer in a patient with symptoms, signs or investigation results which might suggest a lung cancer. Patients with ascites or pleural effusions may have samples of the aspirated fluid sent for examination for malignant cells. Urine from patients with bladder cancer or urothelial malignancy in the upper tracts may show abnormal cells which can be diagnostic. Skin ulcers thought to be malignant, for example cutaneous squamous cell or basal cell carcinoma, can be diagnosed by examination of cells taken from imprints of the ulcer or skin scrapings.

Fine needle aspiration cytology is most commonly used to assess palpable lesions, such as breast lumps, enlarged lymph nodes or a thyroid swelling. It can also be performed under imaging guidance if the lesion cannot be felt; for example, ultrasound can be used to localise impalpable breast lesions. In this procedure, a fine needle (often 23 gauge) is attached to an empty syringe. It is inserted into the lump, and the plunger is withdrawn a little to create a vacuum. Then the syringe and needle is pushed backwards and forwards through the lump, maintaining the vacuum, then the vacuum is released and the needle is withdrawn. The aspirated material is then spread thinly onto glass microscopic slides. Some should be rapidly air dried, and some should be fixed immediately either by spraying with or dipping into an alcoholic fixative. The syringe and needle can also be rinsed with saline and the washing is sent for analysis.

Air-dried and fixed slides are stained with different stains and yield complementary information. Air-dried slides are processed in a similar way to haematology specimens and usually stained with the Giemsa stain. The cells appear larger than with fixed preparations, and the cytoplasmic detail is shown better. With fixed preparations, Pap or haematoxylin and eosin (H&E) staining is used. This shows nuclear detail better than is the case with air-dried smears.

Cytology reports do not just give a "benign" or "malignant" result, but are often graded numerically to indicate the certainty of the result, with C2 indicating definitely benign and C5 meaning certainly malignant. Often, the type of malignancy can be defined with certainty, but in some cases, such as with Hodgkin's disease and other lymphomas, a formal biopsy is still necessary to fully characterise the disease.

HISTOLOGY

Making a diagnosis before treatment

Pathological assessment of tumour type is central to the modern management of patients with cancer. Before a sample is taken for histology, the clinician may already have a good idea that the patient has cancer, and even what type of cancer it is likely to be, on the basis of the history, examination finding and imaging. Nonetheless, these preliminary findings can sometimes be deceptive, and circumstances in which pathological confirmation is not thought to be necessary are now very rare. Often, cytological confirmation of malignancy will have been obtained as an initial procedure.

Sometimes, for example, when a colonic tumour has been shown on barium enema, or a brain tumour has been shown on an MRI scan, the surgeon will undertake a major operation without prior pathological confirmation of malignancy. In such cases, the procedure serves to obtain tissue for pathological confirmation as well as being the definitive initial treatment. More often, however, the diagnosis has been confirmed by cytology or biopsy prior to surgery.

Processing of tissue by conventional histology usually takes at least a couple of days, but "real-time" results can be obtained by frozen section histology. The quality of frozen section histology is not as good as that of conventionally processed specimens, but it is usually good enough to distinguish benign from malignant processes. In the old days, frozen section diagnosis of breast cancer was often undertaken at the time of surgery before proceeding to a mastectomy. This practice – when the patient does not know before her operation whether or not she has cancer and whether or not she will wake up with her breast removed – was inhumane, and nowadays almost all women with breast cancer have the diagnosis made preoperatively by cytology or needle biopsy. Intra-operative frozen section histology is currently used to check that the margins of a resected tumour specimen are free of malignant cells. Frozen section may also be useful, if an unexpected possible malignancy is discovered during an operation for what was thought to be a benign condition.

Tissue samples to confirm the diagnosis of cancer prior to a treatment plan being formulated may be obtained in a variety of ways. Endoscopic biopsy of hollow organs such as the rectum, colon, oesophagus, stomach, bronchi is now routine. Examination under general anaesthesia is still preferred for biopsy of the larynx, pharynx and other parts of the upper aerodigestive tract. The practice of dilatation and curettage (D&C) under general anaesthesia to diagnose endometrial cancer is now being replaced to some extent by aspiration biopsy in the outpatient setting. Abnormal cervical smears are investigated by colposcopically guided biopsy or by cone biopsy which removes the whole of the transition zone of the cervix.

Needle biopsy of breast lumps, soft tissue tumours and visceral abnormalities, such as lung tumours, which are not accessible on bronchoscopy, liver lesions and other abdominal masses are frequently performed. A cutting needle, such as a Trucut, is used which obtains a core of tissue 1 or 2 mm in diameter and about 2 cm long. Often these biopsies are performed by radiologists using imaging guidance to ensure that the tissue is obtained accurately from the abnormal area. This minimises the possibility of false-negative results which might be obtained if adjacent normal tissue was sampled in error. In addition, the use of imaging to guide the route of the biopsy needle will help to avoid unnecessary damage to important anatomical structures.

Taking advantage of all these techniques, the need for open biopsy, that is a surgical procedure which will leave a scar, or a major operation, such as thoracotomy or laparotomy just to make a diagnosis, is now unusual.

Assessment of resection specimens for staging and prognostic features

The modern surgical pathologist will examine a resection specimen very carefully with the naked eye, noting the location and extent of any visible abnormalities. Measurements will be made on the main tumour mass, and the amount of normal tissue surrounding the tumour. Specimens will be cut carefully and many blocks taken for histological processing. Any lymph nodes removed with the tumour will be removed, counted and sectioned for microscopic examination.

The macroscopic and microscopic assessment of a surgical resection specimen has several purposes. It will confirm the diagnosis of cancer. It will provide a pathological stage of both the primary tumour, often the lymph nodes and sometimes if there are distant metastases. This will be an indispensable guide to the need for further treatment, including a further surgical procedure, radiotherapy, endocrine therapy and chemotherapy. It may determine not just whether chemotherapy is indicated, but the intensity or the duration of the course of chemotherapy. The presence or absence of additional pathological and biological features will allow a more accurate prognosis than just the stage, and may also influence treatment. Finally, pathological assessment of surgical specimens allows the quality of surgery to be audited.

To ensure that comprehensive information is obtained, and that results from one pathologist can be compared with results from another, minimum datasets have been defined for some diseases. For example, a national minimum dataset has been defined for colorectal cancer, and agreed by a large number of bodies including the relevant royal colleges and speciality associations. Some of the key features for this standardised reporting are shown in the box below. Similar datasets exist for breast cancer and some other tumours.

For many diseases including breast cancer, colorectal cancer, malignant melanoma and squamous cancer of the head and neck, one of the most important features in guiding the treatment and determining outcome is the lymph node status. Whether any nodes are involved, the number of nodes involved, the size and position of involved nodes and the presence of any extracapsular spread can all be important features. Often, standard surgical practice has been to dissect out the adjacent lymph node areas for pathological assessment. This will be both diagnosis and treatment. Sometimes sampling procedures, assessing just some nodes, has been done.

If an adequate sample is clear, no further treatment is needed, but if the sample is positive further treatment with more surgery or radiotherapy is advised.

Recently, the concept of the *sentinel node* has become important. The sentinel node is the first node to which tumour lymphatics drain. If the sentinel node is not involved, it is unlikely that any other nodes are involved. Surgical clearance, with its associated morbidity, would then be unnecessary. If the sentinel node is involved, clearance of all nodes is appropriate. The sentinel node can be identified in two ways. Preoperatively, the main tumour is injected with either a blue dye or a radioactive substance. The sentinel node is stained blue and can be identified visually at the time of surgery. Similarly, a probe can be used to detect the node which shows the highest level of radioactivity. Detection of the sentinel node is most accurate when both techniques are used. At the moment, although there is much interest in sentinel node surgery, the value is unproven and it remains the subject of clinical trials.

> **COLORECTAL CANCER HISTOPATHOLOGY REPORTING – MAJOR FEATURES**
>
> *Gross description*
> - Site of tumour
> - Maximum tumour diameter
> - Distance of tumour from nearer cut end
> - Presence or absence of tumour perforation
>
> *Histology*
> - Type (e.g. adenocarcinoma or other)
> - Degree of differentiation
> - Local invasion into submucosa (pT1)
> - Local invasion into muscularis propria (pT2)
> - Local invasion beyond muscularis propria (pT3)
> - Tumour cells have breached the peritoneal surface or invaded adjacent organs (pT4)
> - Tumour involvement of cut end
> - Tumour involvement of circumferential resection margin
> - Distance from tumour to circumferential resection margin
> - Number of lymph nodes examined
> - Number of lymph nodes involved
> - Apical lymph node involved
>
> *Staging*
> - Dukes' stage
> - TNM stage

Post-treatment assessment

Increasingly, there is a trend to defer major surgery until after initial medical therapy, sometimes called upfront or neoadjuvant chemotherapy. Sometimes preoperative radiotherapy is given. Common examples are the use of neoadjuvant chemotherapy for locally advanced or inflammatory breast cancer, preoperative radiotherapy for rectal cancer, and initial chemotherapy for embryonal tumours, such as Wilms' tumour, rhabdomyosarcoma and neuroblastoma. The pathologist will then be able to detect changes in the tumour, such as necrosis, maturation or hyalinisation, caused by treatment. A good histological response to initial therapy can be predictive of a more favourable prognosis.

Special techniques

The examination of tissue sections stained with H&E is the cornerstone of diagnostic histopathology. A variety of other traditional histological stains can be used to identify substances, such as collagen, reticulin, melanin, mucin and starch, to aid diagnosis.

Electron microscopy which has a much higher resolution than light microscopy was formerly used as a good deal to study cellular ultrastructure and aid diagnosis in difficult cases. However, processing of specimens for electron microscopy is a specialised area, and to a large extent immunohistochemistry has replaced electron microscopy in routine diagnosis.

> **HISTOPATHOLOGY TECHNIQUES**
>
> - Conventional light microscopy
> - Special stains
> - Electron microscopy
> - Immunohistochemistry
> - Molecular biology assessment

The advent of monoclonal antibody technology in the 1980s has made it possible to look for a wide variety of specific cell markers. This has transformed the pathological assessment of many tumour classes such as lymphoma, which can now be immunophenotyped into B-cell and T-cell varieties. Immunohistochemistry has also aided the differential diagnosis within heterogeneous groups of tumours, such as the so-called "small round blue cell tumours of childhood". All these tumours look similar with conventional H&E staining, but could be Ewing's sarcoma, lymphoma, rhabdomyosarcoma, primitive neuroectodermal tumours or others. Immunohistochemistry is used to identify particular biological features of therapeutic and prognostic importance, such as the presence or absence of oestrogen and progesterone receptors in patients with breast cancer.

Over the last decade a whole variety of different molecular biology techniques have been used to characterise tumours further. These include the identification of chromosomal abnormalities and oncogene amplification.

Many of these have been shown to be of prognostic significance, and in some cases these biological factors are beginning to be used to guide treatment in clinical trials.

PATHOLOGICAL REVIEW

It will be apparent that pathological assessment of tumours can be very complex. It is not surprising that, especially in the assessment of "difficult" tumour groups such as the lymphomas and the sarcomas, there can be differences in interpretation between different pathologists. As the results are of great importance in determining the best treatment for each patient and in predicting outcome, it is important that pathology slides are reviewed at clinico-pathological meetings, and that the pathology of rare and unusual tumours is reviewed by specialist pathologists with particular expertise in that tumour type. It is often a condition of entry into clinical trials of rarer tumours that pathology is reviewed centrally.

Staging of cancer

By "staging", we mean the allocation of patients with a particular type of cancer into sub-groups, depending on the extent of the primary tumour, and the presence or absence of lymph node involvement and distant metastases. Staging is based on an anatomical assessment of the extent of spread based on physical examination, imaging investigations including bone scanning and computed tomography (CT), and pathological examination of any operative specimen. Occasionally, other criteria such as the patient's age, the tumour grade and the presence of specific symptoms are taken into account. Staging is usually undertaken at the time of diagnosis, but investigations may be repeated later to assess response to treatment, and restaging may also be required, if the disease recurs after initially successful therapy.

Staging is undertaken for a variety of reasons. Most important, from the patient's point of view is that the disease stage is usually a key determinant of treatment. For example, while mastectomy may be an important component of treatment for a woman with a large primary breast cancer without evidence of metastases, local excision may be all the surgery that is needed for a small tumour. Similarly, mastectomy is usually inappropriate for women found to have liver or lung secondaries at presentation.

Also important from the patient's perspective is that stage is a guide to prognosis. In general, the higher the stage the worse the outlook. There is, of course, no certainty of a similar outcome between identically designated stages in different diseases. For example, most patients with Stage IV testicular teratoma are curable, whereas Stage IV lung cancer is essentially incurable.

From the cancer specialist's point of view, accurate staging enables a comparison of outcomes to be made between patients with a particular cancer treated in different centres. It is inappropriate to say that survival of patients treated for colon cancer at the general hospital is 10% less good than for patients treated at the Royal Infirmary. Quality of care and real outcome may in fact be better at the general hospital despite the apparently poorer results. The discrepancy may be explained by case mix: there are no emergencies admitted to the Royal Infirmary, as there is no casualty department. Patients with advanced disease, Dukes' category C, and an inherently poorer prognosis who present with intestinal obstruction will all be treated at the general hospital. The elective

surgery only workload at the Royal Infirmary will comprise a larger proportion of earlier, Dukes' category A cancers, which are usually curable.

In comparing results reported by two centres, it is important to ensure that the staging investigations used were similar. This is especially true if comparison is being made between recently treated patients and a historical series. Over the years, increasingly sophisticated imaging has become available, which means that a greater proportion of patients are found to have advanced disease at presentation than was apparent in previous decades. The fact that a patient presenting now may have Stage IV disease, whereas in the pre-CT era the disease would have been designated Stage II known as "stage migration". This can lead to the so-called Will Rogers phenomenon. Will Rogers was a simpleton, who in moving from one country to another was alleged to have raised the average intelligence in both countries. The effect of stage migration on reported results of cancer treatment is shown below. The new staging system results not only in more people having more advanced disease, but stage for stage the outcome appears to be better. The overall survival is, however, identical: there has been no real change.

	Stage				
	I	II	III	IV	Total
Old staging system					
Number of patients	30	30	30	10	100
Percentage cured (%)	80	50	20	10	46
Number cured	24	15	6	1	46
New staging system					
Number of patients	25	25	25	25	100
Percentage cured (%)	84	60	28	12	46
Number cured	21	15	7	5	46

The mirage of the Will Rogers phenomenon has been brought about by the introduction of more sensitive investigations, which up-stage patients (i.e. allocate patients to a more advanced stage than would otherwise have been the case). The same thing sometimes happens when a new staging classification is brought into use. Staging classifications are constantly being reviewed with the laudable aim of making them more accurately differentiate between patients with a different prognosis. For example, it may become recognised that a particular clinical feature is associated with a poorer outcome. In the new classification, patients with that feature are allocated to a more advanced stage. The overall survival may not change, but stage for stage patients appear to fare better.

The other main reason for staging patients is to help in the interpretation of trends over time. For example, the incidence of both testicular teratoma and malignant melanoma is rising, yet mortality from both conditions is declining. For teratoma, the improvement in prognosis has been brought about by tremendous advances in systemic therapy, but the same is not true for melanoma. A greater public awareness of this disease has lead to a larger proportion of cases being diagnosed at an early stage, when treatment may still be curative. Unfortunately, there is no successful treatment for advanced melanoma.

> **REASONS FOR STAGING CANCER**
> - To determine the most appropriate treatment
> - To estimate prognosis accurately
> - To compare treatment results
>   - between different centres
>   - at different times

STAGING CLASSIFICATIONS

The basic requirement is to define in each patient all the factors relevant to the natural history and outcome of the cancer, thereby enabling similar cases to be grouped together. The first subdivision of cancer is by primary site, but histology also needs to be considered. For example, high-grade lymphoma of the nasopharynx needs to be distinguished from carcinoma at this site, and small cell carcinoma needs to be distinguished from squamous carcinoma of the bronchus.

For some tumour types defined in this way, staging classifications established by various groups have been in use for many decades. More recently, there have been international attempts to create a framework for staging tumours, which can be applied universally. This is the "TNM" classification that attempts to describe all tumours in terms of the primary *T*umour, the extent of lymph *N*ode spread, and the presence of haematogenous *M*etastases. The TNM classification often takes earlier staging systems into account, but sometimes it is a very different system from those used previously. Some national organisations and some institutions prefer to use their own classifications, so in certain tumour types various classifications are in use at the same time. They may be broadly similar, but differ in important respects which can lead to a degree of confusion.

THE TNM CLASSIFICATION

The primary tumour is indicated by the letter "T", the status of regional lymph nodes by "N" and distant metastases by "M". In each case, the letter is followed by a suffix, usually an Arabic numeral, to indicate the extent of disease in each category.

The extent of the primary tumour is indicated by the suffixes 1, 2, 3 or 4, representing progressively more advanced disease. Increasing size is usually the sole criterion for categories 1, 2 and 3, while 4 often indicates direct extension from the primary site into adjacent organs. Other criteria are applied in special circumstances, such as fixation of the vocal cord in laryngeal carcinoma. T0 is used when there is no evidence of a primary tumour, Tis when the primary is non-invasive or carcinoma *in situ*, and Tx is used when for some reason the tumour cannot be assessed.

Three lymph node categories, N1, N2 and N3, are usually used for involved nodes, in addition to the designations N0 for uninvolved nodes and Nx for unassessed nodes.

The presence or absence of distant metastases are indicated by M1 or M0, respectively. If the presence of metastases cannot be assessed, the suffix x is used.

While assessment of the tumour, nodes and metastases is usually sufficient for staging purposes, other factors which are sometimes taken into account include the histological differentiation or grade in the case of soft tissue sarcomas, and the patient's age in the case of differentiated thyroid carcinomas of follicular cell origin.

TNM-staging can be performed on data obtained in different ways. At the simplest level, it is a clinical system based on examination findings and radiology. If definitive surgery has been performed on the primary tumour or nodal areas, a post-surgical pathological assessment is used. A prefix can be used to designate the source of the information, "c" for clinical staging, "p" for pathological staging, but often the prefix is omitted and the staging is assumed to be clinically based.

With five principal options for the T-stage, four for the N-stage and two for metastases, there are 40 possible TNM options, more if various subcategories are included. This is clearly too many for easy use. Even in the largest clinical series, there will be some combinations with too few patients for meaningful analysis. Therefore, different TNM categories are aggregated into "stage groupings" designated by Roman numerals. The precise details vary from one tumour site to another, but in general, Stage 0 disease is carcinoma *in situ*, Stage I disease comprises a node negative operable primary, Stage II is an operable primary with operable nodes, Stage III is disease considered inoperable by virtue of either an advanced primary tumour or advanced nodal involvement, and in Stage IV disease distant metastases are present.

Throughout this book, the stage by stage treatment policies for different cancers are referred to. It is not considered appropriate for general practitioners to learn any particular classification in detail. Even cancer specialists working with the staging of tumours on a daily basis often need to refer to books for clarification. Nonetheless, the concept of staging at diagnosis and restaging at relapse to determine treatment and prognosis, and the ways in which staging systems can be misleading, are very important and should be recognised in general practice.

Treatment of cancer

SECTION CONTENTS

The cancer team and shared care

The care of patients with cancer is not the responsibility of any one person. No doctor works in isolation to treat cancer patients, and non-medical colleagues have an equally important rôle. The general practitioner (GP) and the general practice team, who work in conjunction with members of the cancer unit team, specialist staff at the cancer centre and often with hospice and palliative care services, have a pivotal rôle. The GP's team, the cancer unit team, the cancer centre team and the community palliative care team may all be independently organised and funded. Nonetheless, patients and their families perceive them as a single entity designed to meet their needs, and naturally expect a seamless service. Excellent communication is essential between all parties, and successful outcomes are critically dependent on this unified team approach.

KEY LOCATIONS OF THE CANCER TEAM

Community
- General practice
- Hospice and community palliative care team

Hospital
- Cancer unit – district general hospital
- Specialist cancer centre – regional teaching hospital

CANCER UNITS AND CANCER CENTRES

The hub and spoke approach has long existed in the provision of cancer services with regional cancer centres sending consultant oncologists out to associated district general hospitals to run peripheral clinics. The relationship between the hospitals has become more formalised and accountable, since the publication in 1995 of "A Policy Framework for Commissioning Cancer Services" known widely as the "Calman Hine report". This report, which was about equitable standards of care, stressed that all patients should have access to treatment in specialist centres wherever necessary, but that advice and treatment should be given as close to home as possible. Implementation of the report required local health authorities and commissioners to visit and accredit hospitals as comprehensive specialist cancer centres or as units for the management of specified cancers.

The cancer centre is usually part of a large teaching hospital and is often co-located with other regional specialist services, such as neurosurgery. Some cancer centres are free-standing cancer hospitals with an associated research institute. Sometimes a number of hospitals work together as a network to provide services jointly on a number of sites. The cancer centre will provide comprehensive cancer treatment facilities including specialist surgery, radiotherapy, intensive chemotherapy and expertise in the management of rare tumour types. Patients may have to travel some distance to get to their nearest cancer centre.

The cancer unit, often based close to where patients live at their local district general hospital, will usually be recognised for the provision of cancer services for the more common tumour types, such as breast and colon cancer. The cancer centre will usually function as a cancer unit for their local population with common cancers.

TUMOUR SITE-SPECIFIC TEAMS

The Cancer Guidance sub-group of the Clinical Outcomes Group of the NHS Executive has published a series of guidelines for purchasers or commissioners on improving outcomes in various types of cancer. Initial guidance covered breast, colorectal, lung and gynaecological cancers. Other guidelines will follow. These documents stress the importance of multidisciplinary and multiprofessional teams for each cancer type, and the importance of excellent communications between members of the teams, patients and GPs. Establishment of these teams, and demonstration of their effective working, are a prerequisite for designation as a cancer unit.

These teams will usually meet on a weekly basis. They will comprise one or more members from the diagnostic specialities, radiology and pathology, and the treatment specialities, surgery and oncology, along with specialists nurses. New patients will be discussed, and potential management plans formulated in line with local and national treatment policies. Patients who may have relapsed or who have other problems needing discussion will also be mentioned.

GENERAL PRACTICE AND COMMUNITY SERVICES

The GP has many roles in the management of patients with cancer, in conjunction with the hospital-based teams. Effective communication is essential for the system to work best. There must be reliable channels of communication from the GP to the hospital teams, as well as from the hospital to the GP.

It is important for each member of the team to play their full part in helping the patient. It is not acceptable for a team member to deny responsibility for an aspect of care, shifting the responsibility onto another team member without informing them. In this way, shared care can all too easily become shared neglect.

The GP will often be the first doctor to suspect that a patient might have cancer. Maybe some initial investigations, such as a chest X-ray or a full blood count and biochemical profile will be requested, or perhaps the new symptom will be sufficient to merit a referral to hospital for a consultant opinion under the "2-week rule" for patients with suspected malignancy (Chapter 5). Speedy and efficient communication is necessary, and often a faxed referral or telephone call is appropriate.

The patient will often return to the GP after a diagnosis is made, perhaps with a spouse, partner or relative, to discuss the diagnosis and its implications. Of course, GPs cannot reasonably be expected to know all the ins and outs of specialist cancer management, but as the doctors who have known the family longer and better than anyone else, it is not surprising when patients turn to them for help at a difficult and stressful time. A GP is well placed to direct patients towards other sources of help, such as CancerBACUP (Chapter 57).

The GP may be called when a patient is unwell at home during the time of treatment, and will have to decide whether there may be a serious complication, such as neutropaenic sepsis, which requires immediate hospitalisation (Chapter 17), or whether the problem can be managed at home.

GPs are often called upon to prescribe cancer treatments on the recommendation of hospital specialists, the most common examples being adjuvant hormonal therapy, such as tamoxifen for breast cancer. Sometimes these will be parenteral, and the practice nurse may be required to give regular monthly or 3-monthly injections of LHRH agonists, such as goserelin to patients with breast or prostate cancer (Chapter 14). Recognising an adverse family history, the GP may decide to discuss a referral for a genetic assessment (Chapter 4).

A patient who has been successfully treated for cancer is rarely free from worries that it might return. It often falls to the GP to assess whether a new symptom requires investigation, referral back to a specialist or reassurance. Sometimes, as some patients are much more anxious than others, a recommendation for psychological support might be appropriate. Many patients find this extremely beneficial.

If cancer does return, and no further active anti-cancer treatment is thought to be appropriate, the GP is responsible for co-ordinating palliative care services. Sometimes a specialist palliative care opinion may be required for difficult symptoms. Sometimes a hospice referral is appropriate. Often, however, the GP can continue to look after the patient without any additional medical input, with the aid of the practice-based district nurses, community-based Macmillan or Marie Curie nurses, social services and other agencies. New symptoms may develop in the terminal phase of the illness. A GP will need to assess a patient carefully to see if breathlessness, for example, is due to anaemia or a pleural effusion, which may be readily treatable by referral back to the hospital or pulmonary emboli or lymphangitis carcinomatosa, which may be more difficult to manage (Chapters 49 and 50).

The family usually get to know the GP very well during the terminal illness managed at home, and the home visits are usually greatly appreciated, both by patient and family, and in particular within a few days of bereavement.

INTERPLAY BETWEEN HOSPITAL- AND COMMUNITY-BASED TEAMS

The complex relationship of shared care between the GP and hospital-based teams may best be illustrated by one patient's cancer journey. A 45-year-old single mum visits her GP with the recent discovery of a mass in the breast. On examination, there is skin dimpling and axillary lymphadenopathy, features suspicious of malignancy. The GP refers the patient by fax under the "2-week rule" to the breast clinic. There she is seen by a consultant breast surgeon, undergoes mammography, fine needle aspiration for cytology and a core biopsy. The findings are discussed at the multidisciplinary breast meeting. The radiologist demonstrates a malignant looking lesion on the mammogram and the pathologist demonstrates malignant cytology and Grade III invasive ductal carcinoma on the biopsy. The tumour is positive for oestrogen receptors. Subsequent staging investigations show no evidence of metastatic disease. It is decided that the best management would be neoadjuvant chemotherapy followed by surgery with immediate breast reconstruction, then radiotherapy and ovarian suppression.

Following a return visit to the breast clinic, where the patient was informed by the consultant of the diagnosis, some further counselling with the breast care clinical nurse specialist and an initial consultation with the oncologist, the patient returns to see her GP. Her main worries at this time were related to the care of her children, while she is undergoing treatment, and she is put in touch with the social worker.

Ten days after the first course of chemotherapy the patient attends the practice for a routine nadir blood count, which shows that she is neutropenic. At that point she feels well, but the next night she develops a high-temperature and 'flu-like symptoms, and calls her GP who arranges for her admission to hospital for investigation and treatment of suspected neutropenic sepsis.

When in the run-up to surgery, the patient visits her GP to discuss whether or not she should have immediate reconstructive surgery, and which of the available methods of reconstruction might be best for her. While the GP may not know all the pertinent details, he or she can at least listen to the patient, try to understand her anxieties and, if necessary contact the breast care nurse or surgeon to relay the problems he has discovered.

After her surgery at the local hospital, she then has to travel up to the big city for radiotherapy at the cancer centre. Subsequently, she attends her practice regularly for repeat prescriptions of tamoxifen and sees the practice nurse 3-monthly for a goserelin injection.

A year later she returns to her GP worried by back pain. The GP is concerned that this might be a bone metastasis, but a bone scan and some plain X-rays show degenerative disease only and she can be reassured.

When 6 months later she comes back complaining of breathlessness, clinical examination and a chest X-ray showed that she has a large pleural effusion. She is referred back to see the oncologist who organises drainage of the effusion, a pleurodesis and further chemotherapy. Later on she becomes jaundiced. She has an enlarged liver and an ultrasound confirms the presence of liver metastases. The patient is unwilling to believe that the poor prognosis her oncologist has given her, and she asks her GP for a second opinion from a more famous cancer centre, which has seen on television. After discussing this with the original oncologist, the GP arranges for the second opinion.

Finally, no more active anti-cancer treatment can be given. Her GP ensures she is cared for at home as long as possible in accordance with her wishes. Support comes from weekly visits to a day hospice, and close input from the community Macmillan team. Near the end, she is admitted to the hospice where she finds peace.

The above example describes hospital and community interaction at its best. The patient with cancer is sensitively, promptly and efficiently cared for in the context of her family.

The treatment of cancer, radical or palliative?

Before embarking on the treatment of any patient with cancer, it is essential to ask whether or not any treatment directed at the cancer itself will be helpful. For many patients with far advanced cancer, particularly, if they are elderly or also have other serious physical or mental illness at the same time, no treatment is the kindest treatment. This is especially true if their symptoms are minimal and easily controlled by general measures, such as analgesics. From time to time a cancer is discovered incidentally at an early asymptomatic stage when treatment is not required. An example of this is the elderly man with a small localised prostate cancer, which might well not cause problems during his lifetime. It may be sufficient to follow a policy of "watchful waiting" and reserve treatment for symptomatic progression. Exceptionally, there are cancers such as the Stage IVS neuroblastoma of infancy which may not require treatment initially as it may possibly undergo spontaneous remission.

> **TREATMENT INTENT**
> - No treatment
> - Supportive care only
> - Palliative anti-cancer treatment
> - Radical treatment
> - Radical treatment with palliative intent

For those patients who are to have anti-cancer treatment, it is very helpful to decide at the outset on the treatment intent. Will the treatment stand any chance of effecting a cure, or is it aimed solely at relief of symptoms? This divides treatment rather simplistically into radical and palliative categories. There are, however, different degrees of intensity of both radical and palliative treatments, and "radical" treatments may be given with palliative intent. Very occasionally, a patient treated palliatively seems to be cured.

DECIDING BETWEEN RADICAL AND PALLIATIVE TREATMENT

Before making a decision about treatment intent, it is necessary to evaluate the tumour for curability in its own right, and to evaluate the patient for their physical, mental and social ability to tolerate any treatments, which might be offered.

> **FACTORS INFLUENCING TREATMENT INTENT**
> - Tumour-related factors: stage, histology and biology
> - Host factors: physical, mental and social

The principal tumour-related factor influencing the treatment intent is stage. Staging is fully discussed in Chapter 8. Most localised tumours are suitable for an attempt at cure, whereas the presence of distant metastases in most types of cancer indicates incurability and the futility of radical treatments. Exceptions to this are the chemocurable tumours, such as many childhood cancers including Wilms' tumour and neuroblastoma, testicular germ cell tumours, gestational choriocarcinoma and leukaemias and lymphomas. While some or most patients with distant metastases from these tumour types may be cured, the presence of blood-borne spread may still be of sinister significance: for example, even with the most intensive therapy, the overwhelming majority of patients with Stage IV neuroblastoma will die from their disease. Patients without distant metastases but who have locally advanced disease or lymph node involvement have a poorer prognosis than those with early disease, but for many tumour types a substantial proportion of those with intermediate stage disease may be cured by radical treatment.

Other tumour factors to be taken into account along with stage are histological type and grade. Anaplastic carcinoma of the thyroid, for example, is very seldom suitable for radical treatment, whereas few patients with differentiated thyroid carcinoma cannot be considered for radical treatment initially. The few patients who become long-term survivors after treatment for anaplastic thyroid carcinoma usually turn out on review of the histology to have had a lymphoma. In some tumour types, biological factors are increasingly being recognised to have prognostic importance, for example oestrogen receptors in breast cancer and chromosomal abnormalities in leukaemia. While at present this does not often influence treatment intent, it is likely to become increasingly important in the future.

While analysis of tumour characteristics is essentially the province of the cancer specialist, the general practitioner can contribute greatly to assessment of the fitness of the patient to undergo radical treatment. In some tumour types, this is of critical importance. For example, patients with advanced head and neck cancer may require intensive chemotherapy, major surgery with the need for vascular and soft tissue reconstruction, and radiotherapy if they are to be cured. The treatment may extend over 6 or more months, and lead to the requirement for a tracheostomy and nutritional support. To cope with this treatment patients have to be physically fit, mentally and emotionally prepared, and have considerable social support for successful rehabilitation. As these patients are often heavy drinkers and smokers, concomitant alcohol- and tobacco-related morbidity, such as cirrhosis, arterial disease and chronic obstructive airways disease, is frequently found. Less commonly, cardiomyopathy and tuberculosis may be related to alcoholism. In addition, they frequently have social problems, such as unemployment and homelessness. In view of these factors, treatment choice is not easy.

RADICAL TREATMENTS

Radical treatments, as alluded to above, are often time consuming and complex, requiring multidisciplinary teamwork and leading to significant acute and long-term treatment-related morbidity. It is clearly inappropriate to subject patients who are clearly in the last few weeks or months of their lives to futile radical treatments. Nonetheless, there are circumstances where, although the disease is considered to be incurable, the patients life expectancy is sufficiently good to make radical type treatment the best option for successful palliation. An example of this is a young child with a diffuse pontine glioma. Although essentially incurable, the best palliation is achieved by high-dose radiotherapy, which requires daily treatment over 6 weeks. If treatment is given over a shorter period, a higher dose per fraction must be used, which may result in unacceptable late normal tissue morbidity, if the child lives more than a year.

> ### FEATURES OF RADICAL TREATMENT
>
> ◆ Severe acute side-effects
> ◆ Potentially fatal complications
> ◆ Complex
> ◆ Risk of significant late treatment-related toxicity
> ◆ Time consuming
> ◆ Often multidisciplinary
> ◆ Costly

PALLIATIVE TREATMENTS

As life expectancy is limited, palliative treatments should be quick, simple and preferably cheap. It is also important

for them to have few side-effects. While it may be acceptable to put up with severe acute toxicity if cure is sought, it is clearly wrong to destroy the quality of the last few weeks of a patient's life with treatment-related side-effects. The aim of treatment is to make patients feel better, not worse.

> ### PRINCIPLES OF PALLIATIVE TREATMENT
>
> ◆ Quick
> ◆ Simple
> ◆ Cheap
> ◆ Few side-effects

Recently, there has been an increasing research interest in palliative treatments. It has been shown that the same benefit is gained from just one or two radiotherapy treatments for the palliation of primary lung cancer, brain metastases or painful bone metastases as from the 5 or 10 treatments, which were commonly used 10 or so years ago.

Although for most of the common cancers, such as pancreatic cancer and colorectal cancer, chemotherapy has objective response rates only of the order of 20%, randomised trials comparing chemotherapy with best supportive care have shown benefit in terms of survival duration and quality of life for patients receiving active anti-cancer treatment.

In recent years, new techniques such as laser treatment, intubation, and endoscopic and vascular stenting have become available to palliate symptoms, such as dysphagia due to oesophageal cancer, dyspnoea due to endobronchial obstruction, obstructive jaundice caused by bile duct and peri-ampullary tumours and superior vena cava compression. These mechanical techniques can be used in conjunction with conventional anti-cancer agents, such as chemotherapy and radiotherapy.

> ### AIMS OF PALLIATIVE TREATMENT
>
> ◆ Relief of symptoms
> ◆ Prevention of symptoms
> ◆ Rarely prolongation of life

While the principal aim of palliation has always been the relief of distressing symptoms in patients with incurable disease, subsidiary aims are prevention of symptoms, which are likely to arrive soon and possibly prolongation of life, where that is easily possible. For example, a palliative resection of a large bowel tumour may be undertaken in the presence of multiple liver metastases, with the aim of preventing intestinal obstruction. Similarly, oral chemotherapy may be used in a patient with advanced small cell carcinoma of the bronchus to prolong life, even though cure is not a possible outcome.

Handbook of Community Cancer Care

Surgery in the treatment of cancer

ROLE OF THE SURGEON

- ◆ Diagnosis, staging and triage
- ◆ Definitive cancer surgery
- ◆ Reconstruction after ablative surgery
- ◆ Salvage of local recurrence and metastatic disease
- ◆ Supportive care
- ◆ Follow-up
- ◆ Palliation

SURGICAL SPECIALITIES IN THE MANAGEMENT OF CANCER

◆ Breast surgeons	Breast cancer
◆ Coloproctologists	Cancer of the colon, rectum and anus
◆ Gynaecologists	Cervix, endometrial and ovarian cancer
◆ Neurosurgeons	Brain and spinal cord tumours
◆ Ophthalmologists	Ocular and orbital tumours
◆ Oro-maxillo-facial surgeons	Oral cavity cancer
◆ Orthopaedic surgeons	Bone metastases, and bone and soft tissue sarcomas
◆ Otolaryngologists	Head and neck cancer
◆ Paediatric surgeons	Cancer in childhood
◆ Plastic surgeons	Skin, and head and neck cancer; and reconstruction
◆ Thoracic surgeons	Lung and oesophageal cancer
◆ Upper gastro-intestinal and hepatobiliary surgeons	Stomach, pancreas, liver and bile duct cancers, and liver metastases
◆ Urologists	Bladder, kidney, prostate, testis and penile cancers

Surgery plays a number of roles in the management of patients with cancer. Often, the surgeon is the first hospital specialist to see a patient with suspected cancer. Following clinical assessment of the patient the surgeon needs to arrange appropriate investigations including imaging and a biopsy, perhaps in conjunction with an examination under anaesthesia (EUA), before discussion at a multidisciplinary meeting and referral to an oncologist.

Some years ago, there was the concept of "surgical oncology" as a subspeciality within general surgery to complement the role of the medical oncologist and the clinical oncologist. Nowadays, as traditional general surgeons disappear and are replaced with more anatomically specialised surgeons, there is no place for a generic surgical oncologist. Many patients with symptoms potentially due to cancer may in fact have benign disease, and the anatomical site-specific surgeon has to deal with both benign and malignant disease. However, within each surgical discipline there may be some surgeons who specialise in the management of cancer to whom their more general colleagues will refer patients.

DIAGNOSIS, STAGING AND TRIAGE

Patients suspected of having cancer should have very careful assessment before definitive procedures are embarked upon. For example, if on open biopsy is needed for a limb lesion, the biopsy should be planned with the definitive operation in mind so that a badly placed scar does not compromise the major procedure. Patients who present with enlarged lymph nodes in the neck should have a careful EUA and a panendoscopy to ensure that there is no primary malignant tumour in the upper aerodigestive tract before the lymph node biopsy is performed. Radical surgery should not be undertaken unless the presence of distant metastases has been excluded.

DEFINITIVE CANCER SURGERY

Many cancers are localised at presentation, and if this is the case radical surgery may offer the best chance of cure. This is certainly true for most gastro-intestinal tumours, especially those of the oesophagus, stomach and large bowel. Only a small proportion of lung cancers are operable but again this offers the greatest likelihood of long-term survival. In some cases, preoperative therapy may be helpful, for example radiotherapy before surgery for rectal cancer. Sometimes, surgery has minimal functional morbidity, for example removal of part of the colon, but other operative procedures such as major head and neck resections may have dramatic effects on normal bodily functions, such as speech and swallowing. In such cases, non-surgical approaches may be preferred and radical radiotherapy is often an alternative to surgery. Adjacent lymph nodes are often cleared or sampled as part of a radical surgical procedure. This may be both diagnostic and therapeutic, and is considered in the chapters relating to specific tumour sites. The place of sentinel node biopsy has been considered in Chapter 7.

RECONSTRUCTION AFTER ABLATIVE SURGERY

A wide variety of surgical techniques are available to help to restore normal bodily appearances and function after major ablative surgery for cancer. Sometimes this can be done at the time of the major operation, sometimes it is performed as a secondary or subsequent procedure. Often, the reconstructive operation can be performed by the surgeon who undertakes the resection, but sometimes the services of a plastic and reconstructive surgeon are called for. The following are a few examples.

1 At the time of mastectomy, a pedicled myocutaneous flap based on the rectus abdominis muscle can be brought up to replace the lost breast tissue. This results in a horizontal bikini-line scar and is known as a transverse rectus abdominis myocutaneous (TRAM) flap reconstruction. A nipple and areola can be fashioned from skin brought up from the inner thigh or vulva, or an areola can be tattooed onto the skin of the flap. Alternatively, a tissue expander can be placed beneath the skin flaps at the time of mastectomy. This is then gradually inflated with saline to create a breast mound. Often the reconstructed breast is smaller than the contralateral healthy breast, in which case a reduction mammoplasty can be performed to restore symmetry.

   In breast-conserving surgery, the loss of tissue can result in an unsightly dent in the breast. This can be prevented at the time of operation by transposing a pedicled latissimus dorsi muscle flap from the back of the chest wall into the excision cavity. This requires no additional scars and produces a very good cosmetic result with no consequent functional disability.

2 Many reconstructive techniques are possible in patients with head and neck cancer:
   - When small skin tumours are excised from the face, small, local skin flaps can be raised to cover the resultant defect, and the cosmetic results are usually excellent.
   - When larger defects need to be repaired distant muscle, or myocutaneous flaps can be moved on their own pedicle, or free flaps moved with their own blood vessels grafted on to those in the head and neck.
   - A section of mandible and overlying skin removed because of an oral cavity tumour can be replaced with a radial free forearm flap.
   - The pharynx may be replaced with a free jejunal transfer in patients undergoing laryngopharyngectomy.
   - The carotid artery can be replaced with a vein graft if it must be sacrificed during and extended radical neck dissection.
3 Patients requiring major resections for bone tumours can have a custom-made endoprosthesis inserted, avoiding the need for amputation. In this way, the large part or even the whole femur can be replaced. In children who have not yet finished growing, a growing endoprosthesis which is lengthened a little every 6 months or so can be used to maintain symmetry between the limbs. Surgery of this kind is only performed at supraregional referral centres.

SALVAGE OF LOCAL RECURRENCE AND METASTATIC DISEASE

Non-surgical treatments used initially with the aim of avoiding the functional losses which may be associated with surgery are not always successful. In the event of residual or recurrent disease, however, surgery may offer the opportunity for salvage. Examples include:

- combined abdomino-perineal resection of the rectum and anus if radical chemo-radiotherapy for anal cancer fails;
- total laryngectomy following failure of radical radiotherapy to effect a cure for advanced laryngeal cancer;
- mastectomy following local recurrence after breast-conserving therapy.

When metastatic disease develops after successful local therapy for a primary tumour, cure is not usually possible. In carefully selected cases, however, salvage surgery may be possible. Examples include:

- radical neck dissection for lymph node involvement after treatment of a squamous carcinoma of the oropharynx;

- removal of a solitary liver metastasis or metastases confined to one lobe of the liver after primary surgery of bowel cancer;
- resection of lung nodules (or pulmonary metastectomy) in patients with local control of osteosarcoma.

SUPPORTIVE CARE

There are many circumstances when a surgeon undertakes a procedure to help a patient with cancer, in a way which enables other treatments to be used successfully. Some of these procedures now fall within the province of the interventional radiologist. These are considered in more detail in Chapter 17. The following are just a few examples:

- Vascular access by insertion of a Hickman line or insertion of a portal vein or hepatic artery catheter for infusional chemotherapy of the liver.
- Insertion of a percutaneous endoscopic gastrostomy (PEG) or other feeding tube.
- Tracheostomy to prevent respiratory obstruction.
- Stenting of blocked ureters.

FOLLOW-UP

It is important to detect local recurrence early if there is a chance for surgical salvage. Some follow-up requires the help of a radiologist, for example regular mammography after breast-conserving surgery. Other types of follow-up may require the specific skills of a surgeon, for example:

- cystoscopy after treatment of bladder cancer;
- endoscopy or EUA after treatment of laryngeal cancer;
- colonoscopy after treatment of bowel cancer to detect local recurrence, metachronous primary tumours and pre-malignant polyps.

PALLIATION

Sometimes, a patient presents with disease which is too advanced for an attempt at cure, and of course some patients relapse after initial treatment with curative intent. The surgeon may well be able to help in these cases, and occasionally even relatively major procedures may be of benefit to patients with incurable disease. As with all interventions, the clinician must weigh up the advantages and disadvantages with the patient and perhaps any relatives and gain informed consent before proceeding. Examples include:

- colectomy for obstructing or bleeding colon cancers even if metastases are present;
- defunctioning colostomy for inoperable rectal cancers;
- biliary stenting for obstructive jaundice due to advanced pancreatic cancer;
- oesophageal stenting to relieve dysphagia;
- surgical pleurodesis after failed medical pleurodesis for a malignant pleural effusion;
- insertion of a Le Veen shunt for recurrent ascites.

CHAPTER 12

Radiotherapy in the treatment of cancer

Radiotherapy, that is treatment with ionising radiation, has been in use for just over a century. Nowadays, the diseases treated are almost always forms of cancer. Recognition of the hazards associated with the use of ionising radiation, coupled with the development of effective remedies for many benign conditions, means that radiotherapy is now rarely used for non-malignant disorders.

RADIOSENSITIVITY AND RADIOCURABILITY

Radiotherapy could probably cure any tumour, provided a high enough radiation dose could be given to all the cancer cells in the body. There are two principal reasons why radiotherapy does not cure all patients. Firstly, normal tissue tolerance limits the dose that can safely be given to any particular part of the body. In general, small volumes of normal tissue will tolerate a higher dose of radiation than larger areas. With extremely large areas, for example whole body irradiation, only very low doses can be given. Some organs in the body, for example the kidneys and spinal cord, are particularly vulnerable to damage by radiation, and so the dose even to small volumes which include such critical structures is limited. Secondly, cancers spread. This means that although a primary bladder cancer, for example, may be cured by radiotherapy to a small volume of tissue including the tumour, the patient may still die from progression of metastatic disease which was not detectable at the time of diagnosis.

Radiosensitive tumours are ones which respond rapidly following treatment, but this does not necessarily mean that they are more radiocurable, as their propensity for distant spread has to be taken into account. For example, smaller, well-localised tumours, such as early laryngeal cancers or basal cell carcinomas of the skin, are in general easily radiocurable although they are relatively radioresistant. In contrast, small cell carcinoma of the bronchus is radiosensitive but is virtually never cured by radiotherapy because of its widespread dissemination. Tumours which have possibly spread into a large area can be cured only if they are very radiosensitive and have spread in a systematic way, so that all the likely areas of involvement can be encompassed. Thus, it is possible to treat all the supradiaphragmatic lymph node areas with a "mantle" field in a patient with Hodgkin's disease, as the pattern of spread is predictable and lymphomas are relatively radiosensitive, so that the dose required for cure is only about half that needed for a squamous carcinoma of the larynx.

DELIVERY OF RADIOTHERAPY

TYPES OF RADIOTHERAPY

- External beam treatment or "teletherapy"
- Interstitial or intracavitary implants or "brachytherapy"
- Unsealed radioactive isotopes or "radionuclide therapy"

Radiotherapy can be administered in one of three ways. Most commonly, external beam treatment is delivered. The patient lies on a couch and beams of radiation are directed from a treatment machine towards the tumour in, for example the lung or breast. Secondly, radioactive materials may be implanted directly into the tumour or inserted into a natural body cavity, such as the uterus, on a temporary or permanent basis. Finally, unsealed radioactive isotopes may be administered. Given orally or intravenously, some drugs are physiologically or pharmacologically concentrated in tumour tissue. The best example is the use of radioactive iodine in thyroid cancer. Alternatively, unsealed sources may be directly inserted into a tumour cyst or natural space, such as the peritoneal cavity.

External beam radiotherapy

A wide variety of treatment machines is available to deliver external beam radiotherapy. There has been a continuing evolution of radiotherapy technology and modern machines are increasingly sophisticated enabling more precise and complex treatments. Old style machines gradually become obsolescent, although they can continue to provide reliable service relatively cheaply where simple treatments are adequate.

One of the most important attributes of a treatment machine is the energy of the beam produced, as this governs the depth of penetration into the body. The energy is measured in kV (low energy) or MV (high energy). Most commonly, high-energy or "megavoltage" radiation (about 4–10 MV) is used. The radiation usually comprises X-rays or "photons" from a machine called a linear accelerator or "linac". For skin tumours where irradiation of internal organs is not required, low-voltage (about 100 kV) or "superficial" X-rays which penetrate only a centimetre or so are used. "Deep" or "orthovoltage" X-rays (about 250 kV) are more penetrating than superficial X-rays. Until about 40 years ago when linear accelerators were introduced, *D*eep *X*-ray *T*herapy units were the principal radiotherapy machines and the abbreviation DXT is still used (incorrectly) as a synonym for all types of radiotherapy. Orthovoltage treatment is rarely used now because the quality of megavoltage radiation from linear accelerators is preferable in many respects. Orthovoltage radiation is largely confined to palliative treatments where its disadvantages are less important.

Gamma rays produced by cobalt (^{60}Co) units are composed of another type of high-energy photon. They have similar powers of penetration to X-rays produced by a linear accelerator at the low end of the energy range (about 2 MV). Cobalt units were once considered alternatives to linear accelerators, but the increasing capability and sophistication of modern linacs means that cobalt units – although still valuable workhorses for simple treatments – are gradually falling out of favour.

Linacs can be used to provide beams of electrons as well as photons. These have the peculiar characteristic of good penetration to a depth of about 1–7 cm (depending on beam energy) with a greatly reduced penetration at deeper levels compared with X-ray and gamma ray photons. They are valuable for treating relatively superficial tumours, especially where they overlie vulnerable structures which might be damaged by high-radiation doses. Electrons are often used after initial photon treatment of a larger volume to boost the dose to residual tumour masses or the tumour bed. Examples include boosting residual neck node masses, while keeping the spinal cord dose within acceptable limits, and boosting the tumour bed following lumpectomy for breast cancer, while limiting the dose to the underlying lung and heart.

In addition to electrons and X-ray and gamma ray photons, another type of external beam radiotherapy, particle therapy, deserves brief mention. Machines called cyclotrons can be used to accelerate subatomic particles, such as neutrons and protons into high-energy treatment beams. Initially, on the basis of theroretical predictions, neutron therapy was hailed as a great advance. Carefully controlled studies by the Medical Research Council in Britain and by other groups abroad have, however, shown that neutrons offer no great advantage over photons, and can lead to greater normal tissue damage. The particular physical characteristics of the proton beam makes it suitable only for the treatment of certain rare tumours, such as ocular melanoma. There is currently only one particle therapy facility in the UK, at Clatterbridge Hospital in Merseyside.

Interstitial and intracavitary radiotherapy

The principal advantage of intracavitary or interstitial radiotherapy, or "brachytherapy" is that the source gives a very high-radiation dose to the immediately adjacent tissues, but only a small dose beyond a couple of centimetres or so away. This means, for example, that the floor of the mouth may be treated, while sparing the salivary glands that are radiosensitive structures. In addition, small tumour residues may be boosted to a high total dose after external beam radiotherapy has taken a larger area to its tolerance dose. For example, in the treatment of cervical cancer, the cervix and vaginal vault can selectively be given a higher total dose than the whole pelvis would tolerate.

The most common indication for brachytherapy is as part of the treatment of gynaecological malignancy, particularly cancers of the cervix and the endometrium. It is only occasionally the sole treatment modality, for example in women with very early cervical cancer and in women with endometrial cancer who are medically unfit for hysterectomy. More often, it is used in conjunction with external beam radiotherapy. In the old days, radium was used and some people still incorrectly use the word "radium" as a synonym for all types of radiotherapy. Radium is obsolete, however, and has been replaced by caesium and iridium.

TYPES OF EXTERNAL BEAM RADIOTHERAPY

- ◆ Photons: X-rays and gamma rays
  - High energy
    - Megavoltage X-rays from a linac
    - Gamma rays from a cobalt unit
  - Low energy
    - Superficial X-rays
    - Deep X-rays
- ◆ Electrons
- ◆ Heavy particles: neutrons and protons

TYPES OF BRACHYTHERAPY

- ◆ Intracavitary
  - Manual loading with caesium
  - Afterloading with caesium or iridium
    - High-dose rate or low-dose rate
- ◆ Interstitial
  - Iridium wire hairpins
  - Plastic tubes afterloaded with iridium wire
  - Permanent gold grain or iodine seed implants

Intrauterine treatment requires a general anaesthetic and preliminary dilatation of the cervix. Patients who have had a hysterectomy and require insertion of caesium only into the vaginal vault may have this done without anaesthesia. Usually, the sources are an intrauterine tube and two small rugby-ball-shaped objects called ovoids, which are positioned in the lateral vaginal fornices. Packing is positioned around the sources to keep them in place, and to ensure that they are not too close to the rectum and bladder base. The sources are removed when the appropriate dose has been delivered. In most centres, direct manual placement of radioactive sources into the correct position has been superseded by afterloading techniques. For afterloading, empty catheters are positioned in the uterus and vagina and packed into place. As they are not radioactive, plenty of time is available to ensure that placement is optimal. Subsequently, the catheters are connected to a machine, and the radioactive sources are automatically inserted up the catheters into the region of the tumour. The introduction of afterloading techniques has reduced the exposure of operating theatre staff to radiation. Different strength sources are available, which deliver the required dose over different periods of time. High-dose rate afterloading techniques deliver the dose in minutes and the patient may be asleep for the entire procedure. With low-dose rate afterloading, and with manual insertion of sources, the duration of treatment is often a day or two and the patients must stay in isolation until the sources are removed. They are confined to bed and require urinary catheterisation. Patients may require one or two insertions, often a week apart.

Brachytherapy is also useful in head and neck cancer. Iridium wire implants are most often used. Wires shaped-like hairpins may be directly inserted into, for example, a small carcinoma of the tongue and removed after about a week. Alternatively, hollow plastic tubes may be implanted and subsequently afterloaded with iridium wire. Occasionally, radioactive gold grains or iodine seeds may be implanted into a tumour. These radionuclides have very short half-lives, and so decay away completely within a few weeks, so that the implant is permanent and does not require removal.

> **USES FOR BRACHYTHERAPY**
>
> ♦ Intracavitary
>   - Cervix, endometrium and vagina
>   - Bronchus
>   - Oesophagus
> ♦ Interstitial
>   - Tongue, floor of mouth, buccal mucosa
>   - Breast
>   - Prostate

It is usually not possible to re-irradiate a previously irradiated area of the body when a cancer recurs. Brachytherapy offers a possible solution in some circumstances. For example, consider a patient who has previously received radiotherapy to the neck for a laryngeal cancer who later develops nodal disease in the neck. During the radical neck dissection to remove the nodes, empty plastic tubes may be positioned in the tumour bed. The defect in the overlying tissues is reconstructed using a myocutaneous flap from an unirradiated part of the body which will tolerate treatment better than the original skin. The tubes are subsequently afterloaded with iridium wire to irradiate the tumour bed.

Other anatomical sites where interstitial implants may be useful include the anus, the prostate and the breast. Other sites where intracavitary brachytherapy is used include the oesophagus and the bronchus.

Radionuclide therapy

Radioactive chemicals which are selectively taken up by tumour tissue may be injected or ingested. This is sometimes known as biologically targeted radiotherapy. It was hoped that monoclonal antibody technology would enable this form of treatment to be used successfully against previously incurable tumours. Sadly, this dream has not been realised. Radionuclide therapy is rarely used alone, but may form an important part of the strategy against selected tumours in conjunction with other treatment modalities.

> **USES OF RADIONUCLIDE THERAPY**
>
> ♦ Thyroid disorders (^{131}I)
>   - Ablation of thyroid remnant in thyroid cancer
>   - Treatment of distant metastases
>   - Thyrotoxicosis
> ♦ Haematological disorders (^{32}P)
>   - Polycythaemia rubra vera
>   - Essential thrombocythaemia
> ♦ Prostate cancer (^{89}Sr)
>   - Bone metastases
> ♦ Neuroendocrine tumours (^{131}I-mIBG)
>   - Phaeochromocytoma
>   - Neuroblastoma
> ♦ Craniopharyngioma cysts (^{90}Y)

Perhaps the best example is the use of oral radioactive iodine (^{131}I) in the management of thyroid cancer. This radionuclide has two therapeutic roles, in addition to its diagnostic role in imaging the thyroid. After surgery for differentiated thyroid cancer, a small amount of residual normal thyroid tissue always remains. An ablative dose of radioiodine is given which is taken up with great avidity by the remnant and destroys it. Metastatic thyroid carcinoma takes up radioiodine less well than normal tissue, so not much of the ablative dose is taken up by metastases. Second and subsequent therapeutic doses of radioiodine will be concentrated better in metastases, destroying them, as competition from residual normal thyroid tissue has been abolished by the initial ablative dose. Radioactive iodine is also used to subdue or destroy non-malignant but overactive thyroid tissue in patients with thyrotoxicosis.

Patients with haematological disorders, such as polycythaemia rubra vera and essential thrombocythaemia may be treated with injections of radioactive phosphorus (^{32}P) as an alternative to other treatments, such as venesection and cytotoxic drugs.

Strontium acts as an analogue of calcium in bone metabolism. The radioactive isotope ^{89}Sr can be used in patients with pain from osteoblastic bone metastases from carcinoma of the prostate. This treatment provides valuable palliation by alleviating pain, and reducing the likelihood of new symptomatic areas developing.

The catecholamine analogue mIBG when labelled with radioiodine can be used for imaging and therapy of neuroendocrine tumours, such as phaeochromocytoma and neuroblastoma.

Unsealed radionuclides can also be physically (rather than biologically) targeted into a tumour, in much the same way as interstitial therapy with removable implants is given. An example is the instillation of yttrium (^{90}Y) colloid into craniopharyngioma cysts using stereotactic localisation. This can be valuable for patients who continue to have problems after surgery and external beam radiotherapy.

RADIOTHERAPY TREATMENT PLANNING

The basic principle of radical external beam radiotherapy is to give as high a radiation dose as necessary to a tumour to be certain of killing it, while keeping the dose to surrounding normal tissues as low as possible to avoid damaging them. Before deciding whether radiotherapy is a possible treatment option for an individual patient, careful assessment with physical examination and appropriate imaging investigations is necessary to determine the extent of the primary tumour and the presence of metastatic disease. If the tumour is localised, and a course of external beam radiotherapy is decided upon, radiotherapy planning has to be undertaken before treatment can start. This may require upto three or four hospital visits prior to commencement of treatment.

Planning may involve preparation of an immobilisation device, especially for a brain, head and neck or extremity tumour. This device, which is usually a plastic shell made from a plaster cast of the patient, keeps the part of the body in the same position from day to day,

enabling the treatment volume to be kept as small as possible. It bears marks to guide the radiographers who deliver the treatment, and means that the patient's skin does not need to be marked.

In the next part of the planning process, the tumour location is identified from diagnostic imaging, which may include a CT scan specially performed for planning purposes. A number of beams are then chosen, which encompass the tumour completely. These may be shaped to keep them as small as possible. Diagnostic X-rays are taken on a radiotherapy planning simulator to check that the proposed field arrangement gives the desired result. All the data are entered into a radiotherapy planning computer and a final plan is decided upon which ensures that all the tumour and any areas of potential spread which are to be treated receive an adequate dose, while the dose to normal tissues is kept to a minimum, paying special attention to the need to protect critical structures, such as the eyes and spinal cord.

RADIOTHERAPY FRACTIONATION

Radiotherapy works by exploiting differences between normal and malignant cells. Malignant cells are more easily damaged by radiation than normal cells, and normal cells have greater powers of recovery from radiation damage. These differences are greater with relatively small radiation doses. If enough radiation is delivered to kill all malignant cells in one go, then the repair processes of normal cells will be overwhelmed, and all the normal cells will also die. If the same total dose is divided up into a number of fractions given daily, then the normal cells will have a chance to repair themselves, while the malignant cells will perish.

RADIOTHERAPY FRACTIONATION

- Standard radical course
  - One treatment a day
  - Treatment 5 days a week
  - Course comprises 20–30 treatments
  - Course duration 4–6 weeks
- Hyperfractionation
  - Two or three treatments each day
  - Treatment 5–7 days per week
  - Aim is cure
- Hypofractionation
  - Use of a few large treatments
  - Usually given once or twice a week
  - Aim is palliative

Radiotherapy fractionation schedules have been derived empirically over the years, and similar tumours are treated in different ways in different centres. In general, most centres treat patients once a day, 5 days a week, but the number of fractions used can vary considerably. For example, an early laryngeal cancer may be treated in 16 fractions in some places, and in 33 fractions in others. Thus, treatment courses may take from 3 to 7 weeks. Palliative treatments are given in fewer fractions, but the number can vary from 1 to 10 in different centres for the same problem. This use of a small number of radiotherapy fractions with a larger dose per fraction is called "hypofractionation".

Proponents of longer fractionation schedules argue that the damage to normal tissues is likely to be less as the dose per fraction is smaller. The use of a large number of small fractions with the aim of reducing normal tissue damage (or to allow an increased total dose to be given without increasing normal tissue damage) is known as "hyperfractionation". On the other hand, prolonging the overall treatment time may allow tumour cells to repopulate. As most of the radiation-induced damage in normal cells is repaired in 6 hours, treatments two or thee times a day, coupled with treatment at weekends, has been investigated. This may allow 36 fractions to be given in 12 days rather than 7 weeks. Shortening the overall treatment time in this way is called "accelerated" radiotherapy. Such schedules of accelerated hyperfractionation do show some promise, but unfortunately the results of various studies have not shown as much benefit as was hoped for.

RADIOTHERAPY DOSE

The unit of radiation dose is the gray (Gy). Doses are sometimes quoted in centigrays (hundredths of grays), or cGy.

The advantage of using the cGy is that it is the same as the old measure of *R*adiation *A*bsorbed *D*ose, the RAD. A typical dose for radical treatment is 50–66 Gy (5,000–6,600 cGy) in 16–33 fractions. The usual fraction size is approximately 2–3 Gy (200–300 cGy). A typical dose for radiosensitive tumours, such as lymphoma or seminoma, is 30–40 Gy (3,000–4,000 cGy). The dose for total body irradiation is about 10–14 Gy (1,000–1,400 cGy) given in six to eight fractions. For palliative treatments, 10–30 Gy (1,000–3,000 cGy) given in 1–10 fractions are often used.

INNOVATIVE APPROACHES

The therapeutic ratio can be improved in a number of ways. These include stereotactic radiotherapy, conformal radiotherapy and intensity modulated radiotherapy (IMRT). These advanced techniques use modern imaging methods such as MRI/CT fusion to define the tumour more precisely, and beam-shaping methods such as micro-multileaf collimators, to increase the proportion of the dose given to the tumour and lessen the dose to uninvolved normal tissues. Results of treatment may be improved as higher tumour doses lead to a better local control probability, and fewer side effects on normal tissues are encountered.

Chemotherapy in the treatment of cancer

The first use of cytotoxic chemotherapy for the treatment of malignant disease was in the 1940s. More drugs were developed in the 1950s, and by the 1960s combinations were developed which proved to be curative for some chemosensitive cancers. The euphoria of anticipated success in the 1970s led to the establishment of many academic units of medical oncology and fuelled the belief that it would not be long before improvements in chemotherapy would make radiotherapy and even surgery for cancer treatment obsolete. While there have, certainly, been advances in chemotherapy practice in the 1980s and 1990s, especially in the field of supportive care, progress towards the cure of common solid tumours in adults remains disappointing. The principal reason why chemotherapy fails to cure cancer is that malignant cells have either intrinsic or acquired drug resistance. Very few completely novel cytotoxic drugs have been developed in the last decade. Perhaps, the greatest advance has been the recognition that chemotherapy may be used with good effect, not alone, but in combination with radiotherapy.

Chemotherapy is a specialist area of medical practice, and cytotoxic drugs should only be prescribed by oncologists with the relevant expertise. Chemotherapy should only be administered in settings where there are the necessary support staff, such as cytotoxic pharmacists and clinical nurse specialists, and facilities for monitoring of toxicities and supportive care. It is still, however, important for general practitioners (GPs) who refer patients for treatment to know the basics about chemotherapy and its side-effects.

WAYS TO USE CHEMOTHERAPY

For some chemosensitive cancer types, such as lymphoma and testicular germ cell tumours, chemotherapy has an important role. It can be used as the sole radical treatment, and cure is often achieved. In this setting, the real benefits of chemotherapy are easy to appreciate, but unfortunately the use of chemotherapy on its own as a curative treatment applies in only a minority of patients with cancer.

The most frequent use of chemotherapy in patients with the common solid tumours is in the so-called adjuvant setting, when it is given after potentially curative local treatment with surgery and often radiotherapy with the aim of reducing the likelihood of relapse. The value of adjuvant chemotherapy, when the survival rate may be increased by only 5–10% over that which can be achieved by local treatment only, can be difficult to recognise with certainty. Large randomised trials with hundreds or thousands of patients may be necessary to prove any benefit beyond doubt. In some cases, such as in younger women with node-positive breast cancer or following surgery for Dukes' C bowel cancer, the value of adjuvant chemotherapy is known, and the debate centres around which type of chemotherapy is best. In other circumstances, for example patients with Dukes' B bowel cancers, and those with squamous carcinoma of the head and neck, the jury is still out.

WAYS TO USE CHEMOTHERAPY

- ◆ Curative intent
  - Sole therapeutic modality
  - Following definitive local treatment (adjuvant or subsequent)
  - Prior to definitive local treatment (neoadjuvant, upfront or induction)
  - Concurrently with radical radiotherapy (synchronous or concomitant)
- ◆ Palliative intent

In certain circumstances, for example locally advanced tumours of the breast, or in many types of childhood cancer, chemotherapy is used prior to surgery. This will usually shrink the tumour, and may make successful surgery more likely. This practice is commonly called neoadjuvant chemotherapy, and is sometimes referred to as upfront chemotherapy.

Chemotherapy is being used increasingly in conjunction with radiotherapy, although their concomitant use adds to the acute toxicity. There is good evidence that chemoradiation results in improved local control for some tumour types, but the evidence that it may improve survival is less strong. Disease types for which chemo-radiotherapy is assuming greater importance include head and neck cancer, anal cancer, cervical cancer and oesophageal cancer.

OUTCOME MEASURES FOR THE ASSESSMENT OF POTENTIALLY CURATIVE CHEMOTHERAPY

- ◆ Improvement in local control rates
- ◆ Improvement in survival rates

The other common indication for chemotherapy is as a palliative treatment for advanced or recurrent disease. In this setting, where cure is not an outcome, there is often a fine balance between the benefits which may accrue and the drawbacks. On the one hand, there is the inconvenience of frequent hospital attendances for blood tests and the administration of chemotherapy, and the associated toxicity which may be considerable. On the other hand, benefits may include relief of troublesome symptoms, prolongation of survival and the psychological benefit of knowing that something is being done. Palliative chemotherapy is a less attractive option when the response rate is known to be low, when the patient's performance status is poor and when there are no major symptoms to palliate. Studies have been performed in a number of cancer types comparing palliative chemotherapy with the "best supportive care". End points have included symptom control, quality-of-life measurements and survival duration. Many of these studies have favoured active treatment, but that does not mean that chemotherapy should be an automatic choice in these circumstances. The decision to treat (or not to treat) can be a very difficult one, and the patient should always be fully informed of the likelihood of benefit and the nature of the side-effects before consent to treatment is sought.

> **OUTCOME MEASURES FOR THE ASSESSMENT OF PALLIATIVE CHEMOTHERAPY**
>
> ◆ Improvement in distressing symptoms
> ◆ Prolongation of survival
> ◆ Improvement in quality of life

ADMINISTRATION OF CHEMOTHERAPY

Chemotherapy is given most often by the intravenous (i.v.) route, either as bolus injections, short infusions (over minutes or hours) prolonged infusions (over days) or continuously (over weeks). Some drugs may be given orally or by intramuscular (i.m.) injection. These are all systemic methods of administration.

Rarely, regional chemotherapy is given. The most common example of this is the intrathecal injection of methotrexate (and sometimes other drugs, such as cytarabine or hydrocortisone) in the prevention or treatment of central nervous system (CNS) involvement by leukaemia or lymphoma. Other examples include portal vein or hepatic artery infusion of drugs for the treatment of liver disease and isolated limb perfusion for melanoma and sarcomas of the limbs. For some cutaneous malignancies, topical application of cytotoxics, such as fluorouracil or mustine, has been used with good effect. The aim of regional therapy is to get a higher dose of the drug into the target to overcome resistance or to reduce systemic side-effects.

> **ADMINISTRATION OF CHEMOTHERAPY**
>
> ◆ Systemic approaches
>   – i.v. injection or infusion
>   – Oral
>   – i.m. injection
> ◆ Regional approaches
>   – Intrathecal injection
>   – Regional perfusion, for example limb or liver
>   – Topical

Venous access

> **TYPES OF CENTRAL VENOUS ACCESS FOR ADMINISTRATION OF CHEMOTHERAPY**
>
> ◆ Hickman line
> ◆ Portacath
> ◆ Peripherally inserted central catheter (PICC)

Venous access can be a problem in many patients. This is partly because there must be repeated venepunctures and cannulation over a period of months. These are for blood tests, administration of chemotherapy and supportive measures, such as i.v. antibiotics in the event of neutropenic sepsis, and blood or platelet transfusions. It is also because many cytotoxic drugs can cause phlebitis and thrombosis and damage the veins into which they are injected. Central venous lines can overcome these difficulties, but they require meticulous care to minimise the chances of infection. They can also be associated with other complications including blockage and thrombosis of a major vein.

There are a number of different types of indwelling central line in common use in patients receiving chemotherapy. Traditionally, they have been placed by surgeons; but more recently, interventional radiologists, anaesthetists and specialist nurses have become competent in the required techniques.

Hickman lines are tunnelled under the skin of the chest for about 10 cm before they enter a great vein such as the subclavian or less commonly the internal jugular. They continue down into the superior vena cava. Externally, they have a screw cap and clamps. They may have one or two lumens, and can be used for taking blood samples as well as for administering treatment.

Portacaths are completely internal, and are therefore less likely to be accidentally displaced. They terminate in a subcutaneous chamber with a membrane. They are accessed by needling the membrane through the skin.

PICC lines are inserted into a vein in the arm in much the same way as a traditional i.v. cannula, but they extend further inside the body, as far as the subclavian vein or superior vena cava.

SCHEDULING OF CHEMOTHERAPY

Chemotherapy drugs may be used alone or in combination. Single drugs can provide simple treatments in the palliative setting but combination chemotherapy is the basis of almost all potentially curative schedules. By using several drugs with a known activity against a particular tumour type, but with different mechanisms of action, it may be possible to circumvent the development of drug resistance. This is similar to the use of combination anti-retroviral therapy in patients with human immunodeficiency virus (HIV) and multiple drug therapy against tuberculosis. Another reason for the use of combinations is to increase anti-tumour effect without reaching dose-limiting toxicity by using drugs with different toxicity profiles.

For most drugs and combinations, myelotoxicity is the side-effect which limits the dose which can be administered at any one time. Most treatments are scheduled with gaps of 3–4 weeks between courses to allow for haematological recovery. In many courses, an individual course comprises treatment on a single day; sometimes it may involve treatment of 1 day and again 1 week later followed by a 2- or 3-week break. Weekly schedules have been developed for some diseases, such as weekly fluorouracil and folinic acid for colorectal cancer. These are particularly suitable for administration at weekly clinics in cancer units which are not permanently staffed. Wherever possible, outpatient administration is preferred to schedules which need an inpatient stay. Infusional chemotherapy over a few days or a week or continuously can be administered to outpatients who attend only to have a pump connected to (or disconnected from) their Hickman line.

CLASSES OF CHEMOTHERAPEUTIC AGENTS

The 50 or so cytotoxic drugs in general use today have various origins and work in different ways. They also have different patterns of side-effects. They can be grouped together into five classes:

CLASSES OF CYTOTOXIC DRUGS

- Alkylating agents
- Antimetabolites
- Plant derivatives
- Anti-tumour antibiotics
- Miscellaneous

Alkylating agents

These are reactive compounds which exert cytotoxicity by effectively interrupting DNA replication. Other functional cellular molecules can also be alkylated in this way. Examples of drugs in this class are cyclophosphamide, ifosfamide, melphalan, busulfan, chlorambucil and the nitrosoureas, carmustine and lomustine.

Antimetabolites

These are simple chemicals with a structural similarity to normally occurring cellular compounds. They act by interfering with essential cellular metabolism. Methotrexate, for example, is an antifolate compound which acts as a false substrate for the enzyme dihydrofolate reductase, thereby preventing the conversion of dihydrofolate to tetrahydrofolate. Folinic acid bypasses this block and it can be administered to terminate the cytotoxic effect of methotrexate. Blood methotrexate levels can be measured and provide a guide as to whether folinic acid is necessary or not. Other antimetabolites include the purine antagonists mercaptopurine and tioguanine and the pyrimidine antagonists 5-fluorouracil, cytarabine and fludarabine. These drugs act in the DNA synthesis (S) phase of the cell cycle. Folinic acid can be used with 5-fluorouracil to potentiate its efficacy. This is a very different role from its use in conjunction with methotrexate. Newer antimetabolites include raltitrexed, a thymidylate synthase inhibitor, and gemcitabine.

Plant derivatives

Various substances derived from plants are cytotoxic. The vinca alkaloids, namely vincristine and vinblastine have come from the Madagascar pink periwinkle and act by binding to the protein tubulin, preventing spindle formation during mitosis leading to metaphase arrest. Vindesine and vinorelbine are in the same group.

- The vinca alkaloids, namely vincristine, vinblastine, vindesine and vinorelbine are for *i.v. administration only*
- They are *not* for intrathecal administration because of severe neurotoxicity which is usually fatal
- Manslaughter charges have followed the accidental misuse of vincristine in this way

---

The epipodophyllotoxin derivatives etoposide and teniposide are inhibitors of the enzyme topoisomerase II which is involved in DNA processing. The Yew tree derivatives paclitaxel and docetaxel inhibit microtubule disassembly.

Anti-tumour antibiotics

Various naturally occurring drugs have been extracted from bacterial and fungal cultures. They include actinomycin D, bleomycin and the anthracyclines doxorubicin, epirubicin, idarubicin and daunorubicin. Related drugs include mitoxantrone and mitomycin. They work by intercalating between DNA base pairs, preventing cell division.

Miscellaneous drugs

The platinum derivatives carboplatin, cisplatin and the new analogue oxaliplatin form cross links with DNA. Asparaginase breaks down asparagine, depriving some malignant cells of an essential nutrient. Procarbazine is a monoamine oxidase inhibitor, but is also a cytotoxic prodrug which is metabolically activated to produce an alkylating effect on nucleic acid. Irinotecan and topotecan act by inhibiting the enzyme topoisomerase I.

SIDE-EFFECTS OF CHEMOTHERAPY

All cytotoxic chemotherapy drugs are essentially cellular poisons which produce beneficial effects by killing malignant cells. As poisons, they also have the capacity to harm healthy cells and tissues. The skill of the oncologist, based on prior experience and the results of clinical trials, is to select drugs alone or in combination at doses where the benefit exceeds the drawbacks. Even so, in order to maximise benefits, doses often have to be such that there is significant toxicity. Some side-effects are common to most (although not all) cytotoxic agents. These are often due to damage to the stem cell pool of a tissue which is turning over rapidly, such as the bone marrow or gut mucosa. Other side-effects are more specific to particular drugs or classes of drugs. Measures which may be taken to minimise and ameliorate the adverse effects of cancer treatment are described in Chapter 17.

ACUTE SIDE-EFFECTS OF CHEMOTHERAPY

- Neutropenia and infection
- Thombocytopaenia
- Nausea and vomiting
- Alopecia
- Diarrhoea
- Soft tissue necrosis as a result of extravasation

MYELOSUPPRESSION

The bone marrow is one of the most sensitive normal tissues in the body. Almost all cytotoxic drugs therefore will affect the blood count to a lesser or greater degree. For this reason, the blood count is always checked prior to each course of chemotherapy. For most drugs, the low point or nadir in the blood count will occur 10–14 days after administration of the chemotherapy, followed by fairly rapid recovery over the next week or so. For this

reason, many chemotherapy schedules cycles are of 3- or 4-weeks duration. Some drugs such as mitomycin lead to a longer duration of myelosuppression and their scheduling is typically every 6–8 weeks. Some drugs, such as vincristine and bleomycin, are much less toxic to the bone marrow than many others. They are, therefore, sometimes used alternately with more myelosuppressive combinations to enable chemotherapy to be given weekly or fortnightly while still allowing count recovery to take place.

Not all blood components are affected equally. The most common effect is suppression of the white blood cells, particularly the neutrophils. A neutrophil count of $1.0 \times 10^9 l^{-1}$ is usually required before the next course of chemotherapy is given. Neutropenia is more likely if the bone marrow is already compromised by malignant infiltration or prior treatment, such as wide-field radiotherapy.

Severe neutropenia, with a count below $0.5 \times 10^9 l^{-1}$ is often complicated by sepsis, requiring urgent medical treatment. Neutropenic sepsis is usually manifested by a fever, and can be defined as a pyrexial episode when the temperature is elevated to 38°C on two consecutive measurements, or to 39°C on one occasion with an absolute neutrophil count below $1.0 \times 10^9 l^{-1}$. Neutropenic sepsis is more likely if the neutropenia is prolonged, if there is mucositis or ulceration which allows pathogenic organisms easier access to the circulation, or a focus of infection such as urinary catheter, venous cannula or central line. If a patient develops a fever or a 'flu-like episode after chemotherapy they should seek immediate medical attention. Patients with possible neutropenic sepsis should not be treated at home but referred as an emergency to hospital for investigation and treatment. Delay will allow the patient to become sicker, and occasionally neutropenic sepsis may prove fatal.

All patients receiving potentially myelosuppressive chemotherapy will have been warned of the risk of infections occurring when the white blood count is low following chemotherapy. It is good practice for a routine full blood count to be arranged at the time of the anticipated nadir. If the count is low the patient can be contacted to see if they are still well, and to remind them of the need to seek hospital attention, if they develop fever.

Recombinant human granulocyte colony stimulating factor (rhG-CSF) preparations such as filgrastim or lenograstim are given by daily subcutaneous injection to treat or prevent neutropenia. Prefilled syringes enable easy patient self-administration in the community.

Platelets are the blood component next most commonly affected by chemotherapy. It is not usual to give the next course of chemotherapy unless the platelet count is greater than $100 \times 10^9 l^{-1}$. There may be exceptions to this rule, for example if the chemotherapy is being used to treat metastatic breast cancer with bone marrow involvement of which thrombocytopenia is a symptom. Following chemotherapy, platelet counts as low as $20 \times 10^9 l^{-1}$ are not usually a problem, but with very low counts prophylactic platelet transfusions are indicated to prevent bleeding or bruising. Not only are these symptoms unpleasant, but an intracranial bleed, for example, may be fatal. Different thresholds for the use of prophylactic platelet transfusion may be set in various circumstances, but usually they are between 12 and $20 \times 10^9 l^{-1}$. In the presence of evidence of bleeding including petechial haemorrhage, purpura or bruising, platelet transfusions may be necessary even with a higher platelet count. Once transfused, platelets only last for 1 day or 2, so repeated transfusions may be necessary until the count recovers.

Anaemia requiring blood transfusion is not a common consequence of chemotherapy, but milder degrees are often seen. Cisplatin seems to have a greater effect on red cells than other blood components. Patients are often put on iron supplements for this, but this is not beneficial unless there is actually evidence of iron deficiency.

Recombinant human erythropoeitin (epoetin) can be given by subcutaneous injection, usually weekly, to reduce blood transfusion requirements in patients with chemotherapy induced anaemia. Moderate or severe anaemia should be corrected by blood transfusion before epoetin is commenced.

Gastro-intestinal toxicity

> **GASTRO-INTESTINAL SIDE-EFFECTS OF CHEMOTHERAPY**
>
> ◆ Nausea
> ◆ Vomiting
> ◆ Diarrhoea
> ◆ Mucositis

The management of nausea and vomiting, formerly among the most feared side-effects of chemotherapy, has been revolutionised in recent years with the introduction of new and powerful anti-emetics, such as ondansetron and granesetron which act on the 5-hydroxytryptamine-3 receptor (5-HT-3 antagonists). They are usually given in conjunction with dexamethasone before severely emetogenic chemotherapy such as cisplatin. 5-HT-3 antagonists are less good at treating the delayed nausea which sometimes follows chemotherapy. Traditional anti-emetics, such as metoclopramide, can be helpful here and are often sufficient for use with less emetogenic chemotherapy schedules. Premedication with lorazepam can be helpful for some patients who develop severe anticipatory symptoms prior to chemotherapy.

Some drugs, particularly fluorouracil, have an effect on the stem cells in bowel mucosa leading to diarrhoea.

Irinotecan, a new drug used in the management of colorectal cancer, causes diarrhoea through two mechanisms. The early diarrhoea at the time of administration is mediated through a cholinergic response and can be prevented by premedication with atropine. Later diarrhoea developing a week or so after administration requires treatment with loperamide. Occasionally, this can be severe enough to merit hospitalisation.

Several drugs may affect the mucous membranes and cause mucositis and oral ulceration. The most common culprits in this regard are doxorubicin and methotrexate. The mucosal toxicities of chemotherapy and radiotherapy can be synergistic.

Alopecia

Hair loss is common with chemotherapy, although it is not associated with some drugs, such as bleomycin or cisplatin. If alopecia is a possible consequence of treatment, it should be mentioned during the consenting process. Sometimes, the likelihood of hair loss can be reduced by scalp cooling, and this should be offered where appropriate, although it is not always effective, it can prolong the duration of individual treatments and some patients find it too uncomfortable to tolerate. Wigs can be ordered in advance of hair loss for those likely to need them, as this does not usually occur until 3 weeks after the start of treatment. A variety of hats, headscarves and turbans are preferred to wigs by some patients.

Renal and urinary tract toxicity

Renal damage can be associated with drugs, such as cisplatin, ifosfamide and high-dose methotrexate. Baseline renal function should be assessed by glomerular filtration rate (GFR) estimation. Hydration is necessary to promote rapid renal excretion. As methotrexate can precipitate in renal tubules if the urine is acidic, care must be taken to ensure alkalinisation of the urine when high-dose methotrexate is used. Knowledge of the renal function is also required to determine the correct dose of some drugs, such as carboplatin which have complex pharmacokinetics and are largely renally excreted. Various types of nephrotoxicity can be produced, and both cisplatin and ifosfamide can cause renal tubular leakage of elements, such as magnesium and potassium. Affected patients may need long-term mineral supplementation.

Renally excreted metabolites of ifosfamide (and to a lesser extent cyclophosphamide) can damage the urothelium, leading to haemorrhagic cystitis. For this reason, ifosfamide should always be given with the drug mesna, which protects the urothelium. Mesna is sometimes necessary when cyclophosphamide is used, especially, at the higher end of the dose range.

Neurotoxicity

Vincristine can lead to a peripheral neuropathy which often manifests as tingling and numbness in the fingers and toes, and loss of reflexes. There may be a slow but often incomplete recovery after treatment. It can cause transient jaw pain and also an autonomic neuropathy with constipation or even ileus. Vincristine should only ever be used intravenously. Inadvertent intrathecal use is fatal.

Cisplatin and the new platinum analogue, the oxaliplatin, used in the treatment of colorectal cancer, can also produce a peripheral neuropathy, but carboplatin does not. In addition, cisplatin is ototoxic, producing high tone deafness. Patients should have a baseline audiogram and undergo regular monitoring throughout treatment.

Ifosfamide can produce an encephalopathy, and cytarabine can cause spinal cord damage when used in high doses intrathecally.

Cardiotoxicity

The anthracycline drugs, such as doxorubicin, can produce both acute dysrhythmias during administration and potentially fatal cardiomyopathy. This side-effect is related to the cumulative dose. Baseline tests of cardiac function including electrocardiography (ECG) and some measurement of ejection fraction – either a multiple-gated arteriography (MUGA) scan or an echocardiogram – are sensible precautions and are mandatory if there is a history of pre-existing cardiac disease. A cumulative dose of $450\,mg\,m^{-2}$ should not usually be exceeded in adults. The safe limits for children are lower than this. Some sparing of cardiotoxicity without impairing the likelihood of disease control may be achieved either by fractionating the dose per course over 2–3 days or by administering the drug as an infusion rather than as a bolus. Some cardioprotective drugs have been investigated which may be used concomitantly with anthracyclines in those at risk of cardiac damage. Liposomal formulations are available which may similarly be less cardiotoxic.

Fluorouracil is a widely used drug, and occasionally it may cause angina. Its use should be stopped, if a patient does develop angina as myocardial infarction may result.

Pulmonary toxicity

Alkylating agents, particularly busulfan, may cause pulmonary fibrosis after prolonged use. Bleomycin can cause pulmonary infiltrates which can lead to fibrosis. Although idiosyncratic responses can occur at low doses, the likelihood of occurrence is usually dose related, and the cumulative dose should not exceed $300\,mg\,m^{-2}$. Care should be taken in patients with pre-existing lung disease and pulmonary function should be assessed both before and

during treatment. Oxygenation during anaesthesia in patients who have received bleomycin previously, especially within recent months, can lead to respiratory failure. Radiotherapy to the lungs can increase these problems.

If a patient, previously treated with busulfan, has to be referred to hospital for surgery requiring anaesthesia, it is helpful if the GP mentions this fact in the referral letter. This is particularly important in emergencies as previous notes may not be readily available at the hospital.

Extravasation injury

The majority of cytotoxic drugs are given by i.v. injection. If the cytotoxic leaks out into the perivascular soft tissues during administration, local damage can result. At its mildest, this may just be pain and erythema at the site of injection, but at the other extreme there may be tissue necrosis which may need plastic surgery for repair. The drugs, most likely to cause these problems, are vinca alkaloids and anthracyclines. With care, extravasation should be unusual. If it does occur, damage can often be limited if appropriate action is taken immediately. If a patient consults their GP about pain related to an injection site after chemotherapy administration, immediate referral back to the hospital is warranted.

Infertility

Many cytotoxic drugs, especially alkylating agents, can lead to infertility in both men and women. All patients for whom infertility is a potential side-effect of proposed treatment should be warned of this before treatment is begun. Sperm storage is an established way of circumventing infertility in postpubertal males. Much research is going on in the field of reproductive technology, and this is a fast moving area of medicine. Storage of ovarian tissue or eggs is sometimes offered, but is at present an unreliable way of ensuring future fertility. Storage of embryos is a more certain way of achieving a pregnancy in the future, but is dependent upon the woman having a willing partner. All these procedures need time which may not be available if there is an urgent need for treatment. There are no reliable ways of preserving fertility in prepubertal children. There are many ethical and religious issues surrounding reproductive technology, and this field of medicine is also subject to legal regulation by the Human Fertilisation and Embryology Authority. It is entirely appropriate for a patient who is concerned about future fertility to be referred to a specialist with an interest in this area for an opinion prior to treatment, if time permits.

Second malignant neoplasms

It is well recognised that people who are predisposed to one cancer by virtue of exposure to carcinogens (e.g.

smoking) or genetics (e.g. retinoblastoma) may develop second tumours if they survive the first tumour. It is also known that there is a small possibility that radiotherapy may induce a cancer years after treatment, which is one reason for trying to avoid irradiating patients with benign diseases where possible. Chemotherapy also has the ability to damage DNA, and chemotherapy-related second malignancies are seen especially in younger patients who have been treated for Hodgkin's disease, where there is a high likelihood of cure. Alkylating agents and etoposide are the drugs most often implicated. Leukaemia is one of the more common malignancies after chemotherapy. Chemotherapy and radiotherapy may be synergistic in the causation of second malignancies.

GLOSSARY OF CYTOTOXIC DRUGS

Where recent European legislation has substituted recommended international non-proprietary names (rINN) for the former British approved name (BAN), both names are given with the rINN taking precedence.

Glossary of cytotoxic drugs

Drugs	Class	Indications	Route of administration	Major toxicities	Precautions
Bleomycin	Anti-tumour antibiotic	Lymphomas, squamous cell carcinoma, malignant pleural effusions	Intracavitary, i.v. or i.m. injection	Fever and rigors acutely, skin pigmentation, pulmonary fibrosis	Corticosteroids will help 'flu-like symptoms at the time of administration, monitor chest X-ray and pulmonary function, warn anaesthetists to avoid high oxygen concentrations to prevent respiratory failure
Busulfan (busulphan)	Alkylating agent	Chronic myeloid leukaemia, in high dose in conjunction with melphalan as myeloablative therapy prior to bone marrow or peripheral blood stem cell support for neuroblastoma	Oral	Myelosuppression and irreversible bone marrow aplasia, hyperpigmentation of the skin, progressive pulmonary fibrosis	Regular monitoring of the blood count
Capecitabine	Antimetabolite	Breast and colon cancer	Oral	Plantar/palmar erythema (PPE)	Pyridoxine may help PPE
Carboplatin	DNA intercalating agent (platinum compound)	Ovarian cancer, germ cell tumours, lung cancer, paediatric cancer	i.v. infusion	Myelosuppression, particularly thrombocytopenia, nausea and vomiting	Caution in renal impairment, measure renal function (i.e. GFR) to determine dose
Carmustine	Alkylating agent (nitrosourea)	Myeloma, lymphoma, brain tumours	i.v. injection	Myelosuppression (which may be delayed), emesis, renal damage and pulmonary fibrosis	Monitor blood counts and lung and kidney function, use 6-weekly schedule
Chlorambucil	Alkylating agent	Chronic lymphatic leukaemia, low-grade NHL, Hodgkin's disease, ovarian cancer	Oral	Myelosuppression, rarely rashes which can progress to Stevens–Johnson syndrome or toxic epidermal necrolysis	Stop treatment if rash occurs
Chlormethine (mustine)	Alkylating agent	Few nowadays, Hodgkin's disease	i.v. injection	Emesis, tissue necrosis if extravasated	Inject into fast flowing i.v. infusion
Cisplatin	DNA intercalating agent (platinum compound)	Ovarian cancer, germ cell tumours, lung cancer, head and neck cancer, paediatric cancer, as a radiosensitiser	i.v. infusion	Severe nausea and vomiting, nephrotoxicity, neurotoxicity, ototoxicity	Monitor renal function (i.e. GFR), pre- and post-hydration, monitor hearing, electrolytes
Cladribine	Antimetabolite	Hairy cell leukaemiam, refractory chronic lymphatic leukaemia	i.v. infusion	Myelosuppression, neurotoxicity	Monitor use closely
Cyclophosphamide	Alkylating agent	Widely used for lymphoma, lung cancer, breast cancer, paediatric malignancies and other tumour types	i.v. bolus or infusion or oral	Myelosuppression, nausea and vomiting, alopecia, haemorrhagic cystitis	Ample hydration and use mesna for uroprotection with higher-dose schedules or if additional risk factors, such as pelvic radiotherapy
Cytarabine	Antimetabolite (anti-pyrimidine)	Acute leukaemia	Subcutaneous, i.v., intrathecal	Myelosuppression	Monitor blood count
Dacarbazine	Miscellaneous	Melanoma, Hodgkin's disease	i.v.	Intense nausea and vomiting, myelosuppression, hepatic vein thrombosis	Caution in liver disease
Dactinomycin	Anti-tumour antibiotic	Sarcomas and paediatric tumours	i.v. injection	Hepatotoxicity, interaction with radiotherapy	Care with dosing in very young babies and when radiotherapy is also used
Daunorubicin	Anti-tumour antibiotic (anthracycline)	Acute leukaemia, AIDS-related Kaposi's sarcoma (with liposomal formulation)	i.v. infusion	As for doxorubicin	As for doxorubicin

(continued)

Glossary of cytotoxic drugs (*continued*)

Drugs	Class	Indications	Route of administration	Major toxicities	Precautions
Docetaxel	Plant derivative (taxane)	Breast cancer	i.v. infusion	Hypersensitivity reactions, fluid retention, myelosuppression alopecia, nausea and vomiting	Dexamethasone for 5 days with each course starting the day before each docetaxel infusion will limit oedema and hypersensitivity reactions. Caution in hepatic failure
Doxorubicin	Anti-tumour antibiotic (anthracycline)	Breast cancer, sarcomas, paediatric tumours, leukaemia, lymphomas	i.v. infusion	Nausea and vomiting, myelosuppression, alopecia, mucositis, extravasation injury, dysrhythmias and cardiomyopathy	Monitor ECG and cardiac function, limit lifetime dose to 450 mg m^{-2}, caution in patients with pre-existing heart disease, reduce dose in jaundiced patients as the drug is excreted by the liver
Epirubicin	Anti-tumour antibiotic (anthracycline)	As for doxorubicin	i.v. infusion	As for doxorubicin, except it is somewhat less cardiotoxic	As for doxorubicin, except maximum dose is 900 mg m^{-2}
Estramustine	Combination of alkylating agent and oestrogen	Prostate cancer	Oral	Gynaecomastia, impaired liver function	Monitor blood count
Etoposide	Topoisomerase II inhibitor	Lymphomas, paediatric tumours, testicular cancer, lung cancer	i.v. infusion or oral	Nausea and vomiting, myelosuppression, alopecia	Monitor carefully
Fludarabine	Antimetabolite	Refractory chronic lymphatic leukaemia and low-grade NHL	i.v. infusion	Myelosuppression, CNS and pulmonary toxicity	Monitor closely
Fluorouracil	Antimetabolite	Breast cancer, colorectal cancer, skin cancer	i.v. bolus, i.v. infusion, topical	Diarrhoea, skin pigmentation, plantar and palmar erythema, and desquamation	Complex pharmacokinetics and metabolism, action enhanced by folinic acid
Gemcitabine	Antimetabolite	Non-small cell lung cancer, pancreatic cancer	i.v.	Haemolytic uraemic syndrome	Discontinue if microangiopathic haemolytic anaemia develops do not use concurrently with radical radiotherapy
Hydroxycarbamide (hydroxyurea)	Miscellaneous	Chronic myeloid leukaemia, polycythaemia	Oral	Myelosuppression, nausea, skin reactions	Monitor blood count
Idarubicin	Anti-tumour antibiotic (anthracycline)	As for doxorubicin, but the oral formulation makes it especially suitable for the frail and elderly	i.v. infusion or oral	Similar to doxorubicin	Similar to doxorubicin
Ifosfamide	Alkylating agent	Lymphomas, lung cancer, paediatric tumours	i.v. infusion	Urothelial toxicity, renal toxicity	Hydration, always use mesna
Irinotecan	Topoisomerase I inhibitor	Colorectal cancer	i.v. infusion	Acute (cholinergic syndrome) and delayed diarrhoea, myelosuppression.	Premedication with atropine, loperamide for delayed diarrhoea
Lomustine	Alkylating agent (nitrosourea)	Lymphomas, brain tumours	Oral	Delayed myelosuppression, emesis	Monitor blood counts, 6-weekly scheduling
Melphalan	Alkylating agent	Myeloma, lymphomas, high-dose therapy	Usually oral, sometime i.v	Myelosuppression, may be delayed	Monitor blood count
Mercaptopurine	Antimetabolite	Continuing therapy for ALL	Oral	Myelosuppression	Dose should be used if allopurinol is given concurrently as it interferes with mercaptopurine metabolism
Methotrexate	Antimetabolite (inhibits dihydrofolate reductase)	Breast cancer, head and neck squamous cancer, lymphoma, osteosarcoma, choriocarcinoma, leukaemia (CNS directed therapy and	i.v. bolus or infusion, i.m. injection, intrathecal or oral	Myelosuppression, mucositis	Caution in renal or hepatic impairment, GFR should be measured. Avoid use if pleural effusion or ascites is present as it tends to accumulate in these fluids,

Drug	Class	Uses	Administration	Toxicity	Comments
		continuing therapy of ALL). Usually used at low-dose, but high-dose use is possible (see below)			and slow return to the systemic circulation results in enhanced toxicity. High-dose use requires hydration, urinary alkalinisation, monitoring of blood levels and termination of action by folinic acid
Mitomycin	Anti-tumour antibiotic	Upper gastro-intestinal cancers, breast cancer, superficial bladder cancer, anal cancer (with radical radiotherapy)	i.v. infusion, intracavitary instillation	Delayed myelosuppression	6-weekly scheduling
Mitoxantrone (mitozantrone)	Anti-tumour antibiotic (anthraquinone)	Breast cancer, lymphomas	i.v. infusion	Myelosuppression, cardiotoxicity	Cardiac monitoring after doses of $160\ \mathrm{mg\ m^{-2}}$
Oxaliplatin	DNA intercalating agent (platinum compound)	Colorectal cancer	i.v. infusion	Neurotoxicity	Careful monitoring
Paclitaxel	Plant derivative (taxane)	Ovarian cancer, breast cancer, lung cancer	i.v. infusion	Hypersensitivity and anaphylaxis, myelosuppression, peripheral neuropathy, cardiac conduction defects and dysrhythmias, muscle pain, alopecia, nausea and vomiting	Premedication with a corticosteroid, an antihistamine and a histamine-2 receptor antagonist recommended to prevent severe hypersensitivity reactions, as well as usual 5-HT-3 antagonist as an anti-emetic
Procarbazine	Miscellaneous	Hodgkin's disease, brain tumours	Oral	Nausea, myelosuppression, hypersensitivity rash	It is a mild monoamine oxidase inhibitor, and alcohol should be avoided as it causes a disulfiram-like reaction
Raltitrexed	Antimetabolite (thymidylate synthase inhibitor)	Colorectal	i.v. infusion	Myelosuppression, gastrointestinal toxicity	Careful monitoring
Temozolamide	Miscellaneous	Brain tumours	Oral	Myelosuppression	Caution in renal or hepatic impairment
Thiotepa	Alkylating agent	Bladder cancer, malignant pleural effusions, brain tumours	Intracavitary, i.v. injection	Myelosuppression	Blood counts
Tioguanine (thioguanine)	Antimetabolite	Remission induction in acute myeloid leukaemia, continuing therapy for ALL	Oral	Myelosuppression	Monitor blood count
Topotocan	Topoisomerase I inhibitor	Ovarian cancer	i.v. infusion	Acute (cholinergic syndrome) and delayed diarrhoea, myelosuppression	Premedication with atropine, loperamide for delayed diarrhoea
Treosulfan	Alkylating agent	Ovarian cancer	Oral or i.v. infusion	Skin pigmentation	
Vincristine	Plant derivative (vinca alkaloid)	Leukaemia, lymphoma, paediatric tumours	i.v. bolus	Neuropathy	Never give intrathecally
Vinblastine	Plant derivative (vinca alkaloid)	Leukaemia, lymphoma, breast cancer	i.v. bolus	Myelosuppression	Monitor blood count
Vindesine	Plant derivative (vinca alkaloid)	Leukaemia, melanoma	i.v. bolus	Myelosuppression, neuropathy	Monitor carefully
Vinorelbine	Semi-synthetic plant derivative (vinca alkaloid)	Non-small cell lung cancer, breast cancer	i.v. bolus	Myelosuppression	Monitor carefully

Other medical treatments of cancer

In addition to surgery, radiotherapy and chemotherapy, there is a miscellaneous group of established treatments available for patients with cancer. These include endocrine treatments, immunological treatment, drugs affecting bone mineralisation and calcium metabolism and interventional radiology procedures. There are also drugs and other treatment methods, which have not yet found their way into the range of therapeutic options, but remain under investigation in the preclinical setting and in early phase clinical trials. Examples include gene therapy, vascular targeting and anti-angiogenesis drugs. These offer hope for the future, but are not considered further here.

HORMONAL TREATMENTS

The responsiveness of breast cancer to hormonal manipulation has been recognised for over a century since Beatson introduced oophorectomy as a treatment for advanced breast cancer. Since then patterns of treatment have changed as surgical ablative procedures, such as oophorectomy, adrenalectomy and hypophysectomy, have to a large extent been replaced by drug treatments including oestrogen receptor antagonists, progestogens, aromatase inhibitors and luteinising hormone releasing hormone (LHRH) agonists, and treatments found to be effective for advanced disease have been used as adjuvant therapy.

> **HORMONES FOR THE TREATMENT OF PATIENTS WITH CANCER**
>
> - Sex hormones and antagonists in breast, prostate and endometrial cancer
> - Thyroid hormones to suppress thyroid-stimulating hormone (TSH) levels in thyroid cancer
> - Somatostatin analogues for carcinoid tumours
> - Corticosteroids

The use of sex hormones and their antagonists is similarly useful in prostate cancer and, to a lesser extent, in endometrial cancer. Differentiated thyroid cancers grow under the influence of TSH, and can be suppressed by the use of thyroid hormone-replacement therapy. Somatostatin analogues can be used to treat neuroendocrine cancers, such as carcinoid tumours.

Corticosteroids have a very wide rôle in the management of malignant disease including as a cytotoxic agent in leukaemia and lymphoma, ameliorating pressure symptoms due to brain tumours or spinal cord compression, alleviating the side-effects of chemotherapy, such as nausea and vomiting and hypersensitivity reactions, and improving quality-of-life factors, such as appetite and well-being in the palliative care setting.

Corticosteroids, and similarly growth hormone, thyroid hormones, antidiuretic hormone and sex hormones are also used as replacement therapy, when the hypothalamic–pituitary axis or other endocrine organs have been disturbed by the disease or its therapy. Physiological replacement of hormones falls outside the scope of this chapter, which is concerned with treatments for cancer, but is covered in Chapter 19.

OESTROGEN DEPRIVATION IN BREAST CANCER

Oestrogen receptor positive breast cancers (Chapter 20) are stimulated by the physiological levels of oestrogen circulating in pre-menopausal women. Therapeutic oestrogen deprivation through ovarian ablation has benefit in the treatment of advanced disease and as an adjuvant therapy. However, subjecting a woman to an abrupt, early menopause is very unpleasant with the sudden onset of sweats and hot flushes. Also, there may be other menopausal symptoms including mood swings, memory impairment, loss of libido and joint pains. The risk of osteoporosis is brought forward, as the rate of bone density loss is greatest in the first year after the menopause, whether it occurs naturally or is induced artificially. There is also, of course, the loss of fertility.

> **METHODS FOR ACHIEVING OESTROGEN DEPRIVATION IN PRE-MENOPAUSAL WOMEN**
>
> - Surgical oophorectomy
> - Radiation menopause
> - Chemotherapy (not reliable)
> - LHRH agonists, for example goserelin (Zoladex)

Oestrogen deprivation can be achieved in several ways. Surgical oophorectomy is, of course, the oldest method.

It is instantly effective but requires an additional operation and produces additional scars, unless it is done at the same time as another procedure, such as TRAM flap breast reconstruction. Laparoscopic oophorectomy is now often performed, which is a minimally invasive technique.

Pelvic radiotherapy will stop the ovaries producing oestrogen. A radiation menopause, which usually takes only four or five radiotherapy treatments and avoids the need for surgery, can conveniently be administered when the patient attends for chest wall radiotherapy. Results are slow, and it may take months for amenorrhoea to develop. There is a small risk of a second malignancy arising in the pelvic organs.

Chemotherapy is not given with the aim of ovarian ablation, nonetheless amenorrhoea is often a consequence of this treatment. In the adjuvant setting, it may be worth waiting to see if periods stop with chemotherapy, and checking luteinising hormone (LH) and follicle-stimulating hormone (FSH) levels to determine the menopausal status, before using any other form of ovarian ablation.

The use of LHRH agonists, such as goserelin (Zoladex), offers a reversible medical alternative to oophorectomy. A depot formulation in the form of a small pellet is injected subcutaneously into the anterior abdominal wall. Monthly and 3-monthly formulations are available. Two years treatment is thought to be adequate. There is evidence that in pre-menopausal women with oestrogen receptor positive breast cancer 2 years of goserelin in addition to tamoxifen is better than tamoxifen alone. Goserelin therapy is not a cheap alternative, but this approach is especially advantageous in younger women who are keen to retain the option of a subsequent pregnancy.

OESTROGEN RECEPTOR ANTAGONISTS

> **OESTROGEN RECEPTOR ANTAGONISTS AND SELECTIVE OESTROGEN RECEPTOR MODULATORS**
>
> - Tamoxifen
> - Toremifene
> - Raloxifene

Tamoxifen was introduced 30 years ago and very rapidly established a place as a simple and effective treatment with minimal toxicity for the treatment of advanced breast cancer. Subsequently, its value as an adjuvant treatment has been defined.

> **INDICATIONS FOR TAMOXIFEN**
>
> - Adjuvant therapy of early breast cancer
> - Initial treatment of advanced or metastatic breast cancer
> - Chemoprevention of breast cancer in women at high risk

More recently, tamoxifen has been investigated in breast-cancer protection trials in women at greater than normal risk of developing breast cancer. Results so far suggest that chemoprevention with tamoxifen does reduce the incidence of breast cancer, but a consequent reduction in mortality has not yet been demonstrated and trials are continuing.

The likelihood of benefit is greatest in those whose tumours express the highest levels of oestrogen receptor. There is also some benefit in patients with progesterone receptor positive and oestrogen receptor negative tumours. The response rate is very low in patients with tumours known to be completely negative for both receptor types, and most specialists would not recommend its use in this group of patients. It is beneficial in both pre-menopausal and post-menopausal women.

In the post-menopausal woman, the principal side-effects include sweating and hot flushes, but these are often mild. Nausea may be experienced for a few days after starting tamoxifen, but this symptom settles spontaneously. When tamoxifen treatment is started in women with advanced disease, such as bone metastases, there may be a syndrome of tumour flare with increased pain and sometimes hypercalcaemia. Vaginal discharge and pruritis vulvae may occur. Many women complain of weight gain. In pre-menopausal women, the side-effect profile is less favourable: hot flushes and sweating may be more severe, and amenorrhoea or other menstrual disturbance may occur.

With long-term use, there may be some serious side-effects, but these are all rare. Ocular side-effects include corneal changes, cataracts and retinopathy. Any patient on tamoxifen who experiences visual disturbance should be referred for an ophthalmological opinion. Hepatic dysfunction includes changes in liver enzymes, fatty liver, cholestasis and hepatitis. There is an increase in thrombo-embolic events when tamoxifen is used in conjunction with chemotherapy.

> **RARE BUT POTENTIALLY SERIOUS ADVERSE EFFECTS OF LONG-TERM USE OF TAMOXIFEN**
>
> - Ocular symptoms
> - Hepatic dysfunction
> - Endometrial hyperplasia and carcinoma
> - Thrombo-embolic disease

Tamoxifen is a partial oestrogen agonist, and may stimulate the endometrium leading to endometrial hyperplasia, polyp formation, vaginal bleeding and endometrial carcinoma. Women who develop post-menopausal bleeding on tamoxifen, and pre-menopausal women who develop abnormal vaginal bleeding should be referred to a gynaecologist for investigation. A benefit of the partial agonist activity of tamoxifen is that it reduces the likelihood of osteoporosis developing in post-menopausal women, and in pre-menopausal women who have been subjected to some form of ovarian ablation.

The dose of tamoxifen is 20 mg daily. Formerly, higher doses were used, which conferred no additional benefit but increased the likelihood of adverse reactions. Sometimes in women with advanced disease, a high (loading) dose is used for a week, which is then reduced to the standard 20 mg daily. This may shorten the time before benefit is seen, but does not alter the response rate.

In the adjuvant setting, tamoxifen is normally given for a period of 5 years. This duration has been shown to be better than just 1 or 2 years. There is, as yet, no very convincing evidence that to continue tamoxifen indefinitely after 5 years confers additional benefit, but there is, of course, the risk of more adverse effects with prolonged use. Large-scale clinical trials addressing the question of the optimum duration of tamoxifen use are in progress.

Toremifene is another oestrogen receptor antagonist. It is licensed for use in post-menopausal women with hormone dependent metastatic breast cancer. The side-effect profile is very similar to tamoxifen. Once again, it is associated with an increased risk of endometrial changes including hyperplasia, polyps and cancer. Abnormal vaginal bleeding including menstrual irregularities, vaginal discharge or symptoms, such as pelvic pain or pressure should be investigated promptly. It is not widely used as it offers no benefit over tamoxifen.

Raloxifene is a selective oestrogen receptor modulator similar to tamoxifen and toremifene. It is marketed as a form of hormone-replacement therapy (HRT) to diminish the risk of vertebral fractures in post-menopausal women at increased risk of osteoporosis. It does not reduce the menopausal vasomotor symptoms of hot flushes and sweating. It is not licensed as a treatment for breast cancer, and indeed is said to be contraindicated.

OTHER HORMONAL THERAPY FOR BREAST CANCER

When metastatic disease progresses in patients on tamoxifen, or when women who have received adjuvant tamoxifen therapy relapse, second-line (and subsequently third-line) hormonal therapy is often indicated. In the naturally post-menopausal woman, and in pre-menopausal women treated with some form of ovarian ablation, there are still very low levels of oestrogen in the circulation. Oestrogens are created in peripheral fatty tissues by the enzyme aromatase from precursors derived in the adrenal cortex. This was the basis for the now historical procedure of surgical adrenalectomy for metastatic breast cancer. Later, drugs such as aminoglutethimide were developed as a form of medical adrenalectomy. Aminoglutethimide stopped the production of all hormones from the adrenal cortex, and so it had to be used in conjunction with physiological-replacement doses of hydrocortisone. Sometimes mineralocorticoid replacement was also necessary. Initial use of aminoglutethimide and hydrocortisone was often accompanied by a florid rash, but nonetheless it was an effective treatment.

> ### AROMATASE INHIBITORS
> ◆ Anastrozole (Arimidex) (oral, 1 mg daily)
> ◆ Letrozole (Femara) (oral, 2.5 mg daily)
> ◆ Exemestane (Aromasin) (oral, 25 mg daily)
> ◆ Formestane (Lentaron) (deep intramuscular injection, 250 mg every 2 weeks)

The development of aromatase inhibitors has, however, made the use of aminoglutethimide almost obsolete. There are three oral aromatase inhibitors available, anastrozole, exemestane and letrozole, and there is probably little to choose between them in terms of efficacy or side-effect profile. Licensed indications do, however vary, and anastrozole (Arimidex) is the only aromatase inhibitor licensed for adjuvant therapy. Anastrozole is now recommended as adjuvant therapy in women with hormone receptor positive breast cancer, who are naturally or artificially post-menopausal, if tamoxifen is considered undesirable because of the increased thrombo-embolic risk or endometrial abnormalities.

These drugs are very well tolerated and have fewer side-effects than tamoxifen. The principal symptoms relate to oestrogen deprivation, such as hot flushes and vaginal dryness. They should not be used if there is severe renal or hepatic impairment.

Following the use of tamoxifen, aromatase inhibitors are better tolerated and more effective than progestogens as second-line therapy in post-menopausal women. There are some data to suggest that they may be more effective than tamoxifen in the initial treatment of advanced disease. Recent studies have shown that anastrozole has better response rate than tamoxifen, and that the time between starting treatment and tumour progression is longer with anastrozole. Some specialists, therefore, recommend aromatase inhibitors as first-line therapy for advanced disease in post-menopausal women with oestrogen receptor positive breast cancer.

The largest adjuvant breast-cancer study to date, the ATAC trial, which recruited nearly 10,000 post-menopausal women, compared anastrozole with tamoxifen with both drugs in a double blind placebo controlled way. The results of this trial show that anastrozole results in a significantly better disease-free survival at 3 years compared with tamoxifen. There is, as yet no overall survival advantage. There is a significant reduction in the incidence of contralateral second primary breast cancers with anastrozole compared with tamoxifen. The combination of two drugs is no better than tamoxifen alone. The side-effect profiles of the two drugs are different, and this finding may be of greater significance than any difference in efficacy. There is a lower incidence of uterine bleeding requiring investigation with anastrozole, and a lower risk of endometrial cancer developing. There is less chance of potentially fatal thrombo-embolic complications developing with anastrozole compared with tamoxifen. Anastrozole, however, lacks the protective effect of tamoxifen on bone mineralisation, so there are fewer osteoporotic fractures in women treated with tamoxifen. There are also fewer musculoskeletal side-effects observed with tamoxifen.

Formestane was the first available aromatase inhibitor, but it never gained great popularity as it has to be given by fortnightly injections. There may be pain and irritation at the injection site, and occasionally sterile abscesses will result. It is perhaps most suitable for those whose compliance with oral medication may be poor, for example women with mild dementia who live alone in the community.

It is important to remember that aromatase inhibitors only work in post-menopausal women. If there is any doubt about ovarian function (e.g. in a woman who has previously had a hysterectomy with ovarian conservation) laboratory tests for LH and FSH may be helpful.

PROGESTOGENS FOR USE IN BREAST CANCER

- Megestrol acetate
- Medroxyprogesterone acetate
- Norethisterone

Progestogens have been displaced to third-line therapy in post-menopausal women, but they have one advantage over aromatase inhibitors in that they can be used in pre-menopausal women. The most commonly used preparations are megestrol acetate and medroxyprogesterone acetate. These can both be given orally. The side-effects are generally mild and include nausea, weight gain and fluid retention manifested by ankle swelling and dyspnoea. This may lead to congestive cardiac failure requiring diuretic therapy in elderly patients with little cardiac reserve. There was once a vogue for using high-dose medroxyprogesterone acetate by deep intramuscular injection, but this is not recommended as there are additional side-effects, but no additional therapeutic benefit. Norethisterone is another progestogen which can be used for the treatment of breast cancer.

Historically, oestrogens such as stilboestrol and androgenic anabolic steroids, such as nandrolone were used in the treatment of breast cancer. These drugs are now obsolete for this indication as the other drugs mentioned above are more effective and have fewer adverse effects.

HORMONAL THERAPY OF PROSTATE CANCER

As with breast cancer, the hormonal dependence of many prostate cancers has long been recognised (Chapter 35). About 85% of patients with advanced prostate cancer will respond to endocrine therapy, with a response duration commonly in the region of 12–18 months. As was the case with oophorectomy and breast cancer, surgical castration was the first form of hormonal manipulation available, but is not surprisingly associated with some psychological distress. Subcapsular orchidectomy removes all hormone producing tissue, but does not leave the scrotum completely empty.

HORMONAL TREATMENTS IN PROSTATE CANCER

- Bilateral supcapsular orchidectomy
- Gonadorelin analogues (LHRH agonists)
- Anti-androgens
- Total androgen blockade
- Oestrogens

Different types of pharmacological hormone manipulation have the same end results as surgical castration: impotence, infertility, gynaecomastia and testicular atrophy; but they are not perceived in the same way.

Synthetic oestrogens were the first drug treatment used for prostate cancer. They are, of course, complicated by impotence and gynaecomastia, but the most worrying side-effect is the high incidence of thrombo-embolic disease. Indeed, in patients with more favourable prognosis prostate cancer, the death rate from the cardiovascular complications of stilboestrol, especially when used at higher doses, outweighed the mortality of the disease itself. Oestrogens are, therefore, used very little nowadays for this indication. Fosfestrol is a prodrug which following intravenous or oral administration is metabolised by prostatic acid phosphatase to produce stilboestrol. Its side-effects are as for stilboestrol itself, and in addition it can produce unpleasant perineal pain. It too is little used.

ANTI-ANDROGENS FOR PROSTATE CANCER

- Bicalutamide (Casodex)
- Cyproterone acetate (Cyprostat)
- Flutamide (Drogenil)

Anti-androgens are effective in patients with prostate cancer. Several drugs are available in this category including bicalutamide (Casodex), cyproterone acetate and flutamide. They may be beneficial when used alone, either for the initial management of patients with either metastatic or locally advanced non-metastatic prostate cancer, or in patients with metastatic prostate cancer refractory to LHRH agonist therapy. They are indicated to cover the "tumour flare" associated with the initiation of LHRH agonist therapy (see below). Finally, as not all androgens in the body come from the testes (e.g. some androgens may be adrenally derived), anti-androgens may be used in conjunction with orchidectomy or LHRH agonists as "total androgen blockade" which is being investigated in clinical trials to see whether it is in fact better than orchidectomy or LHRH agonist therapy alone.

**USE OF ANTI-ANDROGENS
IN PROSTATE CANCER**

- Monotherapy
- To cover initial tumour flare associated with LHRH agonists
- Total androgen blockade

Production of testosterone by the testes is stimulated by LH. LHRH agonists or gonadorelin analogues, such as buserelin (Suprefact), goserelin (Zoladex), leuprorelin (Prostap) and triptorelin (De-capeptyl) cause initial stimulation, then depression of LH release by the pituitary. Used alone in patients with prostate cancer, LHRH agonists may produce an initial surge of testosterone resulting in a "tumour flare" which, depending on the site of the cancer, may cause bone pain, spinal cord compression, ureteric obstruction and other undesirable effects. Anti-androgens such as bicalutamide (Casodex), cyproterone acetate or flutamide should, therefore, be used for 3 days before a gonadorelin analogue is first given and continued for 3 weeks afterwards.

Gonadorelin analogues are as effective as orchidectomy in the initial treatment of prostate cancer. They lack the psychological trauma associated with castration, however. They cannot be administered orally as, being polypeptides, they would be digested. The formulation of goserelin (Zoladex) is probably the easiest to use. This comes as a pellet, which is injected subcutaneously. Two preparations are available, which are administered either monthly or 3 monthly. Leuprorelin (Prostap) comes as a

powder, which when reconstituted is injected intramuscularly or subcutaneously every month, or every 3 months. Triptorelin (De-capeptyl) comes as a powder, which when reconstituted is injected intramuscularly every month. No 3-monthly formulation is available.

Buserelin (Suprefact) is not available in a depot formulation. Treatment is initiated with subcutaneous injections three times a day for a week, followed by a nasal spray used in both nostrils six times a day. The nasal spray may cause nasal irritation, nose bleeds and an altered sense of smell and taste.

In addition to their use in breast and prostate cancer, drugs such as goserelin may be used to delay the onset of puberty in children with precocious puberty caused by, for example, a hypothalamic tumour.

HORMONAL THERAPY OF ENDOMETRIAL CARCINOMA

Endometrial carcinoma (Chapter 33) is usually a localised disease with a good prognosis treated with surgery and radiotherapy. Response rates to endocrine therapy in patients with recurrent or metastatic disease are reported to be between 15% and 40%. Relapses, where there has been a prolonged interval between initial treatment and recurrence, low-grade tumours, tumours expressing progesterone receptors and disease in the lung or vagina are more likely to show a response. Initial treatment is usually with progestogens, such as medroxyprogesterone acetate or megestrol acetate. Sometimes second-line therapy is tried when there is progression after an initial response to progestogens. In this setting, tamoxifen and goserelin have been used most often. A number of trials have evaluated adjuvant endocrine therapy following local treatment for endometrial cancer, but there is no evidence of benefit even in selected sub-groups of patients.

HORMONAL THERAPY OF RENAL CELL CARCINOMA

Various types of steroid hormone receptor have been identified in renal cell carcinoma. It is, therefore, not surprising that responses have been seen with many different types of hormone therapy. Drugs which have been evaluated include progestogens, anti-androgens and tamoxifen. The response rate is, however, poor at only about 5%. Given the lack of alternative therapeutic strategies, and the very limited toxicity, it is worthwhile offering patients with recurrent or metastatic renal cell carcinoma palliative treatment with oral progestogens, such as megestrol acetate despite the low probability of response. Progestogens have been evaluated in randomised trials as adjuvant therapy for renal cell carcinoma,

---

**FORMULATIONS OF LHRH AGONISTS
(GONADORELIN ANALOGUES)**

Goserelin	Subcutaneous	Monthly/3 monthly
Leuprorelin	Subcutaneous	Monthly/3 monthly
	Intramuscular	Monthly
Triptorelin	Intramuscular	Monthly
Buserelin	Subcutaneous	Three times a day for 1 week then
	Intranasal	Six times a day

but there is no evidence of a reduction in the likelihood of recurrence or of a prolongation of survival.

HORMONAL THERAPY OF THYROID CANCER

The management of thyroid cancers is considered in Chapter 29. Prolonged elevated levels of TSH may cause the development of differentiated thyroid cancers of follicular cell origin, that is papillary and follicular cancer. These cancers, once established, grow under the influence of TSH. After the initial treatment of thyroid cancer with surgery and radiotherapy, the body has lost its ability to produce thyroxine, and without thyroid hormone-replacement therapy the patient would become hypothyroid. The aim of treatment with thyroxine (now to be prescribed by the recommended international non-proprietary name (rINN) levothyroxine sodium) is, however, more than physiological replacement to ensure a euthyroid status. The aim is to give supraphysiological doses, so that TSH is suppressed below the normal range and so that any residual cancer cells are not stimulated to divide. There is evidence that suppressive doses do improve outcome. This mild biochemical hyperthyroidism may unmask any latent tendency for osteoporosis to develop, and measurement of bone mineral density may be appropriate from time to time in selected patients.

CORTICOSTEROID THERAPY

Corticosteroids, such as prednisolone and dexamethasone have many uses in cancer patients, as cytotoxics, immuno-suppressants, anti-inflammatories, replacement and in symptom control and supportive care.

USES OF CORTICOSTEROIDS IN THE MANAGEMENT OF CANCER

◆ Cytotoxic	Leukaemia, lymphoma
◆ Immunosuppressant	Transplantation
◆ Anti-inflammatory	Cerebral oedema
◆ Replacement	Loss of adrenal function
◆ Symptom control	Anorexia
◆ Supportive care	Chemotherapy-induced vomiting

Treatment regimens for acute lymphoblastic leukaemia (ALL), Hodgkin's disease and non-Hodgkin's lymphoma (NHL) contain high-dose steroids given for short courses. The usual drug is prednisolone for Hodgkin's disease and NHL, but dexamethasone has been shown to be superior in ALL. In this setting, steroids act as a true cytotoxic drug. Lymphocytes are exceptionally sensitive to steroids, and steroid therapy alone can be enough to produce

tumour lysis syndrome. Due to this indication, steroids are given for short periods, for example 1 or 2 weeks only, adrenal suppression and Cushingoid side-effects are not common. It is not usually necessary to "tail off" the steroids with each course, but sometimes this is called for, especially in the elderly. Other side-effects, such as osteoporosis, avascular necrosis of bone and cataracts may develop in the long term after the use of treatment regimens containing high-dose steroids.

Patients who undergo allogeneic bone marrow transplant, or who require a solid organ transplant after treatment for cancer, may have steroids as part of their immunosupressive protocol to prevent rejection. Because of the long-term side-effects of steroids, other immuno-suppressants, such as cyclosporin and azathioprine are used in an attempt to reduce the need for steroids.

Some of the pressure symptoms in patients with brain tumours, spinal cord compression and superior vena cava obstruction are not caused directly by the presence of the tumour, but by surrounding oedema. Symptoms of raised intracranial pressure may be alleviated, and sometimes neurological disability will be improved, by the use of steroids in patients with brain tumours.

It is, however, important to keep the dose as low as possible and the duration of use as short as possible. Other measures of reducing intracranial pressure should be used wherever they can. These include the insertion of a ventriculo-peritoneal shunt in the event of obstructive hydrocephalus, surgical debulking of an intracranial mass lesion and radical or palliative radiotherapy. The best use of steroids in the case of brain tumours, spinal cord compression or superior vena cava obstruction is to relieve symptoms in the acute phase and buy time until a diagnosis has been made and plans for a definitive treatment have been put in place.

It is kindest to avoid steroids in the terminal phase of life in patients with recurrent, untreatable brain tumours. Other treatments such as morphine are effective for headaches and avoid the distress of a gross Cushingoid appearance and proximal myopathy, which develops only too quickly in patients on high doses of steroids.

In other palliative care settings, low doses of steroids, such as 10–20 mg enteric coated prednisolone given as a once-daily dose may be helpful. It is always best to try to give a short course, which may be repeated rather than continuous therapy. Steroids given in this way can help to improve appetite and improve the patient's sense of well-being. Sometimes pain, such as that caused by distension of the liver capsule by metastatic disease, may be relieved by steroids.

The use of steroids with anti-emetics for chemotherapy is discussed in Chapter 17. The use of steroid-replacement therapy is covered in Chapter 19.

Patients on steroid therapy should carry a steroid card (see box) which records the personal details of which drug, what dose, and dates in addition to generic advice.

Patients on long-term steroids may benefit from a "tag" stating this fact in case of emergency. This can take the form of a bracelet, watch or necklace. They are available from Hoopers MediTag, 37 Northampton Street, Huckley, Birmingham B18 6DU (telephone 0121-200 1616). Alternatively, they can be ordered from Boots the Chemist, whose larger branches will have a catalogue in store from which to choose.

SOMATOSTATIN ANALOGUES

Somatostatin is the hypothalamic hormone which inhibits the release of growth hormone from the pituitary gland. Two analogues are available, which can be used for the treatment of a number of neuroendocrine tumours including carcinoid tumours, pituitary adenomas causing acromegaly, and neuroendocrine pancreatic tumours, such as VIPomas and glucagonomas.

Octreotide (Sandostatin) is given by subcutaneous injection up to three times a day. The dose will be escalated from a starting dose of 50 μg daily to 200 μg three times a day until symptoms are controlled. A depot preparation for injection every 4 weeks is available. With carcinoid syndrome, if the symptoms of flushing, diarrhoea and bronchospasm are not alleviated after a week, therapy should be stopped.

Lanreotide (Somatuline) has the same advantage as depot octreotide of less frequent administration. It can be given by intramuscular injection every 14 days initially,

thereafter every week to 10 days. A newer preparation offers monthly administration in a small volume from a prefilled syringe.

Side-effects include gastro-intestinal disturbances, such as anorexia, nausea, vomiting, abdominal pain and bloating, flatulence, diarrhoea and steatorrhoea. Post-prandial glucose intolerance may be impaired and rarely persistent hyperglycaemia occurs with chronic administration. Hypoglycaemia has also been reported. Caution should be exercised in diabetic patients. Abrupt withdrawal of octreotide has been associated with biliary colic and pancreatitis, and gallstones have been reported after long-term use. It is helpful to check the gall bladder with an ultrasound at the start of treatment and periodically thereafter with long-term use. Pain and irritation may occur at the injection site, and so rotating sites should be used.

Somatostatin analogues may be radiolabelled and used for diagnostic scanning in patients with known or suspected neuroendocrine tumours. They have also been used for the targeted radionuclide therapy of these conditions.

IMMUNOTHERAPY, MONOCLONAL ANTIBODY THERAPY AND BIOLOGICAL RESPONSE MODIFIERS

There has been much interest over the years in the immunology of cancer. Many cancer cells have a phenotype which expresses particular cell surface markers. These have been extensively exploited for diagnostic purposes with immunohistochemistry (Chapter 7). It has proved less easy to exploit the immunological differences between normal and cancer cells for therapeutic purposes. Reasons for this include the fact that not all malignant cells will express a particular marker, and most so-called cancer antigens are not specific to cancer cells, but also occur on some normal tissues as well.

The technology to produce antibodies of one sort (monoclonal antibodies) in appreciable quantities has been around for more than 20 years, and many attempts have been made to utilise these substances therapeutically. Unfortunately, they have not proved to be the "magic bullets" once hoped for. Nonetheless, they are finding a place in a few limited situations.

MONOCLONAL ANTIBODIES USED AGAINST CANCER

- Rituximab   NHL
- Trastuzamab   Breast cancer
- Anti-GD2   Neuroblastoma

Rituximab (Mabthera) is a monoclonal antibody, which causes lysis of B lymphocytes. It has recently been licensed for the treatment of chemotherapy-resistant advanced B-cell follicular NHL. NICE supports its use for this indication as last-line therapy in prospective case series. Rituximab is also used in the management of high-grade diffuse B-cell NHL. The chemotherapy-combination CHOP (cyclophosphamide, doxorubicin, vincristine and prednisolone) in combination with rituximab is better in older patients than CHOP alone. It can be an effective treatment, but arrhythmias, heart failure, hypotension, allergic reactions, such as rash, pruritis, angioedema, bronchospasm and dyspnoea, and cytokine release syndrome and tumour lysis syndrome may complicate its use. Such adverse reactions may be fatal, and so rituximab should only be used in settings with full resuscitation facilities after premedication with antihistamines, analgesics and corticosteroids. With these precautions, treatment is generally well tolerated, but obviously, treatment should be initiated and supervised by a specialist.

Trastuzamab (Herceptin) offers new hope for women with advanced breast cancer after failure of conventional chemotherapy. Its use is now recommended by NICE in certain circumstances (Chapter 20). It is only used in patients whose tumours express the Her2 antigen (sometimes called Her2neu or CerbB2) at the 3+ level. It may be used alone or in combination with chemotherapy drugs, such as paclitaxel. As with rituximab, there may be infusion-related side-effects with the first dose, such as fever and chills, and anaphylactic reactions are possible. The incidence of moderate or severe cardiac dysfunction is about 5%. Despite the possibility of these toxicities, most patients receiving trastuzamab will tolerate it well. The use of trastuzamab may lead to better outcomes (response rates and survival) than chemotherapy alone in patients selected on the basis of their Her2 status.

There is some evidence that children with advanced neuroblastoma may benefit from treatment with an anti-GD2 monoclonal antibody following conventional therapy. This is unpleasant treatment producing various side-effects including pain severe enough to require a morphine infusion. It is about to be tested in an international multicentre study.

Stimulation of the body's own immune response may help to fight cancer. It may prove to be less toxic than the administration of monoclonal antibodies. The use of BCG as intravesical therapy for superficial bladder cancer has been known to be effective for more than 20 years. Complete remission of carcinoma *in situ* of the bladder occurs in over three-quarters of patients. A number of tumour vaccines are being investigated as adjuvant therapy for a variety of malignancies ranging from osteosarcoma to breast cancer, but their value remains to be proven. Other circumstances where vaccination might help to prevent (rather than cure) cancer are the use of hepatitis B vaccine and hepatocellular carcinoma, and vaccines against human papilloma virus and cervical cancer.

Another reason for the interest in cancer immunology stems from the observation that sometimes (albeit very rarely) some tumours, most noticeably malignant melanoma and renal cell carcinoma, may undergo spontaneous regression. An immunological basis has been postulated to explain this unusual phenomenon, and researchers have sought ways to reproduce this response using naturally occurring biological molecules known to be involved in immunological pathways, such as interferons and interleukins. Collectively, these are known as biological response modifiers, and treatment with these substances is referred to as biotherapy.

Interferons have shown some anti-tumour effect in certain lymphomas and solid cancers. Interferon alpha (leucocyte or lymphoblastoid interferon) is usually used for malignant disease. Interferon beta (fibroblast interferon) is used for multiple sclerosis. The precise role of interferons remains controversial and ill-defined, but indications for interferon alpha are shown in the box. Dose schedules vary, but interferon alpha is most often given by subcutaneous injection three times a week. The side-effects are dose related but often include influenza-like symptoms including fever, chills, myalgia, lethargy and depression. Myelosuppression may also occur.

INDICATIONS FOR INTERFERON ALPHA

- AIDS-related Kaposi's sarcoma
- Hairy cell leukaemia
- Chronic myeloid leukaemia
- Metastatic carcinoid tumour
- Malignant melanoma (adjuvant therapy)
- Myeloma (maintenance of remission)

Aldesleukin is recombinant interleukin-2. It is licensed for use in patients with metastatic renal cell carcinoma. It is thought to work best in patients with a better prognosis, and so it should not be used if all three of the following adverse prognostic indicators are present: performance status 1 or more, more than one organ involved by metastatic disease, and disease-free interval less than 2 years. It is very toxic and although it may bring about a "response" in terms of tumour size, it has not been demonstrated to prolong survival. It is also being evaluated in patients with melanoma.

Differentiating agents are another form of "biological" therapy for cancer. Retinoids and other drugs including interferon have been shown *in vitro* to cause undifferentiated malignant cells to mature into their benign counterparts. The only proven clinical indication is the adjuvant use of the retinoid 13-*cis*-retinoic acid in patients who have successfully completed initial therapy for advanced neuroblastoma. It has been shown in a large randomised trial that this relatively simple oral treatment improves outcome. It is not without its toxicity, however, and symptoms such as dry skin and angular stomatitis may reduce compliance.

DRUGS AFFECTING BONE MINERALISATION AND CALCIUM METABOLISM

Bisphosphonates are a class of drugs which are adsorbed onto hydroxyapatite crystals in bone, slowing both their rate of growth and dissolution, thereby decreasing the bone turnover associated with disease.

> ### INDICATIONS FOR BISPHOSPHONATE TREATMENT
>
> - Paget's disease of bone
> - Post-menopausal osteoporosis
> - Metastatic bone disease

They are indicated in Paget's disease of bone and post-menopausal osteoporosis as well as in metastatic bone disease. There are several bisphosphonate compounds available. Alendronic acid, disodium etidronate and tiludronic acid are licensed only for Paget's disease and/or osteoporosis. Disodium pamidronate and sodium clodronate are used in malignant disease. Both may be given intravenously, but sodium clodronate has the advantage of also being available as an oral formulation.

> ### BISPHOSPHONATES USED FOR METASTATIC BONE DISEASE
>
> - Disodium pamidronate: intravenous administration only
> - Sodium clodronate: intravenous and oral preparations
> - Zolendronic acid: intravenous administration only

In metastatic bone disease, bisphosphonates have several functions including the treatment and prevention of malignant hypercalcaemia, the treatment of bone pain, and the prevention of the development of skeletal complications, such as pain and pathological fracture.

> ### FUNCTIONS OF BISPHOSPHONATES IN METASTATIC BONE DISEASE
>
> - Treatment and secondary prevention of hypercalcaemia
> - Treatment and secondary prevention of bone pain
> - Prevention of other skeletal complications, such as pathological fractures

Hypercalcaemia is a common complication in patients with advanced cancer affecting bone, for example women with multiple bone metastases from breast cancer, and patients with multiple myeloma. Tourniquets should not be used when taking blood for calcium levels. As well as checking the total serum calcium level, it is important to have an albumin measurement so that a corrected value can be derived, and magnesium estimation may also be helpful. Rarely, hypercalcaemia can be a non-metastatic manifestation of cancer, when the tumour secretes a parathyroid hormone-related peptide.

> ### COMMON SYMPTOMS OF HYPERCALCAEMIA
>
> - Thirst and polyuria
> - Tiredness
> - Nausea and vomiting
> - Confusion

Occasionally, hypercalcaemia is the initial presentation of malignancy, but more commonly it occurs as a late event in someone known to have cancer. It is important to bear hypercalcaemia in mind when a patient known to have cancer, especially one with bone metastases, develops non-specific symptoms or is just "not quite right". This is because hypercalcaemia is eminently treatable, but it will not be treated unless the diagnosis is made, and the diagnosis will be delayed if the possibility is not considered early on.

Patients with anything more than the mildest hypercalcaemia are likely to be significantly salt and water depleted and may have a degree of renal failure. The initial treatment is easiest in the hospital setting, where intravenous fluids can be given and blood biochemistry closely monitored. Salt and water replacement are the single most important treatment in the management of acute hypercalcaemia. The use of intravenous sodium clodronate or disodium pamidronate given as a single dose or in divided doses over a few days will usually normalise the calcium rapidly. In the past, a variety of drugs including mithramycin, calcitonin, steroids and phosphate were used, but the development of bisphosphonates has made these treatments essentially redundant.

> ### TREATMENT OF THE HYPERCALCAEMIA OF MALIGNANCY
>
> - Hospitalisation for rehydration
> - Intravenous bisphosphonate therapy
> - Consideration of a change in systemic therapy, for example chemotherapy
> - Maintenance treatment with 3- or 4-weekly bisphosphonate infusions or oral sodium clodronate

Following the initial treatment of hypercalcaemia, the specialist will give consideration to any specific anti-cancer measures, such as chemotherapy or endocrine therapy, which may be appropriate to bring the disease under control. Consideration will also be given to secondary prevention of hypercalcaemia, as without further treatment, hypercalcaemia will often recur within 3–6 weeks. If a patient is proceeding to receive chemotherapy, it is simple to arrange an infusion of sodium clodronate or disodium pamidronate every 3 or 4 weeks when the patient attends for chemotherapy. For patients who do not otherwise need to attend hospital, oral maintenance with sodium clodronate is effective and generally well tolerated. The daily dose is 1,600–3,200 mg in as single or two divided doses morning and evening, 800 mg twice daily is the most commonly used schedule. Sometimes patients may experience mild gastro-intestinal disturbance such as nausea, vomiting or diarrhoea. In this case, the dose can be halved for a few days and gradually increased again by 400 mg increments until the desired dose level is achieved.

As calcium and other minerals bind to this drug making it ineffective, sodium clodronate should not be drunk with milk or calcium-containing mineral water. It should be taken at least an hour (preferably 2) after food, and food should not be taken for at least 1 (preferably 2) hour afterwards.

Drug interactions between sodium clodronate and other bisphosphonates, aminoglycosides, antacids have been described and these drugs should not be co-prescribed. Renal function should be monitored when non-steroidal anti-inflammatory drugs are used with bisphosphonates, as some patients have developed renal impairment.

Localised bone pain due to bone metastases in breast cancer is often amenable to treatment with palliative radiotherapy. However, often patients have multiple sites of bone involvement and the pain can be diffuse making radiotherapy difficult. Of course analgesics are important, but side-effects, such as constipation and mental changes when opiates are used can make them less than ideal. Intravenous bisphosphonate infusions, or oral therapy with sodium clodronate may be beneficial.

Bone is the first site of recurrence in nearly half of all patients with breast cancer, and of course all patients with myeloma have bone involvement. The use of prophylactic oral sodium clodronate in patients with asymptomatic bone involvement significantly lowers the risk of skeletal complications such as hypercalcaemia, vertebral collapse and deformity, pathological fracture and the need for other interventions such as radiotherapy for bone pain. This treatment also lengthens the symptom-free interval.

There are interesting data which suggest that the use of oral sodium clodronate as an adjuvant treatment in women with breast cancer who have not yet developed metastatic disease but are at higher risk of doing so, may reduce the subsequent incidence of both bone and visceral metastases. So far, however, the use of adjuvant bisphosphonates in this way has not become widespread practice.

GUIDANCE FOR PATIENTS PRESCRIBED ORAL CLODRONATE

◆ Sodium clodronate tablets or capsules must be taken on an empty stomach. They can be taken with a small amount of tap water, but do not use mineral water or any milk-containing drink. You should allow at least 1 hour for your body to digest and absorb medication before you eat, drink or take any other medicines. The reason why you need to be so careful about how and when you take it is because the minerals in food and some drinks can stop sodium clodronate from working.

◆ Your doctor will tell you how much of your medicine you should take each day. You can divide this into two doses, taking some in the morning and some in the evening, or take it all at once.

◆ If you are taking two doses, we suggest one in the morning, 1–2 hours before breakfast and one in the evening, 1–2 hours after your last meal of the day, and then nothing else to eat, and no milky drinks, before you go to bed.

◆ If you are taking all your medicine in one dose, then in the evening before going to bed is usually the most convenient, but make sure it is at least 1 hour after your last meal or milky drink.

◆ Remember, you should continue to take your medicine until your doctor tells you to stop, or you might lose the benefit.

◆ You may experience nausea, indigestion or diarrhoea. If this occurs, talk to your GP or hospital specialist.

INTERVENTIONAL RADIOLOGY

In the first half of the last century, radiologists were doctors who used X-rays both for diagnostic imaging and to treat patients with cancer. Practice in radiology then divided into clinical radiology specialists who used X-rays and subsequently other modalities, such as ultrasound and magnetic resonance for imaging for the diagnosis and monitoring of disease, and clinical oncology specialists who used radiation and subsequently other modalities, such as chemotherapy and endocrine therapy for the treatment of cancer. No pattern of practice is ever stable for long and now no cancer centre is complete without one or more "interventional radiologists" who contribute greatly to the management of cancer using image guidance techniques.

Many biopsies for the diagnosis of cancer are now done by the radiologist rather than the surgeon. Often, it is possible to avoid an open operation and obtain cells or tissue for diagnostic purposes (Chapter 7) using percutaneously placed needles guided directly to the tumour with the help of ultrasound, CT or MRI.

Arteriography is sometimes undertaken to delineate the blood supply to a tumour prior to surgical resection. Tumour embolisation, which results in devascularisation and infarction of the tumour, may be performed at the same time as angiography to make the subsequent operation less hazardous.

Obstructed tubes of all sorts may now be stented to relieve the obstruction and palliate the symptoms of advanced cancer. These procedures require very close collaboration between interventional radiologists and the appropriate organ-specific physician or surgeon who often has skills in endoscopic management of obstructive lesions with dilatation and stenting. Examples include:

◆ Stenting the superior vena cava in patients with mediastinal compression, usually as a second-line treatment after failed radiotherapy.
◆ Percutaneous biliary drainage and placement of bile duct stents, when endoscopic procedures have failed.
◆ Insertion of nephrostomies and antegrade ureteric stenting, usually when retrograde cystoscopic approaches have not been possible.

Other examples of stenting a stenosed or obstructed organ fall more commonly in the province of the surgeon or physician who undertakes endoscopic procedures. Examples include the treatment of bronchial, oesophageal, urethral and rectal lesions.

Interventional radiologists may be valuable partners for clinicians in undertaking supportive care procedures, such as the insertion of Hickman lines and other types of vascular access and gastrostomies (PEGs) for nutritional support.

Image guided metastasis ablation has become an important palliative treatment for patients with liver secondaries. Using CT or MRI for guidance needles or catheters are inserted percutaneously into liver lesions and the metastasis is then completely or partially ablated with a variety of techniques including lasers, radiofrequency waves or alcohol injection. The limits of what is considered treatable in this way are increasing. Clearly, a patient needs to be relatively fit, and the presence of untreatable disease at other sites, such as lung metastases, makes local therapy to the liver less valuable. Rules, such as treating only patients with up to three lesions, none greater than 5 cm diameter are likely to be relaxed as more interventional radiologists develop greater expertise. Disease which is initially considered too advanced to be treated with interstitial techniques may become treatable if there is a good but incomplete response to another treatment, such as chemotherapy.

Paramedical disciplines in cancer care

The optimal management of patients with cancer is critically dependent on the input of many groups of health care workers from the professions allied to medicine. The contribution of those in the paramedical disciplines including nursing, radiography, medical physics, pharmacy, speech and language therapy, dietetics, physiotherapy, social work, occupational therapy, counselling, psychology, the chaplaincy and others is considered here. The varied role of doctors in hospital and the community setting as part of the cancer team and in delivering shared care was outlined in Chapter 9.

NURSING

The role of the nurse is one of the most varied and essential in cancer management. In every cancer centre and cancer unit, specially trained nurses are involved in the administration of chemotherapy. All chemotherapy nurse specialists are, of course, skilled and experienced in peripheral venous cannulation and in accessing central venous catheters, such as Hickman lines and Portacaths. In addition, some have also been trained in other aspects of vascular access, such as the insertion of percutaneously inserted central catheters (PICC lines) and the actual placement of Hickman lines. Besides injecting the drugs, these nurses provide a lot of information and support to patients regarding the side-effects they might experience, and they are often the first point of contact for patients in between courses of chemotherapy if there are problems. While most chemotherapy nurses are hospital based and work in an environment where there is immediate access to medical support, there is a growing number of community-based chemotherapy nurses who will give domiciliary chemotherapy.

A clinical nurse specialist with training and expertise in defined cancer types is now the cornerstone of every cancer site-specific multidisciplinary team. The work undertaken by these nurses has evolved a lot over the years. The responsibilities of what used to be called the "stoma sister" have now broadened to include diagnostic and follow-up flexible sigmoidoscopy and colonoscopy in some centres, advice on the risk of a patient having a familial cancer predisposition syndrome and holistic care for the colorectal cancer patient including provision of advice on stoma appliances. The breast-care nurse now does much

more than provide guidance on breast prostheses and bras for women after mastectomy. The role includes support of women newly referred to breast assessment clinics, counselling about the extent of surgery to be undertaken, advice about the available types of breast reconstruction, lymphoedema care and liaison with the oncology team and community services as appropriate. Some breast-care nurses will lead local patient support groups.

Palliative care services, both hospital and community based and are often nurse led, with a clinical nurse specialist making the initial assessment of each patient's needs, providing follow-up and involving the specialist palliative care physician and general practitioner (GP) as necessary. These nurses have detailed knowledge of the physical management of the symptoms of advanced cancer (Chapter 50), but their skill in the psycho-social management of patients and their families is every bit as important as symptom control. Their remit often extends beyond the patient, to the care of relatives during the illness and after bereavement.

These newer specialist nursing roles are in addition to the more traditional inpatient and outpatient and district nurses, who are, of course, essential for the care of cancer patients, and many will have post-registration training and expertise in the management of patients with cancer.

EXAMPLES OF THE TYPES OF NURSES INVOLVED IN CANCER CARE

- Inpatient care on surgical, medical and oncology wards
- Outpatient nurses in clinic areas and radiotherapy and chemotherapy treatment suites
- District nurses
- Chemotherapy nurse specialists and clinical practitioners
- Vascular access nurses
- Breast-care nurses
- Colorectal cancer, lung cancer and other tumour site-specific nurse specialists
- Community- and hospital-based palliative care nurses
- Information, support and counselling nurses

RADIOGRAPHY

Radiographers are an essential, but largely unrecognised professional group in the management of cancer, often erroneously called "nurses" by patients. Diagnostic radiographers play an important rôle in breast-cancer screening through mammography (Chapter 6) and in the diagnosis and staging of almost all cancer types. In addition, patients often undergo repeated imaging investigations to assess the response of their disease to treatment. Therapy radiographers who plan and deliver radiotherapy (Chapter 12) are uniquely dedicated to cancer treatment. As they are the people who see patients day by day as they undergo radiotherapy, therapy radiographers are well placed to provide information and advice on the management of their side-effects and also to give psychological support at what is, for many patients, a difficult time in their cancer journey.

MEDICAL PHYSICISTS

Those working in medical physics are "backroom" staff in that they have little direct contact with patients or community health care professionals such as GPs. Nonetheless, they are vitally important in delivering cancer treatments, such as external beam radiotherapy, brachytherapy and radionuclide therapy (Chapter 12). It may nonetheless be helpful to seek their advice in radiation protection matters, such as regarding the amount of contact an individual can have with someone who has recently received radionuclide therapy, or if a patient dies shortly after such treatment or has had a "permanent" radioactive implant, such as iodine seeds for the treatment of prostate cancer and the body is to be cremated.

PHARMACY

The oncology pharmacist occupies a key position in the cancer centre. The main rôle is, of course, to make up and dispense drugs including chemotherapy, but there is much more to the job than that. The oncology trained pharmacist will scrutinise prescriptions for accuracy and adherence to protocol, warn about potential drug interactions and advise on the prevention and treatment of side-effects, such as emesis, myelosuppression and other aspects of supportive care (Chapter 17). The pharmacist will usually be accessible for advice about medication both directly by the patient and by other health care professionals including hospital doctors and GPs.

SPEECH AND LANGUAGE THERAPY

One of the most dramatic and important things a speech and language therapist (SALT) can do is to help a patient speak again after laryngectomy (Chapter 26). There are now more options for vocal rehabilitation than before. The use of speaking valves inserted into tracheo-pharyngeal fistulae is now more widespread than the development of oesophageal speech. The SALT will be able to counsel the patient preoperatively about the choices available, teach the appropriate techniques and monitor progress. In addition to providing support for speech and communication, SALTs have expertise in dysphagia and swallowing assessment, and are able to advise on the risk of aspiration in patients with swallowing difficulties as well as offer advice on how problems are best dealt with.

DIETETICS

Many patients with cancer are nutritionally compromised, and there are a number of reasons for this including mucositis, dysphagia, vomiting, anorexia and gastrointestinal surgery. The help of a dietician is invaluable in the management of these patients. The dietician will make an assessment of nutritional requirements, present dietary intake and the reasons why this may be inadequate. Solutions may range from recommendations about the type of food which the patient is eating, supplementary nutritional drinks to tube feeding via a nasogastric tube or gastrostomy and the need for total parenteral nutrition (TPN). The dietician will then keep the patient under surveillance to monitor progress.

Nutritional compromise may be acute and self-limiting, for example the mucositis associated with radiotherapy, and long-term follow-up is not required. In this setting, it can be helpful for the dietician to work closely with other patient groups, for example head and neck cancer patients undergoing radiotherapy may be seen weekly in a combined clinic staffed by a SALT and a dietician along with a nurse and a doctor. Sometimes nutritional difficulties may be chronic requiring long-term gastrostomy feeds. In these circumstances, it may be better and easier for the patient to be supervised by a community dietician who will be closer to home and more accessible than the hospital-based counterpart.

Less commonly in the oncology setting, the help of a dietician may be valuable in helping obese patients, most often women with breast cancer on hormonal medication, lose surplus weight.

PHYSIOTHERAPY

Patients may have short-term problems after surgery, for example limited shoulder mobility after mastectomy, for which advice from a physiotherapist and exercises may be beneficial. Other patients, for example those with neuro-disability as a result of brain tumour or spinal cord compression may have longer-term problems. These require physiotherapy input, not just to help mobility and walking rehabilitation, but also to prevent the development of additional disability, for example passive joint exercises to prevent fixed contractures developing. The rôle of the physiotherapist is varied, and may include treatments such as bandaging for severe lymphoedema which has not responded to more simple treatments.

SOCIAL WORK

Cancer and its treatment is stressful not just for the patient but for the whole family. Not only is there the natural distress associated with the diagnosis, treatment and prognosis, but there may well be additional non-medical stresses. For example, the family income may fall if the breadwinner is off work for a prolonged period, or there may be additional expenditure incurred by multiple visits to hospital by the patient or by visiting family for a hospitalised patient. Parents may require help with childcare, if they require either outpatient or inpatient care. Patients who develop neurodisability and unable to cope with stairs may find their present accommodation unsuitable and need help with rehousing urgently. Patients at home, especially those terminally ill and hoping to stay at home to die rather than be admitted to hospital or hospice, may need equipment to facilitate domiciliary care, such as a commode, bathing equipment, a hospital type bed and so on.

Hospital social work departments and community social services are a valuable resource enabling patients to access financial support including state benefits and charitable grants, and for the loan of equipment. Many cancer centres will have their own dedicated social workers, sometimes funded by one of the cancer relief charities.

OCCUPATIONAL THERAPY

The occupational therapists often work closely in conjunction with physiotherapists and social workers as part of a multidisciplinary team for psycho-social support and rehabilitation. The occupational therapist will be able to assess a patient's needs either in the hospital setting or on a domiciliary visit and advise on the use of a wide variety of aids to maintain independence despite disability.

COUNSELLING, PSYCHOLOGY AND PSYCHIATRY

It goes without saying that the diagnosis of cancer, the prospect of treatment and the uncertainties surrounding prognosis lead to a great deal of sadness, stress and worry in every patient. Individual patients and their families vary a great deal in how much they show and share these feelings, and in how well they are able to cope. Some of the anxiety is related to a fear of the unknown, and a sympathetic ear and the provision of accurate information may go a long way to providing relief. Sometimes there are other emotions, such as guilt and anger, which may require greater help. In addition to the information and support offered to their patients by doctors, nurses and other health care professionals in the cancer and in the community, there are a variety of external agencies, such as CancerBACUP, which can provide information, support and counselling (Chapter 57).

Sometimes the natural feelings of anxiety and depression which are part of the cancer experience are more profound and prolonged and should be considered pathological. The GP, who has probably known the patient and the family for years, is usually better placed to provide treatment for these conditions than their hospital consultant. It can sometimes be helpful to enlist the support of a psychologist, and rarely psychiatric help is needed for the profoundly depressed or suicidal. Psychologists also play an important role in psychometric assessment and advising on the educational needs of children with long-term late effects following treatment for brain tumours (Chapter 19).

CHAPLAINCY AND SPIRITUAL SUPPORT

The clergy and other religious leaders are not usually considered as members of the professions allied to medicine, but the needs of patients with cancer are more than just medical and practical. Most people do not think about death on a regular basis, and the diagnosis of cancer in either themselves or their relatives may be the first time some people have had to consider the prospect of mortality. Patients, of course have differing beliefs and faiths and some have none at all. It can be helpful for patients if doctors and nurses discreetly enquire about this aspect when discussing the fact that an illness might not be curable. Even those who have not practised their religion for many years may value contact with an appropriate priest or minister at such a difficult time.

Complementary and alternative therapies

It is important to recognise the distinction between "complementary" and "alternative" treatments for patients with cancer.

COMPLEMENTARY THERAPIES

Some patients may perceive that conventional health care does not address all their emotional needs or recognise all the symptoms of their cancer or the side-effects of treatment, and therefore turn to complementary therapists in addition to standard medical treatment. They may hold a sometimes justifiable view that their doctors and other "official" health care workers merely regard their patients as bodies with cancers requiring eradication and are not interested in them as real people.

These patients find additional, complementary treatments, such as aromatherapy, relaxation, visualisation and massage described below, holistic approaches treating mind, body and soul which reduce stress and enhance well-being. In addition, patients may feel that going out to look for complementary treatment goes someway towards restoring control and overcoming the loss of self-determination that often accompanies the cancer diagnosis.

Most oncologists are very supportive of patients who wish to receive complementary therapies, and most cancer centres now provide some of these treatments, even if not the full range of 60 or so. Some of the more commonly used complementary approaches are briefly described below in alphabetical order, in an attempt not to ascribe any relative importance to one method or another.

ALTERNATIVE TREATMENTS

Other patients, distressed by the lack of effective therapy for many cancers, or choosing to disregard the offer of conventional radiotherapy, chemotherapy and surgery, may turn to alternative practitioners who offer hope through the application of unproven remedies. Such alternative treatment is not subject to any control or regulation and can not only be ineffective but also harmful and expensive. It is important to ensure that those seeking truly alternative therapy for themselves or their relatives are as fully informed as possible about the underlying illness, the prognosis, and the conventional and experimental treatments available.

It can sometimes be very beneficial for patients who may be dissatisfied with the opinion or the service they have received from one individual clinician or cancer centre to be offered a second opinion. If they do decide to go ahead with alternative treatment, they should understand the evidence base or lack of it for the treatment under consideration, and the risks it may pose.

AROMATHERAPY

This treatment involves natural, fragrant essential oils being massaged into the body in a calm and quiet environment. They may also be administered by inhalation or put in bathwater. The smell is detected by the olfactory nerves which are closely related to the limbic system of the brain. The process is very relaxing and does a lot to relieve stress and anxiety, and promote a sense of well-being.

ART THERAPY

Many patients find it difficult to talk about emotional matters or to express complex feelings in words. Some may find it helpful to paint or draw how they feel in the presence of an art therapist. This process may be sufficiently cathartic by itself, or the images used may be used as a basis for discussion and counselling. It is a particularly valuable technique in paediatric practice, as children are already used to playing with paint, and do not have a full vocabulary to express their thoughts and fears.

DIETS

Nutrition is an important concern for patients with cancer, and the rôle of the dietician has been covered in Chapter 15. There is increasing evidence that diet may be an aetiological factor in the development of cancer (Chapter 1), and some argue that a change in diet may help to eradicate cancer. While some patients will benefit from changing to a more healthy diet with adequate vitamins, minerals, calories and protein, there are few grounds to recommend a patient undergoing extreme dietary deprivation if they do not enjoy it.

HERBAL MEDICINE

Many patients seek herbal medicine, believing it to be "natural" by comparison with conventional cancer treatment which they regard as artificial and unnatural. Few realise that many drugs including both chemotherapeutic agents, for example vincristine and paclitaxel, and other medicines, for example morphine, aspirin and penicillin, are derived from plants and fungi. Most herbal remedies used these days are harmless, whereas some herbs are potentially toxic.

HOMEOPATHY

Homeopathy is a form of medical treatment practised by registered medical practitioners which is available in a number of NHS institutions such as the Royal London Homoeopathic Hospital or in general practitioners' (GPs) surgeries where one of the partners has a special interest in homeopathy and arrangements can be made for referrals from other practices. Patients are individually assessed and homoeopathic remedies which have no adverse interaction with standard cancer therapy are prescribed with the aim of improving quality of life in various ways.

MASSAGE

Massage is the systematic and rhythmical use of pressure and movement on the skin and muscles which stimulates the sense of touch. It is often used in conjunction with aromatherapy and reflexology. It can help to relieve stress and tension and enhance quality of life. Its value transcends linguistic and cultural boundaries.

REFLEXOLOGY

Reflexology involves massage of the feet and has its roots in ancient China. Its practitioners believe that the feet are connected by 10 channels to the rest of the body, and that pressure on specific parts of the feet will promote healing in the relevant remote body part.

Supportive care

Patients with cancer may require many types of support, namely emotional, spiritual, social, financial ..., but this chapter refers only to the physical need for treatments which enable the patient to get through the transient, acute side-effects of treatment. It covers all aspects of bone marrow suppression including transfusion of blood and platelets, neutropenic sepsis, growth factor support, blood and marrow transplantation, nausea and vomiting, tumour lysis and nutrition.

BONE MARROW SUPPRESSION

Chemotherapy, as mentioned in Chapter 13, may have toxic effects on the bone marrow which can lower the three principal cellular components of blood. A low white cell count, most importantly, neutropenia defined as an absolute neutrophil count below $1.0 \times 10^9 l^{-1}$, is the most commonly encountered type of myelosuppression. Thrombocytopenia, with a platelet count below the normal range of about $150–450 \times 10^9 l^{-1}$, may also occur. Chemotherapy may also have an effect on the red blood cells and mild anaemia is often seen, profound anaemia due to chemotherapy is less common. Other treatments, for example blood loss during surgery, and radiotherapy, may also lead to abnormal blood counts. Of course, in some patients the disease itself, through haemorrhage, haemolysis or bone marrow involvement may cause anaemia, thrombocytopenia or rarely neutropenia. Mild degrees of myelosuppression can be tolerated without treatment, so when is intervention necessary?

NEUTROPAENIA

Neutropenia occurs during the haematological nadir, most commonly 10–14 days after chemotherapy. Uncomplicated neutropenia is not usually treated, but it is common to arrange for a nadir blood count for two reasons. Firstly, it can be helpful to make contact with neutropenic patients to see if they are feeling well, and to remind them of the need to seek medical attention if they become pyrexial or develop a "flu-like" illness. Secondly, if the degree of myelosuppression is greater than usual it might be wise to reduce the chemotherapy dose in subsequent courses. Patients with suspected or confirmed neutropenic sepsis

as defined in the box above should not be treated at home but should be referred without delay to hospital for urgent treatment. They will require blood and other cultures taking for microbiological assessment and intravenous antibiotics according to local hospital policy.

> **USEFUL DEFINITIONS**
>
> ◆ Neutropenia: absolute neutrophil count below $1.0 \times 10^9 l^{-1}$
>
> ◆ Severe neutropenia: absolute neutrophil count below $0.5 \times 10^9 l^{-1}$
>
> ◆ Neutropenic sepsis: pyrexial episode when the temperature is elevated to 38°C on two occasions 2 hours apart or 39°C on one occasion with an absolute neutrophil count below $1.0 \times 10^9 l^{-1}$

In some cases, antibiotics have been given routinely as prophylaxis in patients likely to develop neutropenia, but this practice is not encouraged as it exposes patients to the risk of side-effects from a drug which they might not need, and it may promote the development of infection with drug-resistant organisms. Clinical trials of this type of approach are continuing.

Patients when warned about the risk of neutropenic sepsis often imagine that it would be prudent for them to stay away from people with colds; but this is unnecessary as the infections are not viral in origin and tend to result from bacteria already within the body. For this reason, gut sterilisation regimens using oral antibiotics which are not systemically absorbed have been tried in people at risk because of prolonged profound neutropenia, but this practice was not found to be useful and is no longer recommended.

In recent years, the development of haemopoietic growth factors, such as recombinant human granulocyte colony-stimulating factor (rhG-CSF) has enabled other approaches to prevent and treat neutropenic sepsis. rhG-CSF is not usually used for the treatment of uncomplicated neutropaenia, but it may be prescribed for an individual patient who has had one or more previous septic episodes while neutropenic which have not been prevented by a dose reduction. Sometimes rhG-CSF is used to allow intensification of chemotherapy.

THROMBOCYTOPAENIA

Unfortunately, specific platelet-stimulating growth factors are not yet available, so thrombocytopenia continues to require blood product support. The platelet count often falls below the normal range after chemotherapy, but thrombocytopenia requiring platelet transfusion does not often occur with most commonly used treatment regimens. Platelet counts as low as $20 \times 10^9 l^{-1}$ in an otherwise well patient are not a problem, but with very low counts prophylactic platelet transfusions are indicated to prevent bleeding or bruising. Different thresholds for the use of prophylactic platelet transfusion may be set in various circumstances, but usually they are between 12 and $20 \times 10^9 l^{-1}$. In the presence of evidence of bleeding including petechial haemorrhage, purpura or bruising, platelet transfusions may be necessary even with a higher platelet count. Once transfused, platelets only last for 1 day or 2; so repeated transfusions may be necessary until the count recovers.

ANAEMIA

Mild anaemia is common in patients with cancer, and in advanced disease may well be related to the cancer itself. Patients may also develop anaemia because of chemotherapy, but this is not usually severe enough to require treatment. More profound anaemia is seen with some drugs, notably cisplatin. Transfusion is usually considered indicated, if the haemoglobin falls below $10 g dl^{-1}$, but sometimes symptoms of anaemia in individual patients mean that a blood transfusion is appropriate at a higher haemoglobin level. Effective radiotherapy is dependent upon tissues being adequately oxygenated, and so often transfusion is used to keep the haemoglobin level at least $12 g dl^{-1}$. Patients with immunosuppression due to leukaemia or lymphoma including Hodgkin's disease should receive transfusion with cytomegalovirus (CMV) negative blood products to prevent transmission of CMV infection.

The red cell growth factor epoetin (recombinant human erythropoietin) is now commercially available and is licensed for the treatment of anaemia caused by chemotherapy, but its use for this indication is not yet widespread.

BLOOD AND MARROW TRANSPLANTATION

Conventional chemotherapy employs doses which, although they may be myelosuppressive, allow recovery of the marrow with time and supportive care. It is thought that, in some cases at least, resistance of cancer cells to chemotherapy which may lead to treatment failure may be overcome by using higher doses of the same drugs which will swamp the cellular drug-resistance mechanisms. The dose-limiting factor in many cases is myelosuppression, and blood and marrow transplant techniques have been developed in an attempt to make high-dose chemotherapy feasible.

Autografts use the patients own haemopoietic stem cells collected before high-dose chemotherapy either directly from the bone marrow, or more commonly nowadays, from the peripheral blood after priming the bone marrow to produce excess cells with a combination of chemotherapy and rhG-CSF. High-dose chemotherapy with peripheral blood stem cell (PBSC) autograft is now standard practice of proven benefit for some diseases like relapsed non-Hodgkin's lymphoma (NHL) and Hodgkin's disease. Unfortunately, it has not been shown to be worthwhile in more common diseases, such as breast cancer. With a PBSC autograft the patient will still have a prolonged period of profound myelosuppression, but recovery usually begins after about 3 weeks.

Allografts, where the bone marrow cells come from another person, either a sibling or a matched unrelated donor (MUD) are more often used in leukaemia after conditioning with high-dose chemotherapy and total body irradiation. In this case, the bone marrow transplant is not just a mechanism for overcoming the otherwise fatal myelosuppression, but it is also hoped that the engrafted donor cells, being foreign to the host, will act against any residual leukaemia cells via an immunological graft versus leukaemia effect.

NAUSEA AND VOMITING

Nausea and vomiting are two of the most feared side-effects of cancer treatment, and in the past some patients have refused the potential benefits of chemotherapy because of this. Nowadays, there are several very effective treatments available, and vomiting can be well controlled in most, if not all, patients. The initial choice of anti-emetic therapy is usually based on the known potential of different chemotherapy schedules to produce sickness.

Metoclopramide given intravenously with dexamethasone prior to chemotherapy is usually adequate for mildly emetogenic schedules, but a 5-hydroxytryptamine-3 (5-HT-3) receptor antagonist, such as granesetron or ondansetron, is used (again with dexamethasone) if this fails or as first-line treatment for moderately or severely emetogenic regimens. Patients receiving outpatient schedules will usually benefit from 2 or 3 days of treatment with oral metoclopramide or domperidone with dexamethasone after each course. Sometimes, a longer period of treatment or 1- or 2-day's treatment with a 5-HT-3 receptor antagonist is needed.

If these strategies fail, then alternative anti-emetic drugs with a different pharmacological mode of action (such as the antihistamine cyclizine) or a phenothiazine (such as prochlorperazine) may be useful. Some patients benefit from transdermal hyoscine. Occasionally, patients who are apprehensive about the prospect of chemotherapy-induced vomiting may develop nausea or actually vomit when they arrive at the hospital before any treatment is given. Such anticipatory nausea and vomiting may be helped by a small dose of lorazepam given as premedication the night before and the morning of chemotherapy.

TUMOUR LYSIS SYNDROME

Patients with a large volume of a disease which is sensitive to treatment, such as lymphoma, may develop a condition known as tumour lysis syndrome following the start of treatment. This is a complex and potentially fatal metabolic problem including renal failure, caused by the release of uric acid, potassium and other chemicals when large numbers of tumour cells break down and release their contents at the same time. Patients at risk should be hydrated well before any treatment which can precipitate tumour lysis, even steroids, is given. The xanthine oxidase inhibitor allopurinol is given to prevent hyperuricaemia. Alternatively, uricozyme, an enzyme which breaks down uric acid, may be used. In severe cases, renal dialysis may be needed for a short period. The prevention and treatment of tumour lysis syndrome is not important in the community, but it is mentioned to explain why some patients are discharged home on allopurinol. This does not need to be continued beyond the first course of chemotherapy.

NUTRITION

Many patients with cancer are malnourished. This may occur for a number of reasons including prolonged dysphagia in the case of oesophageal cancer, mucositis, for example in patients receiving chemotherapy or radiotherapy to the head and neck, or due to the presence of extensive liver metastases. The rôle of the dietician in providing nutritional support has been discussed in Chapter 15, and this may involve advice on the type of food eaten, oral nutrition supplements, tube feeding via a nasogastric tube or a gastrostomy such as a percutaneous endoscopic gastrostomy (PEG) feeding tube and, in extreme cases, the use of total parenteral nutrition.

Dietary support in the form of both complete foods and nutritional supplements are recognised as drugs by the Advisory Committee on Borderline Substances for the treatment of defined conditions, such as dysphagia due to radiotherapy for oesophageal cancers and disease-related malnutrition. As such they can be prescribed by GPs on the standard FP10 form (GP10 in Scotland). Many preparations with a variety of flavours are available, and a comprehensive listing may be found in the British National Formulary. Among those available are: Clinifeed, Ensure, Fresubin, Jevity, Maxijul and Provide.

CHAPTER 18

Assessment of new treatments – clinical trials

Today oncologists, as other doctors, are asked to practise evidence-based medicine. In fact, there has been for many decades a more solid body of evidence supporting the treatments used for cancer than for many other diseases. This is for several reasons, including:

1 Without effective treatment cancer progresses, so there is a simple and robust outcome measure for the failure of treatment – mortality. Other reliable clinical end points, such as local failure, are also relatively unequivocal.
2 When radium was a new and effective treatment for cancer, supplies were scarce and under the control of the Radium Commission. It was one of their conditions of supply that its use was audited, and that patients who had been treated were followed up, so that statistics could be produced.
3 Since the introduction of the technique more than 50 years ago, the randomised controlled trial has been the gold standard for the assessment of new cancer treatments.

Other sources of evidence exist to guide practice, and these can be assigned different values according to the robustness of the methodology. Unfortunately, as with many areas of science and medicine, there is not a single universally accepted classification.

> **LEVELS OF EVIDENCE I**
>
> As used in the Clinical Oncology Information Network (COIN) guidelines
> ◆ Ia: Evidence obtained from meta-analysis of randomised controlled trials
> ◆ Ib: Evidence obtained from at least one randomised controlled trial
> ◆ IIa: Evidence obtained from at least one well-designed controlled study without randomisation
> ◆ IIb: Evidence obtained from at least one other type of well-designed quasi-experimental study
> ◆ III: Evidence obtained from well-designed non-experimental descriptive studies, such as comparative studies, correlation studies and case studies
> ◆ IV: Evidence obtained from expert committee reports or opinions and/or clinical experiences of respected studies

Although it is important to practise evidence-based oncology, there are areas where evidence does not exist. It does not follow that absence of evidence to show that a treatment is beneficial is not evidence of an absence of benefit, and so sometimes a course of action has to be recommended on the basis of logic and first principles without direct evidence that it will help. There is a third way between evidence-based and anecdote-based practice, and that is evidence seeking practice. Health care professionals and patients should be encouraged to participate in clinical research whenever there is the opportunity to do so.

> **LEVELS OF EVIDENCE II**
>
> As used by the National Cancer Institutes CancerNet service
> ◆ 1(i): Double blind randomised controlled clinical trial(s)
> ◆ 1(ii): Non-blinded randomised controlled clinical trial(s)
> ◆ 2: Non-randomised controlled clinical trial(s)
> ◆ 3(i): Population-based, consecutive series
> ◆ 3(ii): Consecutive cases (not population based)
> ◆ 3(iii): Non-consecutive cases
>
> Strength of end points
> ◆ A: Total mortality (or overall survival from a defined point in time)
> ◆ B: Cause-specific mortality
> ◆ C: Carefully assessed quality of life
> ◆ D: Indirect surrogates
>   (i)   Disease-free survival
>   (ii) Progression-free survival
>   (iii) Tumour response rate

ASSESSMENT OF NEW DRUGS

Because of the limited efficacy and significant toxicity of all presently available cytotoxics, new drugs and analogues of existing chemotherapeutic agents are being developed with the hope of improving efficacy or diminishing toxicity. Following initial assessment in *in vitro* and *in vivo* laboratory models, the place of a particular agent is assessed by passing it through a series of clinical trials called Phase I, II and III. It should go without saying that these studies are only undertaken after ethical approval, and that fully informed consent is obtained from the patients or their parents in the case of young children.

CLINICAL TRIALS

- Phase I: To determine toxicity and dose levels
- Phase II: To demonstrate efficacy
- Phase III: Randomised comparison with standard treatment

Phase I studies are usually carried out by or in close collaboration with a drug company to assess dosage levels and toxicity. Heavily pre-treated patients with recurrent untreatable disease are usually used. The prognosis of these patients is usually very poor, and it should be made clear to participants that they are extremely unlikely to derive any personal benefit from the treatment being evaluated, although the information gathered may be of value to future patients. Three patients are treated at one dosage level, and the toxicity and response, if any, are assessed. The dose is then increased by increments on further groups of three patients each, until intolerable toxicity is reached. If the drug shows any signs of activity, it then passes to a Phase II study.

Phase II studies are usually performed on patients with previously treated end-stage disease. The maximum tolerated dose established in a Phase I study is used. The main end point of interest in a Phase II study is the response rate. The size of the tumour is measured before treatment (not always an easy or possible task) and after each course of treatment. If the tumour disappears completely, this is counted as a complete response. If the product of two perpendicular diameters decreases by more than 50% of the original, this is counted as a partial response. Data on the toxicity to various organs is also collected. These studies usually contain 20–50 patients and can be completed in a short time.

Information from Phase II studies is an essential prerequisite for a randomised trial. It is important, however, not to read too much into these early results, as they have not been directly compared with untreated controls. Indirect comparisons, for example, with a historical cohort can be misleading because of selection bias. Results are reported in terms of tumour shrinkage as defined above, but this type of response, although it is a marker of biological efficacy, may have little clinical relevance. Measurement of symptom palliation and quality of life might be more valuable end points. Many reports of Phase II studies compare the survival of responders with non-responders, but one cannot deduce that superior survival rates are attributable to the treatment unless randomised comparisons are made between treated and untreated patients, and that is the aim of Phase III studies.

A Phase III trial has two or more arms and usually compares the best standard treatment with an experimental treatment. In the case of a new palliative treatment for advanced cancer, best standard treatment may be symptom control and best supportive care with no active anti-cancer treatment. Sometimes, two treatments regarded as standard in different centres are directly compared. If possible, both the patient and the clinicians should be unaware of which arm of the trial the patient is in, but this is rarely feasible in cancer treatment. As the principal end point in most Phase III trials is survival of the patient, there is less opportunity for inadvertent investigator bias. Subsidiary end points may include response, local control, toxicity, symptom relief and quality-of-life measurements. This type of trial requires several hundreds or possibly thousands of patients, depending on the magnitude of the anticipated difference in outcome. A statistician will be involved in the trial design to provide guidance on the number of patients required to be confident that the result is reliable. One centre by itself seldom has enough patients and so randomised trials are usually conducted on a multicentre basis, and are often international in rarer cancer types. Trials of this sort, therefore, usually take several years to accrue enough patients, and more time must elapse for adequate follow-up before data can be analysed.

ADVERSE DRUG REACTIONS

When a new drug is licensed, it enters a further phase of clinical assessment called post-marketing surveillance. It is possible that rare but potentially serious adverse effects may become apparent for the first time, and the general practitioner may be the first doctor to know about such a side-effect. Suspected or definite adverse reactions should be reported to the Committee on Safety of Medicines at the Medicine Controls Agency (MCA) using a yellow card. Yellow cards can be found at the back of the British National Formulary or obtained directly from the MCA. This mechanism applies both to old and to new drugs, but is particularly important to file reports on all suspected reactions to new drugs, marked in the BNF with the triangular symbol ▼. Reports should be made despite uncertainty about a causal relationship.

ASSESSMENT OF OTHER TREATMENTS

Other treatments, such as radiotherapy and surgical procedures can be evaluated in a similar way to drugs, but in this case, the opportunities for blinding the patient and the investigator to the nature of the treatment are even less than with drug treatments.

CHAPTER 19

Late effects of cancer treatment – the cost of cure

All treatments for cancer cause side-effects. Often these are short lived, are readily controlled with appropriate medication, and cause no long-term problems. Examples include postoperative pain and wound infections, vomiting and hair loss caused by chemotherapy, and cutaneous erythema and mucositis due to radiotherapy. Many of these side-effects have been covered in Chapters 11–13 and 17. On the other hand, the same treatments may cause organ dysfunction, disability and other effects, which persist for life. These so-called "late effects" are considered in detail in this chapter.

> **SIDE-EFFECTS OF CANCER TREATMENT**
> - Acute effects, occur early and are usually self-limiting and transient
> - Late effects, usually become apparent after years and may be progressive and permanent

Many such problems are insidious in onset and may only be manifested gradually and after a number of years, hence the term late effects. An important example of this is growth failure in children after craniospinal radiotherapy. Others, such as the loss of a limb after amputation, may be immediately apparent and so are not truly "late" effects but are considered here as the consequent disability persists throughout life. Some of the late developing and permanent effects, such as hypothyroidism after neck irradiation for Hodgkin's disease, are relatively easy to treat. Others, such as the neuropsychological sequelae of radiotherapy to the brain in very young children, may be the cause of permanent disability requiring long-term care.

Some of the difficulties encountered will hopefully be seen only in patients treated many years ago, because emerging knowledge of late morbidity and new treatment approaches have enabled strategies to be designed which will avoid similar problems in the future. On the other hand, new treatments may be associated with unforeseen and unpredictable side-effects.

Late effects should not just be considered as an afterthought to be explained to the patient when they develop a complication as the cost of cure for which they should be grateful. Rather the nature, severity and likelihood of possible complications should be explained in a sensitive way to patients or to the parents of children prior to the start of treatment, as part of the process of gaining informed consent. Sometimes, a patient will decline a particular treatment, perhaps reducing the chance of cure by doing so, in order to avoid a potential complication which is regarded as unacceptable.

The contents of this chapter may make disturbing reading, and one may wonder why any patient agrees to receive such damaging treatment. In reality, however, only a small minority of patients will develop distressing or disabling late effects. Knowledge of which treatments cause what effects under which circumstances, and how potential problems may be prevented or minimised, has lead to newer treatment schedules which when applied with care and attention to detail mean that modern cancer treatments are probably safer than ever before.

VISUAL IMPAIRMENT

Of all the senses, vision is often regarded as the most important. Enucleation of the eye or orbital excenteration is sometimes required for ocular tumours such as melanoma or retinoblastoma, or as part of the treatment of extensive sino-nasal cancers. Fortunately, many of these tumour types can be cured without recourse to such disabling and disfiguring surgery.

Radiotherapy is frequently used for tumours in the head including the brain. It is often possible to plan treatment to spare the eye and visual apparatus, but sometimes it is not possible to avoid them. The lens of the eye is one of the most radiosensitive structures in the body, and cataracts may result even after relatively low radiation doses. Steroids, often used in high dose for cancer treatment, may also cause cataracts. Fortunately, cataract surgery nowadays is a straightforward procedure and the use of prosthetic lenses avoids the need for bottle-bottom spectacles. Loss of eyelashes, combined with thinning of the substance of the eyelids, may result from the use of superficial radiotherapy to treat basal and squamous cell skin cancers around the eye, and surgery, if possible is preferred, especially for tumours of the upper lid. The lacrimal gland is more resistant to radiation than the salivary glands, and the gland can often be shielded, so a radiation-induced dry eye is not common. When it does occur, the use of artificial tears during the day and a lubricating ointment at night are required to prevent corneal ulceration. The retina, the optic nerves and the optic chiasm may be damaged by high-dose radiotherapy, but care is always taken so that recognised tolerance levels are never exceeded unless there is no alternative.

Tamoxifen is, of course, a very widely used drug, and ocular side-effects are seen only very rarely. Blurred vision or reduction in visual acuity due to corneal deposits, cataract or retinopathy may be caused by tamoxifen, but only at unusually high doses. Chemotherapy does not usually cause any late visual problems.

AUDITORY IMPAIRMENT

Sometimes, a conductive hearing loss may follow surgery on the external or middle ear. Operations on the petrous temporal bone may involve sacrifice of the inner ear mechanism, and surgery in the posterior cranial fossa may damage the auditory nerve leading to sensorineural deafness.

Radiotherapy alone does not usually cause permanent deafness, but sometimes it can cause crusting or osteonecrosis in the external auditory canal which may be troublesome and require repeated otological intervention.

Cisplatin is an ototoxic drug which may cause a profound sensorineural hearing loss. Auditory function should be monitored with regular audiograms. Special care should be taken in patients such as those with optic pathway gliomas (Chapter 46) who may already have a severe visual handicap, as deafness developing in addition would be devastating. Radiotherapy to the inner ear, if given with concurrent cisplatin chemotherapy, for example, in the treatment of nasopharyngeal cancer (Chapter 26), may lead to a more profound sensorineural hearing loss than chemotherapy alone.

SENSORY IMPAIRMENT

Some surgical procedures may lead to patches of anaesthesia, and patients should be warned preoperatively if this is likely to be the case. A common example is sacrifice of the intercostobrachial nerve during axillary clearance for breast cancer. This leads to a patch of numbness or dysaesthesia on the medial aspect of the upper arm in a T1, T2 dermatome distribution.

DRUGS CAUSING SENSORY NEUROPATHY

- ◆ Vincristine
- ◆ Cisplatin
- ◆ Oxaliplatin
- ◆ Paclitaxel

Vincristine commonly produces a sensory peripheral neuropathy with numbness and paraesthesia of the fingers and toes. This may lead to difficulty with fine finger movements and interfere with buttoning clothes and with knitting, and give a sensation of walking on cotton wool. Loss of autonomic function may result in paralytic ileus or constipation. On examination, loss of the knee jerks and other reflexes may be found. Motor neuropathy is uncommon but ptosis is sometimes seen. Other drugs, such as the cisplatin, oxaliplatin and paclitaxel, may also produce a neuropathy. These side-effects may lessen with time after the treatment has been stopped, but they may be permanent.

NEUROPSYCHOLOGICAL EFFECTS

Radiotherapy is often used in the treatment of brain tumours in children and adults. It was formerly frequently used in patients with acute lymphoblastic leukaemia (ALL) as prophylaxis against central nervous system (CNS) involvement, but it is now only used in patients with established CNS disease, either at the time of diagnosis or relapse. The effects of radiotherapy on the brain are complex. The effects of cranial radiotherapy are more profound in children. They depend, among other factors, on the time since treatment, the age of the patient, the part and proportion of the brain irradiated, the dose given and the simultaneous or subsequent use of drugs, such as methotrexate.

Neuropsychological testing is made more difficult by a poor attention span and difficulty in concentration. Additionally, sensory impairment such as deafness or visual handicap may make testing less reliable. There may be a global reduction in intellectual performance as measured by IQ tests, but often the changes are patchy with worse scores for those tests measuring non-verbal skills such as visual perception and integration, mathematical skills abstract reasoning and sequencing tasks. The National Adult Reading Test (NART) is a standardised, quick and reliable tool for assessing intellectual status in grown-ups.

All children who have had cranial irradiation require extra help and support. They should have regular psychometric assessments by an experienced neuropsychologist as the degree of impairment may worsen with time. It is often helpful to get a Statement of Special Educational Needs from the local education authority at the earliest possible time, but the needs must be reassessed periodically. The Statement may permit additional one-to-one support in schools. Very simple measures can help children with specific difficulties. For example:

- ◆ seating visually impaired children near the front of the class so they can see the blackboard;
- ◆ ensuring that background noise is kept to a minimum to enable deaf children to hear the teacher;

- asking the teacher to attract a deaf child's attention before speaking, and then to speak clearly to the pupil while maintaining eye contact;
- provision of written sheets so that children who find writing slow and difficult are not held back by having to write everything for themselves;
- allowing extra time during examinations for slow writers.

GROWTH AND ENDOCRINE EFFECTS

The pituitary gland and hypothalamus are very sensitive to radiotherapy. All children should have their height and weight checked at regular intervals after radiotherapy to the brain. The first hormone to be affected is usually growth hormone, but there is often a lag of 18 months to 2 years before growth is affected. Recombinant human growth hormone is given to children with established growth hormone insufficiency by daily subcutaneous injection. There is no evidence that this will lead to relapse of a brain tumour, although some patients are pre-destined to have a relapse diagnosed shortly after growth hormone replacement is initiated. Other pituitary hormones are much less commonly affected.

Children, for example those with medulloblastoma, who have had their spines irradiated as well as their heads will develop short stature in time even if growth hormone replacement is given. This is because of a direct effect of the radiation on the growth of the bones in the spine. The legs will grow normally, and there will, accordingly, be a disparity between sitting and standing height.

Hypothyroidism will inevitably result from a total thyroidectomy (Chapter 29), and patients will require lifelong thyroid hormone replacement therapy (HRT). This should be at supraphysiological doses in patients with papillary and follicular cancer to keep thyroid-stimulating hormone (TSH) levels suppressed. Sometimes, transient or permanent hypoparathyroidism may result, and calcium and vitamin D supplementation is needed.

Hypothyroidism may result from radiotherapy to the neck, for example in the treatment of laryngeal and pharyngeal cancer (Chapter 26) or Hodgkin's disease (Chapter 41), and so monitoring of thyroid function should be a regular part of follow-up.

Loss of ovarian endocrine function will accompany surgery or radiotherapy for cervical carcinoma, and so oestrogen-replacement therapy (with a cyclical progestogen, if the uterus is left in position) will be required for at least 5 years in women under the age of 45, and should be offered to women over 45, if pre-menopausal.

ORAL AND DENTAL PROBLEMS

The salivary glands are very sensitive to radiotherapy and a dry mouth commonly follows radiotherapy for head and neck cancer. This is not just unpleasant, affecting quality of life through loss of taste, but may lead to rapidly progressive dental caries. Patients at risk should maintain meticulous oral hygiene and see a dentist regularly for advice and preventive care.

RENAL DYSFUNCTION

Care should be taken to avoid irradiation of the kidneys beyond accepted tolerance levels as hypertension or renal failure may result. Several cytotoxic drugs may lead to renal dysfunction of different types. Both ifosfamide and cisplatin are nephrotoxic, and may cause a tubular leak which requires long-term magnesium and potassium supplementation. Renal function should be checked by creatinine clearance or radionuclide assessment of the glomerular filtration rate (GFR) prior to and during cisplatin use. A GFR assessment is also required before prescribing carboplatin as this drug is renally excreted, and the dose required is dependent on renal excretion. Carboplatin is not, however, nephrotoxic like cisplatin. Methotrexate, especially at higher doses, has the potential to be nephrotoxic. Attention to detail at the time of methotrexate administration, including measurement of the GFR, ensuring adequate hydration with a good output of alkaline urine, and measurement of levels in the blood with use of folinic acid as antidote, should prevent any problems.

> **DRUGS WHICH MAY CAUSE LONG-TERM RENAL PROBLEMS**
>
> - Ifosfamide
> - Cisplatin
> - Methotrexate

CARDIAC DYSFUNCTION

The potential for radiotherapy to cause long-term heart disease has only recently been appreciated. Very long-term reports of patients treated for breast cancer in historic studies have shown an excess cardiac mortality, decades after treatment. This effect seems to be most marked in those with a left-sided cancer whose hearts would have received a higher dose. The mechanism appears to be premature coronary artery disease. Treatment techniques have changed, and it is hoped that current breast radiotherapy techniques will be less likely to cause similar morbidity, but of course it will be many years before data are available. In the interim, the benefits of postoperative breast radiotherapy in individual patients need to be carefully balanced against a possible increased risk of this treatment in women with cardiac risk factors, such as smoking, diabetes, hypercholesterolaemia, or a strong family history of ischaemic heart disease. Similar findings have been reported in patients who have received mediastinal radiotherapy for lymphoma.

Anthracycline drugs, such as doxorubicin, are cardiotoxic. Epirubicin is an anthracycline but is said to be less cardiotoxic. For prevention, it is important to monitor cardiac function, especially in patients with a history of heart disease, and to respect accepted cumulative lifetime limits for anthracycline dose. Children's hearts are more vulnerable and the dose limits are lower for children. The toxicity may be less if the drug is infused slowly over a number of hours rather than given as a bolus, or if the dose is fractionated over 2 or 3 days. Liposomal formulations may spare the heart and there are cardioprotective drugs which may be given at the same time.

Late anthracycline cardiomyopathy usually manifests as intractable heart failure due to a cardiomyopathy. Developing heart failure is treated in the conventional way with diuretics and vasodilators. Cardiac transplantation is, sometimes, considered in end-stage disease if the cancer is thought to be cured.

There can be an interaction between radiotherapy to the heart and anthracycline drugs. In paediatric practice, a lower cumulative limit is used if the patient also requires mediastinal radiotherapy. The effect of the increasing use of anthracycline-based schedules of adjuvant chemotherapy for breast cancer (Chapter 20) on the potential cardiac morbidity of contemporary breast radiotherapy techniques is unknown.

PULMONARY INSUFFICIENCY

Lung surgery will reduce lung volumes. For this reason lobectomy, where feasible, is preferable to pneumonectomy. Patients with lung cancer often have smoking-related chronic obstructive lung disease and very little respiratory reserve. This may preclude surgery even if the cancer is technically operable.

Patients, such as those with breast cancer, who receive radiotherapy to a significant volume of lung tissue may develop pneumonitis about 3 months after treatment. The symptoms are cough and dyspnoea and it usually settles spontaneously after a few weeks. Antibiotics and steroids are often prescribed although there is little evidence to show that they are of benefit.

After radiotherapy to part of the lung, pulmonary fibrosis may develop in the long term whether or not the patient experienced the symptoms of acute pneumonitis after treatment. In the patient who already has some loss of respiratory reserve, pulmonary fibrosis may lead to dyspnoea on less exertion than before.

A large number of cytotoxic drugs have the potential for causing lung damage, but the most commonly implicated culprits are busulphan, bleomycin and carmustine. The problems are often related to the cumulative dose,

but sometimes idiosyncratic reactions may occur at a relatively low dose. Sometimes, the toxicity may be schedule dependent, for example pulmonary toxicity may be encountered with continuous low-dose oral methotrexate but it is exceptionally rare with intermittent intravenous schedules, even with high-dose regimens. The symptoms are cough, dyspnoea and loss of exercise tolerance. The changes may stop if the drug is withdrawn, but sometimes they may be progressive and prove fatal. Particularly following bleomycin use, over-oxygenation during or after anaesthesia may lead to severe and potentially lethal lung toxicity, and anaesthetists must be warned when they are asked to anaesthetise patients who have received bleomycin previously.

MUSCULOSKELETAL EFFECTS

Fortunately, amputation for limb tumours is less often required with modern orthopaedic reconstructive techniques using custom-made bone endoprostheses combined with the use of chemotherapy to shrink the tumour prior to surgery. The situation is more complicated in children who are still growing, but it is sometimes possible to use prostheses which can be lengthened periodically to ensure that limb lengths remain equal.

Radiotherapy can affect the growth of both bone and soft tissue in children even at relatively low doses. It is, therefore, important when treating the spine to treat the whole width of the vertebrae to ensure that scoliosis does not develop as the patient grows. Paraspinal surgery may damage the musculature and cause a scoliosis unrelated to any radiotherapy. It is often possible to treat both sides of the body to ensure symmetrical development. For example, in Stage IA Hodgkin's disease limited to one side of the neck in children, it is usual to treat both sides of the neck, if radiotherapy is used to prevent the development of unsightly asymmetrical growth.

High-dose radiotherapy can lead to avascular necrosis of bone, for example in the hip joints after pelvic radiotherapy, and joint-replacement surgery may be required occasionally. Steroids too can predispose to avascular necrosis.

Radiotherapy to the chest wall in young girls may lead to failure of breast development at puberty, and if irradiation of the breast bud cannot be avoided parents must be warned during the process of seeking consent to treatment. After puberty, breast care nurses can advise about padded bras and breast prostheses if necessary, and surgical breast augmentation may be possible.

SEXUAL DIFFICULTIES

Sexual function is frequently affected in a structural way by cancer treatment. In addition, there are often associated psychological factors which may affect sexual function including anxiety about the prospect of infertility or of dying from the cancer, depression, altered body image after mastectomy or orchidectomy and so on.

In women, pelvic radiotherapy may lead to vaginal dryness and fibrosis which narrows and shortens the vagina. They should be advised early on by their oncologist or gynaecologist about the use of lubricants and regular vaginal dilatation to minimise adhesions and scarring. Telangiectasia may develop within the vagina which cause post-coital bleeding. The loss of ovarian oestrogen production by pelvic radiotherapy and the need for HRT has been mentioned above. Women who find normal sexual relations difficult after treatment of gynaecological cancers should be seen by counsellors skilled in dealing with couples with sexual problems to discuss alternative ways of expressing love and affection with their partners.

TREATMENT FOR IMPOTENCE

- ◆ Sildenafil – given orally
- ◆ Alprostadil – given by intracavernosal injection
- ◆ Alprostadil – given by intraurethral application
- ◆ Surgical implants

In men, prostatic surgery may lead to retrograde ejaculation and sometimes impotence. Medical or surgical castration in the treatment of prostate cancer will of course also cause impotence. Other types of surgery including retroperitoneal lymph node dissection and surgery for rectal cancer can similarly cause impotence. A urologist will be able to advise of the relative merits of medical and surgical treatments for erectile impotence. Fortunately, medical treatments for erectile dysfunction are available on the NHS for men with prostate cancer or after radical pelvic surgery or prostatectomy.

INFERTILITY

Many treatments for cancer, surgery, radiotherapy, chemotherapy and endocrine manipulation may affect reproductive potential. The majority of patients with cancer will be elderly or will have completed their families and so this will not be an issue. However, for children and young adults, especially if there is a good chance that they will be cured, this complication may assume great importance.

Men can give sperm for storage prior to chemotherapy, but it is sometimes found that men are subfertile at the time of diagnosis. Sperm collection can be a very embarrassing topic for young teenagers, and it is probably better if discussions about it are lead by health care professionals in the absence of parents. Even if semen is collected from such patients, the sperm count may be very low. Newer techniques such as intracytoplasmic sperm injection (ICSI) offer the potential of assisted fertility for men with low sperm counts. There are no techniques for storage of gonadal tissue from prepubertal boys which are proven to enable subsequent fertility.

Women can have induced ovulation and cryopreservation of ova. If they have a willing partner, *in vitro* fertilisation (IVF) and cryopreservation of the resultant embryos can be undertaken which is more likely to be successful than subsequent IVF of frozen ova. Alternatively, and in prepubertal girls, strips of ovarian cortical tissue may be taken for cryopreservation, but again the technology for producing functional ova from this are not yet well established.

Reproductive technology is a fast moving area of medicine, and what is unproven or even unthinkable now may well be possible a few years hence. It is also an area where there are many ethical considerations and legal regulation by the Human Fertilisation and Embryology Authority. There are also issues related to obtaining consent for a child who is not Gillick competent to give consent. A parent can, of course, give consent on behalf of a child for treatment of an illness such as cancer. Can a parent, however, ethically or legally give consent on behalf of an incompetent minor for an additional procedure, such as removal of ovarian tissue for storage, to be undertaken when it is not needed to treat the present illness and is of unproven benefit with regard to the long-term aim of treating infertility? Up-to-date specialist advice should always be sought in this area.

Of course, gamete preservation is of no use if there is not a functional uterus. Clearly if hysterectomy is needed, or if the uterus has been damaged by abdominal or pelvic radiotherapy in childhood or by radiotherapy in adult life, then pregnancy may not be possible.

There are concerns about whether a child which is born to parents who have received cancer treatment will be healthy. Despite the theoretical possibility of chemotherapy or radiotherapy causing germ-line mutations which might result in a congenital abnormality or an increased risk of cancer, there is no evidence to show that this is in fact the case. The possibility of children having an increased risk of cancer as the result of a pre-existing gene defect has been covered in Chapter 4. Of course, there is a risk of teratogenesis if chemotherapy or radiotherapy is used in women who are already pregnant, and this possibility must be excluded before starting cancer treatment in women of childbearing age.

SECOND MALIGNANT NEOPLASMS

Both chemotherapy and radiotherapy may lead to an increased risk of second cancers. Of course, patients receiving these treatments may already be at greater risk than normal people of getting another cancer by virtue of either environmental factors such as smoking or genetic predisposition.

Of all the different classes of cytotoxic agents (Chapter 13), it is the widely used alkylating agents including cyclophosphamide, ifosfamide, chlorambucil which are the most often implicated in causing second malignancies. Etoposide is linked with the development of leukaemia. Though there are theoretical grounds for worrying about the potential of drugs such as anthracyclines and platinum compounds to cause cancer, there are no clinical data to show that this is a real risk.

There is much evidence that radiation may cause malignant disease, notably leukaemia, thyroid cancer, breast cancer and sarcomas (Chapter 1), but overall only 1% or 2% of patients treated for cancer will develop a second malignancy related to radiotherapy. The risk is higher when combined modality therapy including alkylating agents is used.

As with all adverse effects, the risk of the development of a second cancer as a result of treatment of the first has to be weighed against the risks posed by inadequate treatment of the first. It is for this reason wise to avoid radiotherapy and chemotherapy unless there is a significant likelihood of benefit, and why their use in benign disease has been dramatically curtailed.

SECTION IV

Management of individual cancers

SECTION CONTENTS

Breast cancer has the highest incidence of any female cancer with about 25,000 new cases each year in Britain, and, consequently, has a high profile both in the public consciousness and the political agenda. Each year about 15,000 women die from breast cancer in this country, and the death rate in most parts of the UK is greater than for any other cancer type. However, in more socially deprived areas, where the prevalence of smoking amongst women is higher than average, the mortality from lung cancer in women exceeds that for breast cancer.

The public perception of breast cancer can overestimate the risk in younger women and lead to an unjustified climate of fear. In the UK, the lifetime risk of a woman developing breast cancer is estimated to be between 1 in 10 and 1 in 12. No one knows for certain the cause of breast cancer in the vast majority of cases, but there are many clearly identified factors, which increase the risk of an individual developing this disease. Most of these risk factors are not easily avoidable. For example, age is the strongest risk factor: the annual incidence is approximately 50 per 100,000 women at 35 years; sixfold greater at about 300 per 100,000 at 70 years; rising to 400 per 100,000 women aged 90. The only way for a woman to avoid this increasing risk is to die young from another cause. As the population ages we can, therefore, expect to see increasing numbers of patients with breast cancer. At present, half of all cases occur in women in the screening age group of 50–64 years, and over a third in older women. Only a minority, therefore, present in women under the age of 50.

RISK OF A WOMAN DEVELOPING BREAST CANCER BY A PARTICULAR AGE

Up to age 20	1 in 43,899
Up to age 30	1 in 2,165
Up to age 40	1 in 220
Up to age 50	1 in 56
Up to age 60	1 in 25
Up to age 70	1 in 16
Up to age 80	1 in 12
Up to age 85	1 in 11

As discussed in Chapter 3, there is a wide geographical variation in the incidence of breast cancer. Rates are highest in the developed countries of Northern Europe and North America, and lower in the Far East and in third world countries. The reasons for this may be partly demographic (the younger age structure in less developed countries compared with the ageing populations of the UK and the US), partly environmental and partly genetic. Although patients are often anxious that their disease may be hereditary, an underlying genetic basis is found in only about 5% (Chapter 4).

A number of reproductive and endocrine factors are associated with an increased likelihood of developing breast cancer. These include a long duration of menstrual life, manifested by an early menarche and a late menopause, nulliparity or older age at first-term pregnancy, failure to breastfeed, use of the oral contraceptive pill and use of hormone-replacement therapy (HRT). None of these increases the relative risk more than twofold, and more modern preparations of the pill with lower oestrogen doses are less likely to be associated with increased risk. The marginal increase in risk, which may be associated with the therapeutic use of oestrogen has to be offset against the benefits, which such treatment may confer.

REPRODUCTIVE AND ENDOCRINE FACTORS ASSOCIATED WITH INCREASED BREAST-CANCER RISK

- Early menarche
- Late menopause
- Nulliparity
- Older age at first-term pregnancy
- Failure to breastfeed
- Oral contraceptive pill
- HRT

THE MANAGEMENT OF BREAST CANCER

It would be helpful if the various stages in the management of breast cancer were self-contained, sequential steps. The various stages are

- diagnosis of a breast abnormality as being cancer,
- pathological typing of the cancer,

- staging of the disease,
- local treatment,
- systemic treatment.

Unfortunately, life is not that simple, and there is often overlap, and some treatments, such as wide local excision and axillary node clearance, are diagnostic procedures also. This means that the treatment for an individual patient is seldom clear at the outset, and the management algorithm is complicated. It is, therefore, difficult to counsel a patient fully before anything is done, and the process of information giving has to be done in a series of stages, depending on the findings of the previous step.

PRESENTATION OF BREAST CANCER

> **PRESENTATION OF BREAST CANCER**
>
> - Symptomatic
> - Screen detected

Patients may present with symptoms, or the disease may be discovered while the patient is still asymptomatic as a result of screening. The majority of patients present with a definite lump in the breast, which is usually painless. Although cancer may arise in any part of the breast, the upper outer quadrant is most commonly affected. Sometimes a patient may notice a change in the shape or size of the breast. Comparison with the opposite breast may be helpful. A crease or dimple may appear, there may be swelling or the nipple may become distorted or indrawn. Sometimes there may be a discharge from the nipple, or the nipple and areola may develop eczema. Skin changes, such as the erythema associated with inflammatory breast cancer, cutaneous nodules, ulceration and *peau d'orange* are all signs of locally advanced disease. Unusually, the disease may present with enlargement of the axillary nodes in the absence of any apparent breast abnormality. Very rarely, the presenting feature may be a symptom attributable to the development of distant metastases, such as bone pain, jaundice or neurological deficit in a patient who is (or who claims to be) unaware of any problem affecting the breast.

As the outcome of breast-cancer treatment is related to the stage at presentation, and delay in diagnosis has been shown to correlate with a worse outcome, there is much pressure to make the diagnosis as swiftly as possible after the patient has presented to her general practitioner. Criteria for early referral to a breast assessment clinic under the "2-week rule" have been given in Chapter 5. Screening for breast cancer is covered in Chapter 6.

DIAGNOSIS OF BREAST CANCER

> **TRIPLE ASSESSMENT**
>
> - Clinical examination
> - Imaging
> - Pathology

When a patient is referred to a breast assessment unit, she will usually undergo "triple assessment" after the history has been taken. This involves clinical examination, some form of breast imaging (usually mammography, but sometimes ultrasound is used in addition or instead), and, if there is a palpable abnormality, some attempt at obtaining cells or tissue for pathology (Chapter 7). This usually involves fine needle aspiration for cytology but core needle biopsy is often used in addition or instead. This is because it is not possible to distinguish reliably between invasive cancer and *in situ* disease on aspiration cytology. If the lesion is small or not easily palpable, imaging may be used to guide the needle biopsy so that one can be confident, if the biopsy is negative, that the abnormality was not missed.

A tissue diagnosis will be made prior to definitive surgery in the majority of cases, but occasionally where this has proved not to be possible, an open (excision) biopsy of the abnormality will be necessary. If the abnormality is not easily palpable and has been identified only on imaging, this is done following the insertion by a radiologist of a guide wire into the abnormal area under ultrasound or mammographic guidance to ensure that the area of concern is not missed. A radiograph of the surgical specimen will demonstrate that the original radiological abnormality has been completely excised.

PATHOLOGY OF BREAST CANCER

The most important pathological distinction to be made in breast cancer is whether the tumour is invasive (or infiltrating), or whether it is purely *in situ* disease. Purely *in situ* disease, which is increasingly commonly diagnosed as a result of breast-cancer screening with mammography, is managed differently from invasive cancer, as discussed below. Of course, *in situ* and invasive disease can (and often do) co-exist, but the management is determined by the invasive component.

Two types of breast cancer are commonly recognised, ductal (which occurs more frequently) and lobular. Sometimes individual cancers show features of both types. Both ductal and lobular cancers can be either invasive or *in situ*. Ductal carcinoma *in situ* is referred to as DCIS and lobular carcinoma *in situ* is referred to as LCIS. Lobular and ductal cancers are usually treated in similar ways, and stage for stage have a similar prognosis, but there are important distinctions. Lobular cancers are more likely to be multifocal within the breast and are more likely to be bilateral, either at the time of original diagnosis or subsequently. Lobular cancers more often show atypical patterns of metastasis, such as diffuse intraperitoneal disease with ovarian deposits.

Less common types of breast cancer include tubular, mucoid and medullary. These may be associated with a better prognosis and require less intensive treatment.

The pathologist will also comment on other features of the cancer which are important in determining stage, treatment and outcome. These include the size of the tumour, which can be measured more accurately by the pathologist than either clinically or radiologically. The degree of differentiation, or histological grade, relates to the metastatic potential and is used to guide adjuvant treatment. Similarly, the observation of invasion of lymphatic or vascular channels within the breast by tumour cells is an indication of a more malignant tumour. Completeness of excision should be commented on, and usually further surgery will be called for if resection margins are positive for either invasive or *in situ* cancer. It is of both prognostic and therapeutic importance to know whether any resected lymph nodes are free of tumour, and if they are not, how many are involved. Immunohistochemical techniques will be used to see if tumour tissue expresses steroid hormone receptors for oestrogen and progesterone. This information will be used to guide the need for treatments, such as tamoxifen and ovarian ablation. With the recent introduction of trastuzamab (Chapter 14), testing for Her2neu is becoming important for selected patients.

PATHOLOGICAL FEATURES GUIDING TREATMENT AND PROGNOSIS

- Type of cancer, invasive or *in situ*
- Histological grade
- Tumour size
- Completeness of excision
- Vascular or lymphatic invasion
- Number of lymph nodes involved and total number examined
- Oestrogen/progesterone receptor (ER/PR) status
- Her2neu

STAGING OF BREAST CANCER

The principles of cancer staging have been described in Chapter 8. In the case of breast cancer, the TNM classification is used. The TNM classification, however, does not tell you all you need to know about and individual patient's cancer, and it has been condemned as a two-dimensional description of a three-dimensional phenomenon. Nonetheless, it is still helpful to know the stage. The clinical stage (cTNM) is less accurate than the pathological stage (pTNM), and so patients are not fully staged until after their definitive surgical procedure(s). The main points (but not the full details) of the staging system are shown in the boxes.

T-STAGES OF THE TNM CLASSIFICATION FOR BREAST CANCER

- TX: Primary tumour cannot be assessed
- T0: No evidence of primary tumour
- Tis: Ductal or lobular carcinoma *in situ* or Paget's disease of the nipple with no tumour
- T1: Tumour 2 cm or less in greatest dimension
  - T1mic: Microinvasion 0.1 cm or less
  - T1a: More than 0.1 cm, but less than 0.5 cm
  - T1b: More than 1.5 cm, but less than 1.0 cm
  - T1c: More than 1 cm, but not more than 2 cm
- T2: Tumour more than 2 cm but not more than 5 cm in greatest dimension
- T3: Tumour more than 5 cm in greatest dimension
- T4: Tumour of any size with direct extension to chest wall or skin
  - T4a: Extension to chest wall
  - T4b: Oedema (including *peau d'orange*), or ulceration of the skin of the breast, or satellite skin nodules confined to the same breast
  - T4c: Both 4a and 4b, above
  - T4d: Inflammatory carcinoma

T-STAGES OF THE TNM CLASSIFICATION FOR BREAST CANCER

- NX: Regional lymph nodes cannot be assessed
- N0: No regional lymph node metastases
- N1: Metastasis to moveable ipsilateral axillary lymph nodes
- N2: Metastasis to ipsilateral axillary lymph nodes fixed to one another or to other structures
- N3: Metastasis to ipsilateral internal mammary lymph nodes

There is controversy about how hard one should look for metastatic disease in newly diagnosed patients. It is unusual to find distant metastases in patients with early operable invasive breast cancer at the time of diagnosis.

Routine liver ultrasound examinations and bone scans are likely to reveal more false-positive than true-positive results at this time. It is, therefore, sensible to limit staging investigations to a chest X-ray and full blood count and biochemical profile, reserving other scans for patients with abnormal results or worrying symptoms.

> ### M-STAGES OF THE TNM CLASSIFICATION FOR BREAST CANCER
>
> ◆ MX: Distant metastasis cannot be assessed
> ◆ M0: No distant metastasis
> ◆ M1: Distant metastasis

In patients with locally advanced disease, there is a higher likelihood of distant disease at presentation, and it is prudent for them to be fully staged.

TREATMENT OF BREAST CANCER

It is clear from the above that women presenting with breast cancer form a heterogeneous group. Most present with a breast lump, but some are truly asymptomatic and have screen-detected cancer. Some have only *in situ* disease, but the majority have invasive cancer. Some have small, localised tumours, while others have locally advanced disease. A minority will have overtly disseminated disease at presentation. Because of this variety, there is no single answer to the question "how should a woman with breast cancer be treated?" It is necessary to divide patients into a number of groups, and talk about treatment options for each group. To some extent these groups are arbitrary, and there will always be borderline cases which do not fit easily into the groups. For the purposes of this chapter, we will consider the following groups:

◆ *in situ* disease,
◆ early invasive carcinoma,
◆ locally advanced invasive carcinoma,
◆ metastatic disease.

TREATMENT OF *IN SITU* DISEASE

Ductal carcinoma *in situ* used to be a rare diagnosis, accounting for only about 1% of cases. With the introduction of routine mammographic screening, the incidence has increased greatly, and it now accounts for about one in five cases. DCIS may present with the nipple appearing eczematous, so-called Paget's disease of the nipple. Historically (as with invasive breast cancer) the treatment for all forms of DCIS including Paget's disease was mastectomy, which was curative for all patients. As surgical practice for patients with invasive cancer has evolved to offer breast conservation wherever possible, so it has in DCIS. Most cases are impalpable, and for these, image

guided wide local excision with specimen radiography to ensure that the mammographically abnormal area has been completely excised, and pathological confirmation of complete excision is adequate surgery. No surgery is needed for the lymph nodes in the axilla. If the lesion has not been completely excised by the initial operation, re-excision is required. In the case of very extensive DCIS mastectomy (which can be of the skin-sparing type with immediate reconstruction) is still the best surgical option.

Studies commenced in the early days of local excision for DCIS showed that postoperative radiotherapy was beneficial, and it became the recommended management for all. However, gradually it has become apparent that DCIS is a very heterogeneous entity, and no single treatment approach is suitable for all patients. The pathologist will measure the tumour size, assign a nuclear grade to DCIS, note the presence or absence of necrosis (often referred to as comedo pattern) and comment on completeness of excision. These factors can be combined into a score called the Van Nuys Index, which is predictive of recurrence after local excision. Patients with low scores have a low risk of recurrence after surgery alone and do not require radiotherapy. Patients with intermediate scores benefit from radiotherapy. Patients with high scores should be offered mastectomy, as wide local excision and radiotherapy is associated with unacceptably high rates of local recurrence.

> ### PATHOLOGICAL FEATURES OF DCIS GUIDING TREATMENT AND PROGNOSIS
>
> ◆ Tumour size
> ◆ Nuclear grade
> ◆ Presence of necrosis
> ◆ Completeness of excision

Adjuvant tamoxifen is often prescribed after initial treatment for DCIS, and improves outcome. Overall, the likelihood of recurrence in patients treated for DCIS is about 7%, but in half of these cases, the disease is invasive when it recurs.

Lobular carcinoma *in situ* is often multifocal and bilateral. It can be helpful to take "blind" trucut biopsies from apparently uninvolved areas of the affected breast and also from the opposite breasts. In some cases, bilateral mastectomy is recommended. If the disease appears localised, wide local excision of the abnormal area, tamoxifen treatment and careful follow-up should be sufficient.

TREATMENT OF EARLY INVASIVE BREAST CANCER

Most patients fall into this category. It includes patients with T1–T3, N0–1, M0 disease, whether the presentation was with symptoms or through screening. Some patients with T3 disease are better considered as having locally advanced disease; the dividing line between these categories is not clear cut.

SURGICAL MANAGEMENT OF EARLY INVASIVE BREAST CANCER

The definitive surgical treatment of breast cancer is not normally undertaken without prior histological confirmation of the diagnosis. The era of the brutal practice of getting patients to consent to "frozen section of breast lump? proceed to mastectomy" is fortunately over. Preoperative discussion is very important. Most patients, these days wish to be empowered to share some of the decisions, which will affect their lives. Patients value the opportunity to talk through issues, such as whether to have only a wide local excision or a full mastectomy, and whether or not reconstruction should be performed, with the breast-care nurse as well as the surgeon. It is essential to allow the patient enough time to consider all the issues, and for her to involve family and friends if she so wishes, before the type of surgery and date of the operation is decided. In this way, the patient will know she has been involved in decision-making, she will have agreed to the extent of surgery prior to the operation being performed, and she is likely to have fewer regrets later.

SURGICAL OPTIONS

◆ Breast-conserving treatment, wide local excision
◆ Mastectomy, immediate or delayed reconstruction

There is now sufficient evidence that, in appropriately selected patients, breast-conserving surgery with postoperative radiotherapy results in the same survival as mastectomy, although the possibility of local recurrence remains higher. The term "wide local excision" is preferable to "lumpectomy" when describing breast-conserving surgery for a cancer as it indicates that the cancer should be removed with a clear margin of normal tissue. The pathologist will report whether or not the margins around the tumour are adequate. If there is evidence of tumour at the resection margins, then a further excision should be performed to reduce the likelihood of local recurrence. If this does not completely clear the disease, mastectomy may be necessary.

CLEAR INDICATIONS FOR MASTECTOMY

◆ Patient preference
◆ Large (>4 cm) tumours
◆ Involvement of skin or chest wall
◆ Multifocal tumours
◆ Widespread ductal carcinoma *in situ*

Even when wide local excision is deemed to be an appropriate surgical option, some patients will still prefer to undergo mastectomy. They may feel greater reassurance, if all the breast has been removed, or they may wish to avoid the need for radiotherapy, if possible.

Mastectomy is still the best option for those with locally advanced tumours (greater than 4 cm diameter, or involving the skin or pectoral muscles or chest wall, multifocal tumours, centrally placed tumours where adequate local excision would involve sacrifice of the nipple, and in patients with widespread ductal carcinoma *in situ*. If mastectomy is necessary, reconstruction can be performed at the time of the principal procedure or subsequently. For some carefully selected patients, such as those with extensive ductal carcinoma *in situ*, skin sparing or subcutaneous mastectomy with reconstruction may be an option, which gives a better cosmetic result.

Management of the axilla has always been controversial. Traditionally, the choice lay between no surgery (in which case radiotherapy was often used), axillary node sampling, or axillary node clearance. Most surgeons nowadays will perform axillary node clearance at the same time as the definitive procedure on the breast. This has the advantage of allowing complete pathological assessment of the axillary lymph nodes, which gives important information about prognosis and is important for making decisions about the type of adjuvant systemic therapy, which should be offered. In addition, axillary clearance is the best treatment for involved nodes. If node sampling only is performed, the axilla will require no further treatment if an adequate sample (four or more nodes) is negative. If the sample is positive, then a further surgical procedure to clear the axilla, or axillary radiotherapy will be required. The practice of sentinel node biopsy has been introduced recently (Chapter 7), but this should still be regarded as an experimental technique not established practice. If the sentinel node is negative, no further surgery should be necessary, but if it is positive full axillary clearance is required.

BREAST RECONSTRUCTION

It should now be standard practice to offer breast reconstruction to women undergoing mastectomy. It may be performed at the same time as the mastectomy, or at a later date. Various techniques are in use. Some of the best results are seen when a pedicled myocutaneous flap is brought up from the lower abdomen. This is based on the rectus abdominis muscle and results in an easily concealed horizontal scar below the bikini line. It is, therefore, known as the transverse rectus abdominis myocutaneous (or TRAM) flap procedure. A similar operation can be done using a myocutaneous flap based on the latissimus dorsi muscle, but this results in a more obvious and unsightly scar across the back. Neither of these techniques involves the use of any artificial materials. Alternative techniques involve the use of implants. Initially, a tissue expander is placed under pectoralis major and gradually inflated with saline injected at intervals through a port. Because of the controversy surrounding the possible ill-effects associated with the use of silicone gel filled breast endoprosthesis which may leak, saline or oil filled implants are now more commonly used. It is difficult to reconstruct a very large breast, so a contralateral reduction mammoplasty may be offered to restore symmetry in these cases.

POSTOPERATIVE RADIOTHERAPY

Radiotherapy is given after definitive surgery for early breast cancer with the principal aim of improving local control, that is to say to reduce the likelihood of recurrence in the residual breast tissue or on the chest wall. It has long been believed that the use of radiotherapy in this setting had no influence on survival, but there are now some data, which suggest that in node-positive patients, radiotherapy may reduce the likelihood of death from breast cancer.

Postoperative radiotherapy to residual breast tissue is generally recommended for all patients who have undergone wide local excision of an invasive breast cancer. Maybe it can be avoided in some carefully selected patients. For example, those with small, well-differentiated, ER-positive tumours have a good prognosis anyway and systemic therapy alone may be adequate. In very old patients and those with serious intercurrent illness, the risk of recurrence may be perceived to be small in relation to other factors and lead to the avoidance of radiotherapy. These are still areas of uncertainty, and clinical trials are in progress which will in time provide us with more evidence to guide our practice.

When radiotherapy is given after breast-conserving surgery, it is usual practice to treat the entire ipsilateral breast, and then give a boost to the tumour bed. The tumour bed boost may not be necessary in older women with favourable histological features. Fractionation schedules vary. At one extreme, 25 treatments will be given to the breast with a five fraction boost, making a total of 30 attendances for treatment 5 days a week over 6 weeks. In other centres, only 15 treatments may be given, either daily over 3 weeks, or only two or three times a week over a longer overall period. At the moment, we do not know for sure whether one approach is better than the other, and clinical trials are underway, which will hopefully give us more information.

Following mastectomy, radiotherapy is not always necessary. It is considered indicated, if the risk of local recurrence is high, that is in the case of large (more than 5 cm diameter) or multifocal tumours, if the overlying skin or the chest wall is involved, if the tumour was not completely excised or if there was heavy lymph node involvement. In doubtful cases, factors such as the grade of the tumour and the presence or absence of vascular invasion may guide decision-making. Fractionation schedules vary, as in the case of radiotherapy after breast-conserving surgery, but a boost is not required.

After both wide local excision and mastectomy, radiotherapy is not given to the axilla, if there has been a complete dissection, regardless of whether or not the nodes were involved. In the unusual case, where for some valid reason, there has been no axillary surgery, or if a node sample only was positive, radiotherapy will usually be offered. The supraclavicular fossa is usually treated in continuity when axillary radiotherapy is delivered. Following axillary dissection, the supraclavicular fossa alone may be treated, if there is heavy lymph node involvement.

Patients undergoing radiotherapy should be warned in advance that they may well find the process tiring. As the weeks go by, the skin will become pink or red (erythematous reaction), and flaking of the skin (dry desquamation) or blistering (moist desquamation) may occur, especially in the inframammary fold. hyperpigmentation of the skin may occur, especially in individuals with a darker skin to start with. It is usual to treat the acute skin reaction with a moisturiser, such as aqueous cream, and many patients find *aloe vera* preparations helpful. Sometimes hydrocortisone cream is prescribed, but this may well not confer any benefit. If moist desquamation occurs, dressings with colloid gel will promote healing. Sometimes, topical antibiotics may be needed for secondary infection. This acute reaction will settle down within a few weeks after treatment is complete.

POSSIBLE ACUTE SIDE-EFFECTS OF BREAST RADIOTHERAPY

- Tiredness
- Cutaneous erythema
- Flaking of the skin
- Blistering of the skin
- Increased pigmentation

Late side-effects of radiotherapy may take months or years to develop. A small volume of lung tissue is included in the field of irradiation and a small proportion of patients, usually fewer than 5%, will develop symptomatic pneumonitis manifested by cough and dyspnoea, about 3 months after treatment. This will usually settle spontaneously, but antibiotics and steroids are commonly prescribed. Later, limited pulmonary fibrosis may develop. This is usually asymptomatic, but may show up as an incidental finding on a chest X-ray requested for another purpose.

The breast may be oedematous for some time following surgery and radiotherapy, but this usually settles eventually. Then there may be some fibrosis apparent, which gives the breast a diffuse or localised firmer texture. Persistent breast discomfort is a common feature after breast-conserving treatment. It can cause a lot of anxiety, but it is rarely a sinister sign and not usually severe enough to warrant medication. Telangiectasia may develop over the breast or chest wall, especially at the site of the tumour bed boost. Again the apparently sudden appearance of red marks can make a woman anxious about recurrence unless the possibility has been explained to her. Rarely changes of osteonecrosis in the underlying ribs may make them more prone to fracture after minimal trauma.

There has been concern, supported by data from old randomised trials, that radiotherapy to the breast, especially to the left breast, may be associated with an excess cardiac mortality due to premature coronary artery disease. More modern radiotherapy techniques and fractionation schedules should reduce this risk, but the very long-term effect of the increasingly widespread use of anthracycline chemotherapy in conjunction with radiotherapy to the breast is at present unquantified.

Second malignant neoplasms may result from radiation exposure. Sarcomas of bone and soft tissue arising on the chest wall or around the shoulder may arise many years after radiotherapy, but this is rare. Many thousands of women undergo this treatment without developing this complication, for every patient who does. Second cancers in the opposite breast are more common, and it seems that some of these, at least may be related to previous radiotherapy.

LYMPHOEDEMA

Lymphoedema of the arm is a potential complication of breast cancer and its treatment, which is a source of much anxiety among patients. Fortunately, severe lymphoedema is less common than previously, thanks to changing surgical and radiotherapeutic practice. Mild and easily treated swelling of the arm is not uncommon after axillary node clearance. Radiotherapy of the clinically uninvolved axilla does not cause lymphoedema, if there has been no axillary surgery. The risk of lymphoedema is high, however, if radiotherapy is administered to the axilla after surgical clearance. It is, therefore, contraindicated following clearance except in exceptional situations where there is a very high probability of disease recurrence, when the patient must be fully informed of the risk of lymphoedema, and be prepared to accept this in an attempt to prevent disease progression. Nowadays, severe lymphoedema is seen most commonly in the context of progressive uncontrolled axillary recurrence of cancer, rather than as a treatment-related complication. Breast-care nurses are trained in lymphoedema management and have various useful techniques including massage, bandaging and compression hosiery at their disposal.

BRACHIAL PLEXUS NEUROPATHY

The nerves of the brachial plexus which supply sensation and motor function to the arm, pass through the axilla where they are vulnerable to damage by radiotherapy and surgery. Many patients in the past have sustained severe damage as a result of treatment, however, the risk is now recognised, and radiotherapy treatment techniques and fractionation schedules have been modified in a way which makes neuropathy very uncommon these days. The only neurological damage commonly encountered presently is anaesthesia and parasthesia of the medial aspect of the upper arm caused by surgical division of the intercostobrachial nerve at the time of axillary dissection. Brachial plexus neuropathy arising after modern era treatment is more likely to be due to axillary recurrence of breast cancer. This can sometimes be difficult to diagnose clinically and MRI can be helpful.

ADJUVANT CHEMOTHERAPY

Adjuvant chemotherapy means cytotoxic drug treatment given after definitive and potentially curative local treatment with surgery and possibly radiotherapy with the aim of eliminating occult foci of metastatic cancer to improve the chance of cure. It is now well recognised that chemotherapy following local treatment for breast cancer improves the likelihood of survival, perhaps by about 10%. This means that at least 90% of patients receiving this treatment will get no personal benefit from it. Either they are destined to be cured regardless of chemotherapy, or their cancer cells will be resistant to chemotherapy and they will still relapse and die from their disease.

As chemotherapy has well-recognised toxicities (Chapter 13), we try to select only those patients who have the best chance of benefit from chemotherapy for treatment, sparing those with a good prognosis and hormone sensitive tumours for endocrine treatments only. As there are still some uncertainties about which groups of patients stand to gain most from chemotherapy, and other areas of uncertainty within the field of breast-cancer adjuvant chemotherapy, such as whether an individual chemotherapeutic regimen is better than another, this is a focus of much clinical trial activity.

Different cancer centres may have slightly different protocols for deciding which patients should be offered adjuvant chemotherapy, and a large number of different regimens are in common use. In general, these are all simple to administer outpatient schedules. Perhaps, the gold standard is six cycles of cyclophosphamide, methotrexate and fluorouracil (known as CMF), but even with one combination of drugs, there are various schedules which differ in dose and frequency of administration, and in whether the cyclophosphamide is delivered orally or by intravenous injection. There are some data, which suggest that anthracycline drugs, such as doxorubicin and epirubicin may be more potent than CMF, so four courses of doxorubicin and cyclophosphamide are probably equivalent to six courses of CMF, and more prolonged anthracycline-based regimens, such as six courses of fluorouracil, epirubicin and cyclophosphamide (FEC), or four courses of epirubicin followed by four courses of CMF are often favoured for patients with poor prognosis disease. The use of high-dose chemotherapy with peripheral blood stem cell support has been investigated in women at high risk, but so far no additional benefit over standard schedules has been shown. Current research focuses on the place of taxanes, especially docetaxel (Taxotere), known to be valuable in the treatment of advanced disease, in the adjuvant setting.

In deciding which patients should be offered chemotherapy, and which chemotherapy schedule should be used, factors to be taken into account include:

- the age of the patients (younger patients have more years at risk ahead of them, are more likely to have biologically unfavourable disease and are generally better able to tolerate chemotherapy);
- the presence and extent of nodal involvement (in general, lymph-node negative patients have a good prognosis, and this worsens with increasing numbers of involved nodes, such that those with four or more involved nodes constitute a high-risk group);
- the size of the tumour (larger tumours are associated with higher risk);
- the grade of the tumour (less well-differentiated tumours have a higher metastatic potential).

GUIDELINES FOR THE USE OF ADJUVANT CHEMOTHERAPY

Age 49 years or less

No nodes involved, tumour less than 1 cm and favourable histology	No chemotherapy
No nodes involved, tumour 1 cm or greater or unfavourable histology	Standard chemotherapy
1–3 nodes involved	Standard chemotherapy
Four or more nodes involved	Intensive chemotherapy

Age 50 to 59 years

No nodes involved	No chemotherapy
1–3 nodes involved, ER positive	No chemotherapy
1–3 nodes involved, ER negative	Standard chemotherapy
Four or more nodes involved	Standard chemotherapy

Age 60 years or greater

No nodes involved	No chemotherapy
1–3 nodes involved	No chemotherapy
Four or more nodes involved	Standard chemotherapy

Notes

- Standard chemotherapy is, for example, CMF six courses or doxorubicin/cyclophosphamide four courses
- Intensive chemotherapy is, for example, doxorubicin four courses followed by CMF four courses
- Favourable histology is Grade I or tubular or mucoid
- Unfavourable histology is Grade II or III or vascular invasion or lobular or medullary
- In addition, adjuvant endocrine therapy will be used depending on hormone receptor status

The presence of ERs and PRs is also important. Tumours responsive to endocrine therapy may additionally respond to chemotherapy, but if a tumour is likely to respond to hormone manipulation, is the additional toxicity of chemotherapy still warranted? Co-morbidity may also influence decisions about chemotherapy. For example, anthracyclines should be avoided in patients with heart failure. Possible guidelines for the use of adjuvant chemotherapy are given in the box, but different centres may use a slightly different approach.

Finally, the attitude of the patient herself may play a significant part, and decisions about adjuvant therapy often require much discussion, sometimes spread over several consultations. It is often helpful for the patient to have the breast-care nurse present, and it may, in addition, be valuable for her to have the opportunity to discuss the practicalities of chemotherapy administration and side-effects with a chemotherapy clinical nurse specialist in advance of the decision to give chemotherapy being made.

Chemotherapy side-effects have been discussed in Chapter 13. All commonly used schedules may cause nausea and vomiting, but modern anti-emetic drugs are usually successful at preventing vomiting. Nonetheless, most patients will still feel a bit "off colour" for a few days after each chemotherapy administration. The risk of alopecia is greater with anthracycline-based regimens than with CMF. The use of scalp cooling is sometimes helpful in preventing hair loss. Patients should be warned about the possibility of myelosuppression, and given clear instructions about seeking medical help, if they develop a pyrexia or a 'flu-like illness at the anticipated time of the haematological nadir, 10–14 days after chemotherapy. The full blood count should be checked, and they may require hospital admission for supportive care (Chapter 17). Mouth ulcers are not uncommon, particularly, if anthracyclines are used. Cardiotoxicity is very rare, but all patients receiving anthracyclines should have cardiac function checked prior to treatment.

ADJUVANT ENDOCRINE THERAPY

The use of adjuvant endocrine therapy and chemotherapy is not an either/or choice. Some patients will require one, some patients the other, some both and some neither. The key factors in deciding about the place of adjuvant endocrine therapy (Chapter 14) are the receptor status of the tumour and the menstrual status of the patient.

Usually tumours will be tested for both ER and PRs, but information about PR status is really only helpful in ER-negative patients. All patients with early invasive ER-positive cancer should be considered for endocrine therapy of some sort. Those with ER-negative, but PR-positive tumours, may derive some benefit from hormonal manipulation. Patients with ER- and PR-negative cancers should not receive hormone treatment.

Pre-menopausal ER-positive patients can be considered for some form of ovarian ablation (surgical oophorectomy, radiation menopause or LHRH agonists, such as goserelin (Zoladex or Zoladex LA)). If they are also receiving chemotherapy, one can wait to see if this renders them post-menopausal prior to undertaking additional treatment. Selective ER modulators, such as tamoxifen (Nolvadex) can be used in pre-menopausal women in addition to or instead of ovarian suppression.

In post-menopausal women with ER-positive tumours, tamoxifen 20 mg daily is usually prescribed for 5 years. Whether a longer duration of tamoxifen use might give additional benefit is presently the subject of clinical trials. The use of anastrozole (Arimidex) 1 mg daily and other drugs in place of tamoxifen is similarly being explored. Anastrozole can only be used in women who are naturally or artificially post-menopausal. If it is difficult to know whether there is still ovarian function (e.g. in women who have had a prior hysterectomy with ovarian conservation) LH and FSH levels can be measured. Anastrozole is now licensed as adjuvant therapy in women with hormone-receptor-positive breast cancer who are naturally or artificially post-menopausal, if tamoxifen is considered undesirable because of the increased thrombo-embolic risk or endometrial abnormalities.

SEQUENCING OF ADJUVANT THERAPIES

Typically, a patient undergoes surgery, then chemotherapy, then radiotherapy followed by the introduction of endocrine therapy. There is, however, no magical order, and sometimes treatments are given in a different sequence. There are anxieties that local control may be compromised, if radiotherapy is long delayed after surgery, and similar worries that systemic control may be prejudiced, if chemotherapy is delayed by radiotherapy. Radiotherapy is often given at the same time as CMF chemotherapy, but if anthracyclines are used they are given first to minimise toxicity. Usually, tamoxifen (or anastrozole) is not started until chemotherapy is complete, as the risk of thrombo-embolic disease is greater, if the two are used concurrently. Occasionally, non-surgical treatment used preoperatively to shrink the tumour. This so-called neoadjuvant therapy is more common in the case of locally advanced disease (see below).

FOLLOW-UP

It is widely held that women are followed up too much after treatment for breast cancer. Regular clinical examination of the breasts, together with annual mammography of the affected breast for 5 years after conservation treatment is probably useful for detection of local recurrence. Mammography after treatment can be difficult to interpret, and other investigations, such as ultrasound, magnetic resonance imaging and sestamibi scintimammography may also be helpful in selected patients. If local recurrence is confirmed, careful evaluation for metastatic disease is important because the recurrence is localised to the breast (and, therefore, potentially curable with further surgery) in only 50% of cases. In the other half, local recurrence is an indicator of metastatic relapse. After 5 years, mammography of the treated and contralateral breasts is indicated only every 2 or 3 years.

Routine evaluation for dissemination as part of follow-up is not worthwhile, because metastatic breast cancer is incurable, and the patient gains nothing from its diagnosis at a time when it is asymptomatic.

TREATMENT OF RELAPSED DISEASE

In the case of isolated local recurrence after breast-conserving surgery, further surgery may be curative. In most cases, mastectomy will be necessary, but for some carefully selected patients, a further wide excision may be feasible. After mastectomy, local excision of a chest wall recurrence is not always feasible. Radical radiotherapy can be administered if it was not used initially, but it cannot be given again to the same side. There is logic in using adjuvant chemotherapy after local recurrence, but few data to prove its worth. If the disease is positive for hormone receptors, a change in endocrine therapy may be worthwhile, for example a switch to anastrozole from tamoxifen (or vice versa) in post-menopausal women.

If the disease is metastatic at relapse, treatment is as described below, obviously taking into account any prior systemic therapy, which may have been administered. It is important to take into account specific symptom control measures, as well as giving appropriate systemic anti-cancer treatment. The psycho-social management must not be overlooked, and it may well be wise to enlist the help of the community palliative care team at this stage.

TREATMENT OF LOCALLY ADVANCED DISEASE

Patients in this category include those with T4 cancers, especially inflammatory carcinoma. Inflammatory carcinoma of the breast is characterised by diffuse brawny induration of the skin with an erysipeloid edge. The whole breast is often swollen and oedematous, and sometimes no discrete mass can be felt. Some centres would also include all patients with a breast carcinoma unsuitable for breast-conserving surgery, for example those with tumours greater than 4 cm diameter or multifocal disease. There is a continuum of disease between early invasive cancer and locally advanced cancer, and the dividing line is not entirely clear cut. Also in the category of locally advanced disease are those patients, sometimes with only a small breast tumour or no clinically detectable primary cancer, who have extensive, fixed nodal disease.

These patients have a high risk of metastatic disease at presentation or subsequently, and local control can be difficult to achieve. Following biopsy and full staging investigations, primary medical treatment is given. This is usually with an intensive anthracycline-based schedule. Surgery can be undertaken after a few courses of chemotherapy. It will usually entail a mastectomy and axillary node clearance. Often in the case of T4 tumours, it is wise to remove more skin than would be necessary with an early cancer, in which case a myocutaneous flap may be required to close the defect, not just for cosmetic breast reconstruction. Postoperative radiotherapy should always be used. If the disease is considered to be inoperable even after primary medical therapy, radical radiotherapy without mastectomy can be used, but the likelihood of local control is not as great as when it has been possible to perform radical surgery. Adjuvant endocrine therapy will also be given, as with early breast cancer.

Elderly patients with hormone-receptor-positive disease who are not fit enough for chemotherapy may be managed with primary endocrine therapy with anastrozole or tamoxifen instead of chemotherapy.

TREATMENT OF METASTATIC DISEASE

Patients whose breast cancer is metastatic at the time of diagnosis will not be cured, but nonetheless survival with good quality of life for a number of years can often be achieved. Obviously, symptom control measures, such as analgesia, where necessary, go hand in hand with active anti-cancer treatment in the care of patients with metastatic breast cancer. This diagnosis, in a patient who was previously well is devastating, even though it may be possible to temper the bad news with some therapeutic optimism. It is, therefore, often wise to involve the palliative care team (Chapter 49) at an early stage for psycho-social support, even if there are no pressing symptoms and the prognosis may be measured in years. Management of particular metastatic problems, such as bone metastases, hypercalcaemia and pleural effusion is described in Chapter 50, this section concentrates on specific anti-cancer treatment.

NICE GUIDANCE ON THE USE OF TAXANES IN BREAST CANCER

- The use of docetaxel in combination with an anthracycline in first-line treatment of advanced breast cancer is not currently recommended. As paclitaxel is not licensed for first-line use with anthracycline, its use has not been considered in this indication.
- Docetaxel and paclitaxel are recommended as an option for the treatment of advanced breast cancer where initial cytotoxic chemotherapy (including an anthracycline) has failed or is inappropriate.
- The taxanes are not currently licensed in the UK for adjuvant treatment of early breast cancer, therefore, their use in this indication should be limited to randomised clinical trials.

If the metastatic disease is not extensive, limited, for example, to one or two sites in bone, then it may still be worthwhile treating the breast and nodes "radically" to ensure that uncontrolled local disease does not result. Systemic treatment similar to that which might be used in the adjuvant setting can be used to control metastatic disease. In patients with metastatic disease, both endocrine treatment and chemotherapy offer the possibility of multiple sequential systemic treatments. Assessment of hormone receptor status is predictive of response to endocrine therapy (Chapter 14). In hormone-receptor-positive patients, tamoxifen has traditionally been the first line of treatment, followed (in post-menopausal women) by an aromatase inhibitor, such as anastrozole, and then by a progestogen, such as megestrol acetate. However, better results may be obtained, if anastrozole is used as first-line treatment. Ovarian suppression can be used in pre-menopausal women. It is important to monitor response to treatment carefully. Serial measurements of tumour markers, such as CEA, CA125 and CA15-3 can add to measurement of soft tissue masses or measurements made on chest X-ray or liver ultrasound.

NICE GUIDANCE ON THE USE OF TRASTUZAMAB FOR ADVANCED BREAST CANCER

- Trastuzamab in combination with Paclitaxel (combination trastuzamab is currently only licensed for use with paclitaxel) is recommended as an option for people with tumours expressing human epidermal growth factor receptor 2 (HER2) scored at levels of 3+ who have not received chemotherapy for metastatic breast cancer and in whom anthracycline treatment is inappropriate.
- Trastuzamab monotherapy is recommended as an option for people with tumours expressing HER2 scored at levels of 3+ who have received at least two chemotherapy regimens for metastatic breast cancer. Prior chemotherapy must have included at least an anthracycline and a taxane, where these treatments are appropriate. It should also have included hormonal therapy in suitable ER-positive patients.
- HER2 levels should be scored using validated immunohistochemical techniques and in accordance with published guidelines. Laboratories offering tissue sample immunocytochemical or other predictive tests for therapy response should use validated standardised assay methods and participate in and demonstrate satisfactory performance in a recognised external quality assurance scheme.

In patients with receptor-negative cancers, or if the metastatic disease is more advanced with symptomatic visceral involvement, such as lung or liver metastases, chemotherapy is called for. Cytotoxic therapy is usually associated with a higher response rate, but a shorter duration of palliation than endocrine agents. A variety of schedules is in use. Often combinations, such as CMF or doxorubicin and cyclophosphamide are used as in adjuvant therapy. Taxanes such as docetaxel and paclitaxel are not used for first-line therapy of metastatic disease, but the National Institute for Clinical Excellence (NICE) recommends their use for treatment of disease, which has progressed or relapsed after an anthracycline-containing regimen. Again it is important to monitor response carefully, so that patients are not subjected unnecessarily to the toxicity of ineffective treatment.

The monoclonal antibody trastuzamab (Herceptin) is used alone or in combination with chemotherapy for the management of metastatic disease in patients whose tumours express high levels of Her2neu (Chapter 14). The NICE has published guidance on its use in this setting. Trastuzamab also offers hope in the adjuvant setting, but at the moment it does not have an established place for this indication and so its use as an adjuvant is still a subject for clinical trials.

TREATMENT OF BREAST CANCER IN ELDERLY WOMEN

The principles of cancer management in elderly patients are discussed in Chapter 48. In general, if a patient is fit, her breast cancer should be managed in the same way as if she were younger. This is because, even though she may be old, her life expectancy is long enough for the cancer to cause problems, if it is not treated optimally. The natural tendency to minimise treatment for elderly patients out of kindness often leads to increased problems later on.

This means that the indications for surgery, whether wide local excision or mastectomy should be the same as for younger women. For relatively early disease, mastectomy may, however, sometimes be preferred to local excision, if it reduces the need for radiotherapy in addition. Age, by itself, should not be considered a bar to reconstructive surgery.

Radiotherapy is probably indicated in the same circumstances as it is in younger women. There is the possibility that some carefully selected elderly women who have undergone wide local excision for a small, well-differentiated, ER-positive tumour can be managed by adjuvant endocrine therapy without radiotherapy, and the safety of this approach is currently being tested in clinical trials. Patients with more advanced disease have a significant risk of local recurrence and should receive radiotherapy. If radiotherapy is given, then the same dose and fractionation schedule should be used.

Adjuvant chemotherapy offers much less benefit in the elderly, and is probably not routinely indicated in patients over the age of 70. There are, however, inadequate data from clinical trials in this group of patients and further research is done to define more clearly the place of adjuvant chemotherapy. Nonetheless, chemotherapy can be very beneficial in carefully selected patients with advanced disease, which is no longer responding to hormonal treatment.

In patients who are disabled by diseases, for example severe congestive cardiac failure, which might make conventional treatment dangerous or difficult to administer and which already limits life expectancy, more conservative treatments is an acceptable compromise. Similarly, some fit elderly patients refuse offers of surgery and radiotherapy. In these cases, endocrine therapy alone in the first instance is often very successful.

MANAGEMENT OF BREAST CANCER IN PREGNANCY

Breast cancer is the most common malignancy arising in pregnant and postpartum women, with an incidence of about one in 3,000 pregnancies. Because of the changes which occur in the breast during pregnancy and lactation, diagnosis is often delayed and cancers arising in pregnancy or postpartum are typically more advanced at the time of diagnosis than in non-pregnant women of the same age. Pregnant women, and those who have recently been delivered, who develop breast abnormalities should be referred to a breast clinic for investigation without delay.

The overall survival of patients with breast cancer diagnosed during pregnancy is worse than that of non-pregnant women. If the cancer is diagnosed early in pregnancy, the woman may wish to consider termination of pregnancy, but she must understand that this will not improve her prognosis. Surgery is possible during pregnancy, and mastectomy may be preferable, if it avoids the need for radiotherapy. If indicated, radiotherapy should be given postpartum to avoid radiation exposure of the unborn child. Chemotherapy is potentially teratogenic and so should be avoided in the first trimester. Women receiving chemotherapy should not breast feed. Most cancers diagnosed during pregnancy are receptor negative, so that endocrine therapy would not be beneficial.

Pregnancy does not appear to worsen the prognosis of previously diagnosed breast cancer, but it is wise to suggest that women should wait for 2–3 years after treatment of breast cancer before becoming pregnant. As chemotherapy and other treatments are potentially harmful to unborn children, women on treatment should take contraceptive precautions.

BREAST CANCER AND THE ORAL CONTRACEPTIVE PILL

There has been a natural concern that the hormones in the oral contraceptive pill might lead to an increased incidence of breast cancer. Many studies have been performed, which indicate that the excess risk of the modern combined oestrogen/progestogen pill is very small during the time of pill use and in the 10 years after. More than 10 years, after stopping the pill, the risk has returned to the baseline. Cancers diagnosed in pill users tend to be less advanced and have a better prognosis. Any possible increase in risk from breast cancer has to be offset against the protective effect of the pill against the development of endometrial and ovarian cancer, and the medical risks of pregnancy. It is possible that use of the progestogen only mini-pill may be protective against the development of breast cancer.

It is generally recommended that women with a history of breast cancer avoid exogenous oestrogens and use non-hormonal methods of contraception. However, there is no clear evidence that the use of the oral contraceptive pill will promote relapse of breast cancer. In emergencies, use of the morning pill is permitted, as it seems unlikely that a single exposure to oestrogen would be harmful.

BREAST CANCER AND HRT

As with use of the pill, there have been concerns that oestrogen-based HRT in post-menopausal women may lead to an increased incidence of breast cancer. Studies indicate that the excess risk of HRT is small, and this needs to be put in perspective with the potential benefit.

> **RULE OF THUMB FOR HRT DURATION AND BREAST-CANCER RISK**
>
> ◆ Up to 5 years HRT – no increased risk of breast cancer developing
> ◆ 5–10 years of HRT – slightly increased risk
> ◆ More than 10 years of HRT – greater increase in risk

As in the case of the pill, cancers diagnosed in HRT users tend to be less advanced and have a better prognosis. Non-oestrogen-containing forms of HRT, such as the selective ER modulator raloxifene may be protective against the development of breast cancer.

The use of HRT in women with a history of breast cancer is controversial. Women who are using HRT when breast cancer is diagnosed are recommended to stop it, many pre-menopausal women with breast cancer are deliberately made post-menopausal by ovarian suppression, and others may undergo a premature menopause as a result of chemotherapy or tamoxifen. The resultant sweats, hot flushes and other symptoms can be a source of great distress and morbidity.

There is a natural reluctance to prescribe oestrogen-containing HRT in case it promotes a recurrence of the breast cancer, but there is, in fact, very little evidence that it will do so. Women with vasomotor menopausal symptoms can try clonidine or evening primrose oil in the first instance, although many gain no benefit. Otherwise a low-dose progestogen such as norethisterone may be helpful. Vaginal dryness can be treated with lubricants, topical oestrogens can be used for short periods, but long term use is best avoided because of the risk if systemic absorption. If these measures fail, and the symptoms are sufficiently severe, HRT can be used, providing that the patient accepts that there may be a small risk. Clinical trials of HRT in women with breast cancer and menopausal symptoms are underway in an attempt to quantify the risk–benefit ratio. Bone mineral density loss can be minimised by the use of tamoxifen or raloxifene, along with the use of weight-bearing exercise, bisphosphonates and calcium supplementation.

MALE BREAST CANCER

About 1% of breast cancer arises in men. Because of the lack of awareness of the possibility of the diagnosis in most men, and the small volume of breast tissue surrounding the lump, the disease is more often staged as T4 at the time of diagnosis. Mastectomy and axillary node clearance with chest wall radiotherapy are usually recommended for local control. There is a lack of data surrounding the value of adjuvant treatments in men, but chemotherapy is usually offered in the same way as it is for women. Tamoxifen is usually prescribed in addition, but is probably of no value in ER-negative cases. Stage for stage, the prognosis is similar to that of breast cancer in women.

Bowel cancer

Cancers of the colon and rectum cause nearly 20,000 deaths per year in the UK, second only to lung cancer and exceeding breast cancer in terms of cancer mortality. Two-thirds arise in the colon, most commonly in the left side (descending and sigmoid colon) and one-third in the rectum. The sex ratio for colon cancer is approximately equal, but rectal cancer is more common in men. Colorectal cancer is rare in those under the age of 45 years and becomes increasingly common each decade. The median age at diagnosis is just under 70 years.

AETIOLOGY OF BOWEL CANCER

For the most part the causes of bowel cancer are not known. It is much more common in developed countries and the possible protective effects of factors, such as diet and exercise, are discussed in Chapter 1. There is, undoubtedly, a genetic basis in a minority of cases, and this is also outlined in Chapter 1, and the management of patients and their relatives with suspected or proven family cancer syndromes is described in Chapter 4. It is important for the general practitioner (GP) to remember that familial cases often present at an unusually early age. Patients with inflammatory bowel disease, especially ulcerative colitis, are at increased risk of bowel cancer. The risk is greatest when the whole large bowel has been affected for many years.

In many cases, carcinomas develop in pre-existing adenomas which may have been present for years. There is a typical transition from hyperproliferative epithelium, to focally dysplastic crypts, to macroscopically evident tubular adenoma, to progressively dysplastic and or villous adenoma and finally to invasive adenocarcinoma.

SCREENING AND PREVENTION

There is at present no national population screening programme as there is for breast and cervix cancer, despite evidence that it might reduce mortality by between 10% and 30%. Studies are being undertaken to investigate the feasibility and cost-effectiveness of population screening by faecal occult blood testing with or without some form of endoscopy (usually flexible sigmoidoscopy), and these are discussed in more detail in Chapter 6. Patients at high risk by virtue of ulcerative colitis or one of the defined family cancer syndromes should undergo regular colonoscopy. Ideally, lesions will be identified at the pre-malignant adenoma stage, but hopefully screen-detected carcinomas will still be at an early stage and potentially curable by surgery.

The risk for individuals with a family history of colorectal cancer but without a definite "syndrome" depends on the strength of the family history and the age of the individual. The strength of family history can be divided into no affected relatives, one affected FDR over the age of 45, one affected FDR under the age of 45 and two or more affected FDRs. The table below shows the level of risk for an individual depending on age and family history, relative to that of someone of 45 with no family history.

RISK OF COLORECTAL CANCER RELATED TO AGE AND FAMILY HISTORY				
Age	45	55	65	75
No family history	1	5	7	11
1 affected FDR age >45	2	9	12	19
1 affected FDR age <45	4	18	25	38
2 or more affected FDRs	6	28	38	57

Some care has to be exercised when considering relative risk data, as the absolute risk can still be quite small even if the relative risk is elevated. For example, for 45-year olds the population incidence is only 2 per 100,000, so a fourfold increase in relative risk gives an incidence of 8 per 100,000. This means that more than 10,000 people at this level of risk would need to be screened to pick up a case. Given that invasive screening techniques are at best unpleasant and at worst may be associated

CAUSES OF BOWEL CANCER IN INDIVIDUAL PATIENTS

- No cause identified – the majority
- Single first-degree relative (FDR) (15%)
- Hereditary non-polyposis colon cancer (5%)
- Familial adenomatous polyposis (1%)
- Inflammatory bowel disease (1%)

with complications, one would not wish to undertake these lightly.

For some patients, those with long-standing total ulcerative colitis and familial adenomatous polyposis, prophylactic surgery may be undertaken. This, nowadays, usually entails pan-proctocolectomy with ileo-anal anastomosis and formation of a neo-rectum (or ileal pouch) rather than the need for either a permanent ileostomy or the retention of a rectal stump which would require regular surveillance for the development of cancer.

For the general population, the GP can use any suitable opportunity to reduce the likelihood of patients developing colorectal cancer by promotion of a healthy lifestyle. This includes avoidance of obesity, regular exercise and a diet rich in fibre, and fresh fruit and vegetables, and has the added benefit of protecting against other cancers and cardiovascular disease as well.

There is some evidence that non-steroidal anti-inflammatory drugs (NSAIDs), such as aspirin, may have a protective effect against the development of colorectal carcinoma, and there may be opportunities in the future for primary chemoprevention in high-risk patients and secondary chemoprevention in those who have been successfully treated for a first bowel cancer. At the moment, however, there are inadequate data about the safety and cost-effectiveness of this approach and it remains a subject of continuing clinical trials and is not yet recommended practice.

PRESENTATION

About one in five patients with colorectal cancer presents as an acute abdominal emergency, usually with intestinal obstruction. Less commonly there may be perforation with generalised peritonitis or nausea, vomiting, fever and abdominal pain due to the formation of a localised pericolic abscess. Very rarely do such symptoms come completely out of the blue, and in most patients the acute surgical emergency comes after months of prodromal symptoms which may have been ignored by the patient or not adequately investigated by the GP. As there is a significantly higher early mortality among patients operated on as emergencies, patients with symptoms which might be due to bowel cancer should be investigated promptly.

> ### RECTAL BLEEDING
>
> Rectal bleeding, either fresh or mixed with stool, and change in bowel habit should never be ignored even if there is other benign pathology present

Symptoms due to bowel cancer can be rather non-specific, but rectal bleeding and change in bowel habit

must be taken seriously, even if another possible cause, such as haemorrhoids are found. Rectal bleeding is not often apparent in patients with caecal or right-sided colonic tumours, these more often present with anaemia. Fortunately, they are less common.

Criteria for urgent referral for specialist investigation under the "2-week rule" are given in Chapter 5, although there is some controversy surrounding these guidelines.

> ### PRESENTING SYMPTOMS OF BOWEL CANCER
>
> - "Acute abdomen" with pain, vomiting, tenderness
> - Change in bowel habit
> - Bleeding per rectum
> - Anaemia
> - Abdominal pain
> - Weight loss
> - Tenesmus

Patients who have previously had a benign condition, such as diverticular disease or irritable bowel syndrome diagnosed following investigation for colonic symptoms, must be alert for the development of new symptoms or for a change in the pattern of previous symptoms. Similarly, their doctors must not forget that even though neither irritable bowel syndrome nor diverticular disease is associated with an increased risk of bowel cancer, the two diseases may still be associated by chance.

While some symptoms such as change in bowel habit and bleeding per rectum clearly draw attention to the bowel, it may be more difficult to pinpoint the origin of other presenting features such as weight loss and anaemia. In these cases, an initial referral for investigation may be to a general physician, haematologist or geriatrician.

Sometimes, presentation is with much more advanced local or metastatic disease, such as pneumaturia due to the development of a vesico-colic fistula, right upper quadrant pain or jaundice due to liver metastases or ascites due to peritoneal seeding. In these cases, there may have been no previous symptoms caused by the primary tumour. More often a careful history will elicit symptoms which were ignored by the patient, overlooked by doctors or sometimes missed by appropriate investigations.

INVESTIGATIONS

Physical examination is often unrewarding, but there may be pallor, jaundice or signs of weight loss. In the abdomen, there can be tenderness, hepatomegaly or a mass. Very rarely a Sister Joseph nodule, a metastasis at the umbilicus, is found. Rectal examination must be performed as

90% of rectal cancers, and 25% of all bowel cancers can be directly palpated. Sometimes, an extra-rectal "shelf" of tumour can be felt due to peritoneal spread of tumour from the colon or another abdominal primary site such as the stomach.

A barium enema is often requested when a patient presents with bowel symptoms, but a normal barium enema cannot be relied upon to exclude disease unless rectal examination and sigmoidoscopy are also both normal, as distal tumours can be missed. If a tumour in the distal colon is identified on barium studies or sigmoidoscopy, it is important to make sure that the more proximal bowel is also normal as synchronous polyps and cancers are not uncommon. A colonoscopy is an alternative to a flexible sigmoidoscopy and double-contrast barium enema. It is recommended practice to perform cross-sectional imaging (usually computed tomography (CT), but sometimes magnetic resonance imaging (MRI)) prior to definitive surgery where feasible. This is, especially, helpful in patients with rectal cancer to delineate the extent of local disease, and it may also show nodal or hepatic metastases. Lung metastases are unusual at presentation, but a chest X-ray is needed for staging as well as for routine preoperative assessment of fitness for anaesthesia. Endorectal ultrasound may be helpful in patients with rectal cancer, along with findings at examination under anaesthesia (EUA), to decide on operability.

A histological diagnosis should be made preoperatively in all patients with rectal cancer. Many patients with colonic cancer will have had a biopsy at the time of colonoscopy which provides preoperative histological confirmation, but often it is necessary to proceed to laparotomy on the basis of imaging appearances alone.

SURGERY FOR COLON CANCER

For patients who present electively, a good deal of information should be available preoperatively following the investigations described above. For fit patients with confirmed or suspected colon cancer and no evidence of distant metastases, surgery is undertaken as the initial and definitive treatment. The disease is operable in about 80% of patients. A colostomy is not normally needed, and the stage of the primary tumour and any associated lymph nodes as determined by the pathologist is used to guide decision-making about adjuvant non-surgical treatments.

SURGERY FOR RECTAL CANCER

For fit patients with rectal cancer which is localised and non-metastatic on imaging, and felt to be mobile at EUA,

there is controversy about the best treatment. Traditionally, surgery was undertaken first in this group of patients with operable tumours. A restorative anterior resection was performed for mid and upper rectal tumours which avoided the need for a permanent end colostomy, although sometimes a temporary colostomy was needed if there was doubt about the integrity of the anastomosis. Low rectal tumours which are too close to the anus for sphincter-conserving surgery were usually treated by synchronous combined abdomino-perineal resection which removed the lower rectum and anus, leaving a permanent colostomy. Carefully selected patients with localised disease may be suitable for transanal local excision with postoperative radiotherapy.

Sometimes, when it was felt that a single sphincter-preserving operation would be too difficult, a staged procedure or Hartmann's operation was performed. The initial procedure removed part of the rectum with the tumour, and the proximal end of the bowel was fashioned into a colostomy. The rectal stump was oversewn. At this stage, the patient still had an anus although it was non-functional. Subsequently, if there was no evidence of residual or recurrent tumour and no pelvic sepsis, a second procedure could be undertaken to join the proximal part of the bowel to the rectal stump. Usually this was accompanied by a temporary colostomy to protect the anastomosis and allow healing to take place. When the anastomosis was confirmed to have healed satisfactorily, the temporary colostomy could be closed, and the bowel contents were allowed to leave the body by the normal route. Although a return to physiological normality was the aim, too often patients never progressed beyond the first stage of a Hartmann's procedure.

Local recurrence is a common problem after surgery for rectal cancer. As a patient with local recurrence is usually incurable, every effort should be made to prevent this. Wide variations in the rate of recurrence between different surgeons suggest that the operative technique is of critical importance. Recently, the need for total mesorectal excision (TME) has been emphasised by some surgeons. Another way of reducing the possibility of local recurrence is radiotherapy. This may be given preoperatively to all patients or postoperatively to selected patients on the basis of the pathology report.

PATHOLOGY AND STAGING OF COLON AND RECTAL CANCER

The pathological type of cancer found in the colon and rectum is adenocarcinoma in 95% of cases. It may be well, moderately or poorly differentiated. Other tumour types are rare and include squamous cancer, carcinoid tumours, sarcomas and lymphomas. The important features of colorectal cancer histopathology reporting have been mentioned in Chapter 7. The pathological finding in rectal adenocarcinoma which best predicts for local recurrence is involvement of the circumferential resection margin.

Patients with colorectal cancer need to be fully staged before all aspects of treatment can be decided on, and before a prognosis can be given. The principles of staging have been set out in Chapter 8. Full staging for colorectal cancer involves both pathological assessment of the operative specimen and clinical staging (sometimes, with histological confirmation) for metastatic disease.

DUKES' CLASSIFICATION

- A: The tumour does not invade beyond the muscularis propria. There are no involved lymph nodes
- B: The tumour invades beyond the muscularis propria into the subserosa or beyond. There are no involved lymph nodes
- C: Lymph nodes are involved by tumour deposits

The first staging classification was introduced by Dukes, a pathologist, 70 years ago. It is still in use today although there have, of course, been attempts to refine and modify it. The original Dukes' system had three categories, namely A, B and C, as shown in the box. As it was based on the study of resected cancers no reference was made to the absence or presence of distant metastases, but some have used the term Dukes' D for patients with distant metastases.

The TNM classification and the stage grouping (see box) which is commonly used nowadays alongside Dukes' system is more detailed, but clearly correlates with the traditional method. It should be noted that Stage II (Dukes' B) is a composite of better (T3 N0 M0) and worse (T4 N0 M0) prognostic groups, as is Stage III (Dukes' C) (any T N1 or N2 M0).

T-STAGES FOR THE TNM CLASSIFICATION OF CANCER OF THE COLON AND RECTUM

- TX: Primary tumour cannot be assessed
- T0: No evidence of primary tumour
- Tis: Carcinoma *in situ*: intra-epithelial or invasion of the lamina propria
- T1: Tumour invades submucosa
- T2: Tumour invades muscularis propria
- T3: Tumour invades through muscularis propria into subserosa or into non-peritonealised pericolic or perirectal tissues
- T4: Tumour directly invades other organs or structures and/or perforates visceral peritoneum

---

N-STAGES FOR THE TNM CLASSIFICATION OF CANCER OF THE COLON AND RECTUM

- NX: Regional lymph nodes cannot be assessed
- N0: No regional lymph node metastasis
- N1: Metastasis in 1–3 regional lymph nodes
- N2: Metastasis in 4 or more regional lymph nodes

M-STAGES FOR THE TNM CLASSIFICATION OF CANCER OF THE COLON AND RECTUM

- MX: Distant metastasis cannot be assessed
- M0: No distant metastasis
- M1: Distant metastasis

STAGE GROUPING FOR COLORECTAL CANCER AND APPROXIMATE 5-YEAR SURVIVAL RATES

- Stage I   T1 or T2 N0 M0   Dukes' A   90%
- Stage II   T3 or T4 N0 M0   Dukes' B   60%
- Stage III   Any T N1 or N2 M0   Dukes' C   30%
- Stage IV   Any T Any N M1   <5%

ADJUVANT CHEMOTHERAPY

There is evidence that the use of fluorouracil-based adjuvant chemotherapy after potentially curative surgery for Dukes' C colon cancer will improve outcome (measured as the 5-year survival rate). There is uncertainty to what extent survival will be improved by this, but it is estimated as being between a 2% and a 10% benefit, 6% improvement can be taken as an average figure. This, of course, means that between 90 and 98 people out of each 100 treated will not benefit, and other factors such as co-morbidity, age and the patient's own wishes should be taken into account. On the basis of this small benefit it is recommended that adjuvant chemotherapy is offered to patients with Dukes' C colon cancer.

INDICATIONS FOR POSTOPERATIVE ADJUVANT CHEMOTHERAPY

- Certain: chemotherapy indicated in fit and willing patients
  - Dukes' C colon cancer
- Uncertain: clinical trial entry encouraged in fit and willing patients
  - Dukes' C rectal cancer
  - Dukes' B colon and rectal cancer
- Chemotherapy not indicated
  - Dukes' A colon and rectal cancer

There is less evidence for a benefit in patients with the same stage of rectal cancer, nonetheless it is usually offered.

At the moment, evidence to support the routine use of chemotherapy in all patients with Dukes' B disease is not available. Patients with Dukes' B colon and rectal cancer have a higher chance of survival anyway, so even if the proportionate benefit from the use of adjuvant chemotherapy is the same, the absolute gain in survival in percentage terms will be less. Clinical trials investigating the place of chemotherapy in this area of uncertainty are continuing. Given the doubt it is entirely reasonable to offer chemotherapy to young, fit patients with Dukes' B cancers, especially those with the worse prognosis of T4 N0 M0 disease, who, understanding the uncertainty, still wish to have the treatment.

Chemotherapy is not recommended for patients with Dukes' A cancers.

There is no consensus about the best type of adjuvant chemotherapy. Greatest experience has been gained with fluorouracil-based regimens. This is most commonly given as a bolus into a peripheral vein. Various schedules have been used including a single injection weekly for 30 weeks (about 6 months) and daily injections for 5 days in 1 week, repeated every month for 6 months (again a total of 30 attendances). There is no evidence that either approach is better in terms of outcome, but the weekly injections are less toxic. Usually, fluorouracil is given with folinic acid which is not itself cytotoxic but modulates fluorouracil metabolism. There is no evidence that the much more expensive high-dose folinic acid schedules are better than low-dose ones. It was once thought that the antihelminthic drug levamisole improved the outcome of fluorouracil-based chemotherapy by immunomodulation, but this has not been supported in large-scale clinical trials.

ADJUVANT FLUOROURACIL AND FOLINIC ACID CHEMOTHERAPY OPTIONS IN BOWEL CANCER

- Weekly bolus for 6 months
- Daily bolus for 1 week each month for 6 months
- Infusional treatment 2 days every 2 weeks for 6 months
- Portal vein infusion for 1 week postoperatively

Alternatively, infusional fluorouracil may be given. Usually this means systemic venous infusion via a Hickman line or a peripherally inserted central catheters (PICC) line. Systemic fluorouracil infusions are usually given for 2 days each fortnight for 6 months. Alternatively, portal vein infusion is used to effect regional perfusion of the liver (which is the organ at greatest risk of harbouring occult micrometastases) with higher doses of fluorouracil than

is achieved by peripheral infusion for the same drug level in the systemic circulation. Portal vein infusion requires surgical placement of a line at the time of definitive surgery, but is only given for a week postoperatively.

The principal side-effects of standard fluorouracil and folinic acid schedules include diarrhoea and plantar and palmar erythema. Hair loss is not a feature. Myelosuppression is uncommon and most often mild when it does occur.

Newer agents such as raltitrexed, irinotecan, oxaliplatin and capecitabine (Chapter 13) all have activity against cancers of the colon and rectum, but there is as yet no evidence to justify their routine use in the adjuvant setting. Clinical trials are in progress which will clarify whether adjuvant regimens containing any of these newer drugs give better results than standard schedules comprising fluorouracil and folinic acid.

ADJUVANT RADIOTHERAPY

Radiotherapy is not routinely used after surgery for colon cancer, but may be offered in exceptional circumstances where there is thought to be an unusually high risk of local recurrence.

RADIOTHERAPY FOR RECTAL CANCER

- Operable disease
  - Short-course low-dose preoperative radiotherapy or
  - Long-course higher-dose postoperative radiotherapy for selected high-risk patients
- Inoperable disease
  - High-dose radical radiotherapy with or without subsequent surgery (see below)

Radiotherapy is commonly used in rectal cancer. A short course (1 week) may be given preoperatively to all patients with mobile, operable tumours. An alternative strategy is to use surgery as the initial treatment for mobile and easily operable tumours, reserving radiotherapy (sometimes, given in conjunction with chemotherapy) for those patients in whom the pathology report signifies a high chance of local recurrence such as positive circumferential margins or lymph node involvement.

FOLLOW-UP AFTER POTENTIALLY CURATIVE TREATMENT OF BOWEL CANCER

Patients should be followed up carefully after definitive treatment of colon and rectal cancer to pick up local recurrence or metastatic relapse at a stage when intervention may still be helpful. Clinically detected signs of recurrence or metastatic disease such as jaundice, anaemia, hepatomegaly or an abdominal mass are likely to herald incurable disease, and so additional investigations are warranted. These include CT scanning (or ultrasound examination) 6 monthly for 2 years after surgery to detect operable liver metastases, and regular endoscopic examination of the bowel perhaps 6 monthly for the 1st year or 2, thereafter every 1–3 years indefinitely to detect anastomotic recurrence and metachronous primary tumours. The value of regular carcino-embryonic antigen (CEA) measurements is controversial, and most authorities do not recommend routine tumour marker surveillance.

TREATMENT OF LOCALLY ADVANCED DISEASE

If resection is not possible because of the extent of local spread of a colon or rectal cancer, or if the patient is too frail to undergo a major procedure, formation of a defunctioning colostomy may provide valuable palliation for an obstructing lesion.

> **TREATMENT OPTIONS IN LOCALLY ADVANCED BOWEL CANCER**
>
> - Palliative surgical resection
> - Defunctioning colostomy
> - Stenting
> - Palliative radiotherapy

Bowel obstruction caused by some bowel cancers can be relieved palliatively by insertion of an expanding metallic stent.

For patients with locally advanced rectal tumours, usually indicated by fixation on EUA, high-dose radical radiotherapy may be given. It may be helpful if a defunctioning colostomy is fashioned prior to radiotherapy. If there is a good response to treatment, surgery may then become possible. If reassessment after radical radiotherapy shows the tumour is still inoperable, the treatment will probably have been only palliative, but some patients are cured with radiotherapy alone.

TREATMENT OF METASTATIC DISEASE

Some patients with cancers of the colon and rectum have metastatic disease, usually in the liver, at the time of presentation. It is still beneficial for these patients to be considered for resection of the primary tumour to prevent symptoms such as obstruction, perforation and bleeding.

Patients with liver metastases used to be considered incurable, but there have been a number of therapeutic advances in this area recently. Patients with controlled primary tumours who develop metastatic disease confined to the liver may be considered for surgical resection of their liver disease. Similarly, newly diagnosed patients who have metastatic disease confined to the liver may also be considered for surgery to the liver either at the same time as the definitive procedure on the primary tumour or subsequently. This type of surgery is best suited to those with a solitary lesion confined to one lobe of the liver situated well away from the central structures. Approximately 20% of those undergoing partial hepatic resection for bowel cancer metastases will be cured by this procedure.

Various interventional radiology procedures have been developed for the treatment of liver metastases (Chapter 14). Probes are inserted percutaneously under imaging guidance directly into the metastases, and ablation is attempted using one of a number of methods including radiofrequency waves, laser or alcohol injection. These techniques are still developing, and it is likely that the proportion of patients with liver metastases considered suitable for this type of treatment will increase.

> **TREATMENT OPTIONS IN METASTATIC BOWEL CANCER**
>
> - Symptom control measures and supportive care
> - Palliative chemotherapy (systemic or regional)
> - Resection of liver metastasis
> - Interventional radiology procedures for liver metastases
> - Palliative radiotherapy

The likelihood of both successful surgical resection and interventional radiology procedures may be improved, if chemotherapy is given first to reduce the number and size of the metastases. Chemotherapy is, of course, often used as the principal treatment for metastatic disease.

For patients who have not previously received chemotherapy, fluorouracil- and folinic acid-based schedules are usually used as first-line treatment of metastatic disease. If patients relapse after previous adjuvant chemotherapy, or if there is disease progression after first-line therapy for metastatic disease with fluorouracil and folinic acid, one of the newer drugs such as irinotecan or oxaliplatin (mentioned above) may be used either alone, or more often in combination with fluorouracil and folinic acid.

Regional chemotherapy techniques have been investigated for patients with disease confined to the liver, as well as with adjuvant therapy. Chemotherapy infused into either a portal vein or hepatic artery catheter will result in higher doses to the liver for equivalent systemic toxicity compared with normal intravenous administration. There is, however, no evidence that this theoretically attractive technique achieves better results.

Chemotherapy is not necessarily appropriate for all patients. Patients with poor performance status due to very advanced disease, old age or co-morbidity may have a better quality of life if they receive symptom control measures and supportive care without any active anti-cancer treatment. Similarly, some generally older patients who would be fit enough for chemotherapy may prefer supportive care to the inconvenience and toxicity of chemotherapy. Nonetheless, there is evidence that both quality of life and survival duration are better in actively treated patients than in those receiving symptomatic care only.

PALLIATIVE RADIOTHERAPY

Palliative radiotherapy often utilises simple short courses or single treatments, and is well tolerated even by frail patients with a poor performance status. It can be used to provide symptomatic relief for patients with bone, soft tissue or brain metastases. The pain of locally recurrent disease in the pelvis or perineum and other symptoms of uncontrolled local disease, such as bleeding, are frequently alleviated by palliative radiotherapy.

Lung cancer

Lung cancer is a disease with a high incidence and a high mortality – the age standardised 5-year survival rate for England is just 5.5%. It is, therefore, the most common cause of cancer death in the UK, accounting for about 35,000 deaths each year.

Tobacco smoking is the direct cause of lung cancer in over 80% of cases (Chapter 1). There may be a genetic susceptibility to the carcinogenic effects of tobacco smoke. Industrial exposure to other carcinogens, such as asbestos and environmental exposure to radon are other aetiological factors responsible for a small minority of cases. Decades ago, there were at least four cases in men for every woman affected, but changes in smoking habits have lead to a gradual reduction in the incidence in men, whereas the incidence in women continues to rise so that the sex ratio is now closer to 2:1. It is disturbing that smoking among young women and teenagers appears to be increasing.

There is a five fold variation in the likelihood of developing lung cancer depending on social class: the standardised mortality ratio is 206 in men of Social Class V compared with only 45 in Social Class I men. This is largely attributable to class differences in the prevalence of smoking.

PREVENTION OF LUNG CANCER

A reduction in smoking has for decades been the greatest opportunity for primary prevention of premature death from cancer. It is regrettable that our society has so far failed to rise to this challenge, but the government's strategy *Our Healthier Nation* aims to reduce lung cancer death rates by at least 30% in men and 15% in women below 75 years of age by 2010, principally through reduction in smoking. Opportunities for preventing cancer have been discussed in detail in Chapter 2, but some key points relevant to lung cancer are reiterated here.

General practitioners (GPs), practice nurses and other health care professionals should identify all patients who are current smokers. They should use every opportunity to emphasise the importance of stopping smoking, and offer advice, encouragement and structured support for smokers who wish to give up, and to those who have given up, particularly during the year immediately after stopping.

> **ROUTES OF ADMINISTRATION OF NICOTINE REPLACEMENT**
>
> - Sublingual tablets
> - Chewing gum
> - Transdermal patches
> - Nasal spray
> - Inhaler device

Smokers who need additional support, particularly heavy smokers, should be advised to try substituting other sources of nicotine (see box) for cigarettes. Explicit information should be given on the use of these devices. Nicotine replacement is a useful adjunct to structured counselling, advice and support. Nicotine replacement should not, however, replace these interventions as it has only been shown to be effective when used in conjunction with them. Women often cite weight gain after stopping smoking as a reason for not giving up. The weight gain is partly as a result of eating more, and partly from a decreased basal metabolic rate. Patients should be advised that nicotine replacement may help to prevent weight gain, and that although about half their weight gain will be lost within 6 weeks of cessation the remainder will have to be worked at if they are to return to their earlier weight.

Treatment with a nicotine-replacement product should be continued for only 10–12 weeks with gradual withdrawal over this period. Unfortunately, although GPs are well placed to advise on their use, nicotine replacement is not available as an NHS treatment. Bupropion is, however, a prescription-only medication which helps with smoking cessation.

Patients are usually most amenable to stopping smoking when they face other health issues, such as during pregnancy, after their first myocardial infarction or during a chest infection.

GPs who provide occupational health services should encourage their employers to implement smoking cessation programmes within the workplace, and encourage no-smoking policies at work. Health care workers should take advantage of any training opportunities designed to help them practice smoking cessation interventions and to improve the effectiveness of their advice to patients.

Screening programmes based on chest X-rays and sputum cytology have not in the past shown benefit, and so there is no accepted evidence base to support screening. There is, nonetheless, a renewed interest in screening based on low-dose computed tomography (CT) scans in carefully selected groups at high risk (Chapter 6).

PRESENTATION OF LUNG CANCER

Lung cancer may present with a variety of symptoms. Few if any of these give an early warning of localised disease, most are markers of local disease progression or metastases and so the cancer is usually advanced at the time of diagnosis. Rarely, the disease may be an incidental finding, for example a shadow on a chest X-ray performed for another indication. In such cases, the disease is more likely to be localised, and the prognosis may correspondingly be better.

PRINCIPAL PRESENTING SYMPTOMS OF
LUNG CANCER

Cough	90%
Dyspnoea	80%
Haemoptysis	50%
Chest pain	50%
Dysphagia	10%

Symptoms such as

- cough (usually non-productive),
- haemoptysis (which may be intermittent or continuous),
- stridor,
- wheeze and
- dyspnoea

may be directly due to the primary tumour itself. Patients with pre-existing lung disease may have had cough or dyspnoea for years, and the GP must be vigilant as to the possible sinister significance of a change in long-established symptom patterns. Chest infections, particularly localised pneumonias associated with collapse or consolidation, found clinically or on chest X-ray may be due to infection distal to an obstruction caused by cancer in a bronchus. Rarely, a deep vein thrombosis or a pulmonary embolism may be the presenting feature.

A COUGH IN A SMOKER

- Any smoker or ex-smoker presenting with a new cough which does not settle after one course of antibiotics should be referred for a chest X-ray

Direct local extension of the cancer or metastatic lymph node involvement may cause:

- a pleural effusion leading to dyspnoea,
- a pericardial effusion associated with dyspnoea or a dysrhythmia,
- pleuritic or constant chest pain,
- hoarseness due to a cord palsy,
- supraclavicular fossa lymph node enlargement or oesophageal compression leading to dysphagia,
- Pancoast's syndrome and
- superior vena cava obstruction.

The last two specific presentations, namely Pancoast's syndrome (which is caused by direct local extension of an apical (superior sulcus) lung tumour) and superior vena cava compression (which is most often caused by mediastinal lymph node spread from a primary lung cancer, but may occasionally be due to other malignancies or rarely benign disease), deserve special mention.

The syndrome caused by superior sulcus tumours was first described in 1838, although it now bears the name of Henry Pancoast who reported a series of seven patients in 1932. The tumour causes pain radiating down the medial aspect of the arm, weakness and wasting of the small muscles of the hand, trophic changes and Horner's syndrome as a result of invasion of the lower part of the brachial plexus and nerve roots containing sympathetic fibres. There is often erosion of the first rib and the T1 vertebral body. Tumour may extend through the vertebral foramina into the spinal canal and occasionally result in paraplegia. When a Pancoast tumour is suspected on clinical grounds, histological confirmation is necessary as benign diseases may cause a similar picture.

Mediastinal compression or superior vena cava obstruction is characterised by dilatation of collateral veins and venules over the chest wall and neck, upper body, and oedema and plethora, conjunctival suffusion and headache. It occurs in about 5–10% of patients with lung cancer either at presentation or later in the course of the illness.

Lung cancer may, sometimes, present with symptoms due to haematogenous metastases including bone pain or spinal cord compression due to skeletal metastases, jaundice and right upper quadrant pain due to liver metastases and focal neurological signs, ataxia or personality change due to brain metastases.

PARANEOPLASTIC SYNDROMES

- ◆ Finger clubbing
- ◆ Hypertrophic pulmonary osteoarthropathy
- ◆ Proximal myopathy
- ◆ Dermatomyositis
- ◆ Peripheral neuropathy
- ◆ Cerebellar degeneration
- ◆ Myasthenia gravis
- ◆ Hypercalcaemia
- ◆ Cushing's syndrome
- ◆ Ectopic antidiuretic hormone (ADH) secretion

Lung cancer is associated with a large number of paraneoplastic syndromes or non-metastatic manifestations which may be the presenting feature. Each individual with paraneoplastic syndrome is relatively rare, but collectively they are not uncommon. Some of the more common syndromes are listed in the box, but this is not a comprehensive list.

Criteria for urgent referral under the "2-week rule" are set out in Chapter 5. Patients who present to their GP with symptoms which could be caused by lung cancer are usually referred for a chest X-ray in the first instance. Patients with suspicious X-ray appearances, or with persistent haemoptysis, signs of superior vena cava obstruction or stridor will be referred for specialist investigation and subsequent management to a chest physician who is usually the gatekeeper for the lung cancer multidisciplinary team (Chapter 4).

DIAGNOSIS AND INVESTIGATION OF LUNG CANCER

All patients in whom the history, clinical examination and chest X-ray indicate a reasonable probability of lung cancer as a cause of their symptoms should be considered for bronchoscopy with biopsies for histology and brushings, and washings for cytology. This will include, for example, smokers over the age of 40 years with persistent haemoptysis, even if the chest X-ray is normal, as there may be a centrally situated cancer. Exceptions may include the very old or frail and those who, clearly, have widespread metastatic disease. In these cases, sputum cytology or biopsy of an accessible metastasis may

confirm the diagnosis in a less invasive manner. Some cancers, for example Pancoast tumours, are not usually accessible by bronchoscopy but a needle biopsy can be performed percutaneously under radiological guidance. Rarely, a patient with a small solitary peripheral lung tumour often referred to as a "coin" lesion because of the radiological appearances, will, after further investigation, proceed to thoracotomy and undergo definitive resection without prior histological diagnosis.

DIAGNOSTIC TESTS FOR LUNG CANCER

- ◆ Is there a suspicion that the patient has lung cancer?
  - History, clinical examination and chest X-ray.
- ◆ Does the patient has lung cancer and if so, what is the histological type?
  - Bronchoscopy and pathological assessment of specimens, sputum cytology (when invasive investigation is not acceptable), fine needle biopsy of tumours which cannot be accessed by bronchoscopy.
- ◆ What is the stage of the cancer and what treatment is appropriate?
  - Blood tests (including tests for liver function and alkaline phosphatase), lung function tests, assessment of performance status.
  - CT scan if surgery or radical radiotherapy is being considered; mediastinal biopsy if CT scan shows enlarged nodes in non-small cell lung cancer NSCLC but surgery seems feasible.

PATHOLOGY OF LUNG CANCER

There are several different histological types of lung cancer, but they are divided into just two groups for the purposes of treatment: small cell lung cancer (SCLC) and NSCLC.

HISTOLOGICAL TYPES OF LUNG CANCER

- ◆ SCLC (25%)
- ◆ NSCLC (75%)
  - Squamous cell carcinoma (50%)
  - Adenocarcinoma (15%)
  - Large cell anaplastic (10%)

STAGING OF LUNG CANCER

The extent of staging investigations appropriate for an individual with proven lung cancer depends on the histological type. The staging system for patients known to have SCLC is straightforward, patients are allocated to one of two categories: limited disease and extensive disease. The limited disease stage was originally defined on the basis that all known sites of disease could be encompassed with a single radiotherapy field, but the classification has been shown to be of value with other treatments as well.

STAGING OF SCLC

- Limited disease (30% of patients)
  - Disease confined to one hemithorax, including involvement of ipsilateral and/or contralateral hilar, mediastinal and supraclavicular lymph nodes. Patients with ipsilateral pleural effusion, regardless of pleural cytology, may be included in this group.
- Extensive disease (70% of patients)
  - Any disease beyond the definition of limited stage

There is evidence that, in SCLC, a simple prognostic index is better than staging alone in guiding treatment and predicting prognosis. Patients have a relatively good prognosis if they have a good performance status (WHO 0 or 1) and not more than one of the following factors: extensive disease, low serum sodium, raised alkaline phosphatase, raised aspartate aminotransferase (AST) or raised LDH. This group has a 1-year survival rate of about 50% and includes all 2-year survivors. Those who have a WHO performance status of 2 or greater and more than two of the above factors have a median survival of 6 months or less.

GOOD PROGNOSTIC GROUP IN SCLC

Performance status 0 or 1 and not more than one of

- extensive disease
- low serum sodium
- raised alkaline phosphatase
- raised AST
- raised LDH

Staging of NSCLC is more complex. As surgery is the principal curative option, it is important to identify all those patients for whom surgery is appropriate, and to select out those for whom surgery would be of no benefit, to spare them an unnecessary procedure. Patients who appear on initial examination and investigation to have potentially curable disease should have a contrasted CT scan of the thorax and upper abdomen. This will image the primary tumour, intrathoracic nodes, the liver and adrenal glands. Enlarged lymph nodes in the mediastinum do not necessarily indicate metastatic involvement, and mediastinoscopy and lymph node biopsy may be useful prior to thoracotomy. In the absence of clinical suspicion of metastases or abnormal

---

PRIMARY TUMOUR T-STAGE IN NSCLC

- T1 A tumour that is 3 cm or less in greatest dimension, surrounded by lung or visceral pleura, and without bronchoscopic evidence of invasion more proximal than the lobar bronchus (i.e. not in the main bronchus)
- T2 A tumour with any of the following features of size or extent:
  - More than 3 cm in greatest dimension
  - Involves the main bronchus, 2 cm or more distal to the carina
  - Invades the visceral pleura
  - Associated with atelectasis or obstructive pneumonitis that extends to the hilar region but does not involve the entire lung
- T3 A tumour of any size that directly invades any of the following:
  - Chest wall (including superior sulcus tumours)
  - Diaphragm
  - Mediastinal pleura
  - Parietal pericardium or
  Tumour in the main bronchus less than 2 cm distal to the carina but without involvement of the carina
  or associated atelectasis or obstructive pneumonitis of the entire lung
- T4 A tumour of any size that invades any of the following:
  - Mediastinum
  - Heart
  - Great vessels
  - Trachea
  - Oesophagus
  - Vertebral body
  - Carina or
  Separate tumour nodules in the same lobe or
  Tumour with a malignant pleural effusion

REGIONAL LYMPH NODES N-STAGE IN NSCLC

- N0 No regional lymph node metastasis
- N1 Metastasis to ipsilateral peribronchial and/or ipsilateral hilar lymph nodes, and intrapulmonary nodes including involvement by direct extension of the primary tumour
- N2 Metastasis to ipsilateral mediastinal and/or subcarinal lymph node(s)
- N3 Metastasis to contralateral mediastinal, contralateral hilar, ipsilateral or contralateral scalene, or supraclavicular lymph node(s)

serum biochemistry, the chance of finding unsuspected metastases by routine organ scanning is too low (less than 5%) to make brain or bone scans worthwhile.

The TNM system (Chapter 8) is used for NSCLC. The principal categories (but not all the details) are shown in the boxes.

TREATMENT OF LUNG CANCER, RADICAL OR PALLIATIVE?

Lung cancer is usually locally advanced or metastatic at the time of diagnosis. The median age at presentation is about 70 years so the majority of people with lung cancer are elderly. As smoking causes many other health problems including chronic obstructive lung disease and cardiovascular disease, many newly diagnosed lung cancer patients have significant co-morbidity.

These three factors, advanced disease, age and associated diseases often mean that patients are unfit for a radical approach to treatment. Even though the disease may, therefore, be incurable from the outset, an active approach to palliation can do much to control symptoms and improve quality of life. For effective delivery of care, there must be excellent communication between the GP, the hospital diagnostic and treatment services, and community- and hospice-based palliative care teams, not to mention, of course, patients and their families.

However, the poor prognosis of the majority of patients must not be allowed to obscure the fact that some carefully selected patients are suitable for radical treatment and of these a significant proportion will be cured. Therapeutic nihilism may lead to some potentially curable patients being denied active treatment, and may also lead to inadequate use of active treatment aimed at palliation, and so must be avoided in lung cancer.

The distinction between radical and palliative treatments is less clear-cut in SCLC. Although the proportion of patients cured by radical treatment is very small, it does offer improvement in quality of life and prolongation of survival.

TREATMENT OF LIMITED STAGE SCLC

Even in limited stage disease, the presence of occult metastases means that purely local treatments, such as surgery or radiotherapy, are very rarely curative in SCLC. Surgery, therefore, is not normally part of the treatment for patients known to have small cell carcinoma. Occasionally, a patient will be discovered to have SCLC after surgery for a radiological abnormality when a preoperative tissue diagnosis could not be obtained. In these cases, postoperative chemotherapy will be used.

Fortunately, this type of lung cancer is very chemosensitive. Moderately intensive regimens give better results than less toxic single agent schedules. For these reasons, combination chemotherapy is the mainstay of treatment. Various agents are used, most combinations include two to five of the following drugs: cisplatin, carboplatin, etoposide, cyclophosphamide, ifosfamide, doxorubicin and vincristine. There is no additional benefit for courses of treatment longer than 3–6 months, for maintenance chemotherapy, or for high-dose chemotherapy with autologous stem cell or bone marrow support.

Myelosuppression is a common complication of this type of chemotherapy. Patients will have been warned about symptoms, such as fever, for which they should seek immediate medical attention. GPs must be alert to the possibility of neutropenic sepsis developing in a patient receiving chemotherapy and arrange emergency hospital admission for assessment and treatment.

A combined modality approach, using early thoracic radiotherapy in addition to chemotherapy, produces a small improvement in survival compared with chemotherapy alone. Patients who achieve a complete remission with chemotherapy and thoracic radiotherapy can be considered for administration of prophylactic cranial irradiation (PCI). This reduces the risk of developing brain metastases by more than half, and may also improve overall survival.

Current protocols for limited stage SCLC result in response rates of 65–90% and complete response rates of 45–75%. The median survival is of the order of 18–24 months and 40–50% are alive at 2 years.

EXTENSIVE STAGE SCLC

As with limited stage disease, combination chemotherapy is the principal treatment for extensive stage SCLC. Many schedules of similar efficacy are available which use the same drugs listed above for limited disease. Best results are obtained when relatively intensive radical schedules, associated with significant toxicity especially myelosuppression, are used. Up to four courses of chemotherapy will usually be adequate.

Impaired performance status is common at the time of diagnosis of extensive stage disease. These patients have a poor prognosis and do not tolerate aggressive chemotherapy well. Simple low-toxicity palliative regimens have been developed for these poor prognosis patients, although life expectancy is better with conventional radical treatment. It is often helpful for patients to be introduced to community palliative care services.

The addition of thoracic radiotherapy to combination, chemotherapy does not improve survival compared with chemotherapy alone in extensive stage disease. As with limited stage disease, PCI may be used in complete responders to initial chemotherapy to reduce the subsequent appearance of symptomatic brain metastases. Radiotherapy plays an extremely important role in palliation of symptoms of the primary tumour and of metastatic disease.

Treatment of extensive stage small cell carcinoma produces overall response rates of 70–85% and complete response rates of 20–30%.

RECURRENT SCLC

The prognosis of patients with SCLC which progresses following chemotherapy is exceedingly poor regardless of stage. Symptom control and simple palliative treatments, such as radiotherapy, are usually the best approach. Further chemotherapy is unlikely to be of value except in those who initially responded well and relapse after a disease-free interval longer than 6 months. If they have not already been involved, the assistance of community palliative care teams should be sought.

RADICAL TREATMENT OF NSCLC

The thoracic surgeon is a key member of the lung cancer multidisciplinary team. About 20% of patients with NSCLC have disease suitable for surgical treatment. Patients require careful staging as described above to enable decision-making regarding surgery. With detailed staging investigations and careful preoperative assessment, the open and close thoracotomy rate should be less than 5%. Those with early disease, that is T1 or T2 N0 M0 or T1 N1 M0 disease, providing they are medically fit, should be considered for surgery. Those with advanced disease, either T4 or N3 or M1 are not suitable for surgery. Surgery may, sometimes, be appropriate for those with disease between these two extremes, and patients in this category require individualised expert clinical assessment.

SURGERY IN NSCLC

- Early disease, surgery recommended
  - T1 N0 M0
  - T2 N0 M0
  - T1 N1 M0
- Intermediate disease, surgery appropriate in some carefully selected cases
  - Patients with disease not in categories above or below
- Advanced disease, not suitable for surgery
  - T4 any N any M
  - Any T N3 any M
  - Any T any N M1

Lobectomy is the preferred operation where this is feasible, pneumonectomy is sometimes required. Surgery for lung cancer carries a 5% operative mortality risk. Ten per cent of patients have major complications from surgery. Quality of life usually deteriorates immediately after surgery, but returns to the baseline within 3–6 months. Postoperative pain may last for years.

Some patients, perhaps 70% of those with T1 N0 M0 disease, and between a quarter and one-third of all those undergoing resection, may be cured by surgery alone. The ability of adjuvant non-surgical treatment to improve survival rates is not well established.

There is no place for radiotherapy prior to surgery, and radiotherapy is not recommended after surgery for N0 or N1 disease. In patients with N2 disease or with residual macroscopic disease after surgery, postoperative radiotherapy should be considered.

Neoadjuvant chemotherapy to down-stage disease prior to surgery is not proven to be beneficial, but may be considered in the context of a clinical trial. Postoperative chemotherapy may offer a minor improvement in survival following surgery, but is not yet established practice. It is recommended that willing and eligible patients should be enrolled into clinical trials where appropriate. The most active agents in NSCLC include cisplatin, vinorelbine, gemcitabine and paclitaxel.

Some patients have early NSCLC which, on the basis of the disease extent, would normally be considered for surgery but operation is precluded by age, frailty, intercurrent illness or patient refusal. Radical radiotherapy is a potentially curative option for many patients in this group. Radical radiotherapy may also be considered for patients in the intermediate group who are not suitable for surgery, but still have a good performance status and no significant weight loss. Patients in the advanced disease category are not suitable for radical treatment.

The results of radical radiotherapy are not as good as those of surgery, but there are no contemporary clinical trial data directly comparing the two treatments. The perceived differences in outcome between surgery and radiotherapy are due at least in part to disparities in stage (a greater proportion of patients with more advanced disease and a worse prognosis treated in the radiotherapy group) and in part to varying host factors (surgically treated patients have a better prognosis as they are more likely to be relatively young, fit, free of other serious diseases and have a good performance status).

Conventional radical radiotherapy for lung cancer is given with daily treatments: 5 days a week for 4–6 weeks. The innovative technique of continuous hyperfractionated accelerated radiation therapy (CHART) involves treatment three times a day for 12 days without a break (Chapter 12). CHART has been shown in a large clinical trial to produce better results in lung cancer than the traditional approach (survival at 2 years 29% compared with 20%), but it is not universally available. Conformal radiotherapy is an approach which, by individually tailoring the shape of the treated volume to each patient's tumour, seeks to minimise normal tissue damage and possibly give scope for improving outcome by dose escalation.

Chemotherapy is sometimes given in conjunction with radical radiotherapy. Current clinical trial data suggest that cisplatin-based regimens may lead to a 2% improvement in survival at 5 years. Given that this involves exposing 49 patients to the toxicity of treatment for each life saved, it remains controversial whether chemotherapy confers a real advantage. In view of this uncertainty, the use of chemotherapy in this setting should still be the subject of clinical trials with an emphasis on quality-of-life assessment. Gemcitabine should not be used with radical radiotherapy because of enhanced and potentially fatal toxicity.

PALLIATIVE TREATMENTS FOR LUNG CANCER

It remains a sad fact that the majority of patients with lung cancer are not suitable for treatment with curative intent, and most of the minority who are treated radically will still relapse and die from their disease. Effective palliative care must, therefore, be embedded in the foundations of any lung cancer service. The general practice team is the cornerstone of this care, and there must be effective liaison between patients and their families, the hospital-based lung cancer multidisciplinary team, specialist palliative care provision including hospice support, and less specialised community care.

While lung cancer patients, in common with others suffering from advanced malignancy, require generic palliative care measures (Chapter 50), there are a number of palliative interventions specific to lung cancer.

NICE GUIDANCE ON PALLIATIVE CHEMOTHERAPY FOR NSCLC

- Chemotherapy for NSCLC should be considered as an option in patients who are unsuitable for, or considered unlikely to respond to an attempt at curative treatment.
- Gemcitabine, paclitaxel, and vinorelbine should each be considered as part of first-line chemotherapy options for advanced (Stages III and IV) NSCLC patients. Combination of these three agents individually with platinum-based chemotherapy, where tolerated, is likely to be the most effective approach.
- Docetaxel monotherapy should be considered where second-line treatment is appropriate for patients with locally advanced or metastatic NSCLC when relapse has occurred after prior chemotherapy.
- Chemotherapy regimens should be administered under the supervision of appropriately trained health professionals experienced in the use of cancer and chemotherapeutic agents, should be accompanied by best supportive care. Informed decisions regarding appropriate chemotherapy should take account of side-effect profiles, use of concurrent radiotherapy, performance status of the individual being treated and patient and carer preferences. Total cost differences between the various chemotherapy regimens should also be taken into account.

Palliative radiotherapy can be offered to all those with locally advanced lung cancer and symptoms, such as haemoptysis, chest pain and dyspnoea due to bronchial obstruction. There is good evidence that in most patients one or two radiation treatments produce an outcome which is as good as that conferred by the more protracted schedules (e.g. 10 treatments in 2 weeks) which were used previously. In carefully selected patients with a relatively good prognosis, as indicated by a good performance status and no significant weight loss, longer palliative schedules over, say, 3 weeks may be associated with better outcome in terms of both symptom control and survival.

Palliative chemotherapy is probably underused in advanced and metastatic NSCLC. It is estimated that only between 5% and 20% of patients will receive chemotherapy. The most commonly used schedules, until recently, have been cisplatin-based regimens, such as MIC (mitomycin, ifosfamide, cisplatin) and MVP (mitomycin, vindesine or vinblastine and cisplatin). The National Institute for Clinical Excellence (NICE) has recently published guidelines on the use of newer drugs for the palliative treatment of NSCLC. This guidance is summarised in the box, and may be found in full on the NICE website, www.nice.org.uk

A variety of endobronchial treatments can be given which may open up compressed proximal airways and relieve haemoptysis. They include:

- Endoluminal brachytherapy, a radiotherapy technique involving remote afterloading of a radioactive source into a catheter placed bronchoscopically adjacent to the tumour. The advantage of this technique is that a high radiation dose is delivered in a single session directly to tumour which is bleeding or causing an obstruction. There is a rapid fall off of dose away from the source, which means negligible irradiation of lung parenchyma or other thoracic structures, such as the spinal cord. This technique is, therefore, especially suitable as re-treatment after earlier external beam radiotherapy.
- Insertion of an expanding metal wall stent. Again using a bronchoscope, a device like a compressed spring can be inserted into a compressed bronchus. Once the stent is at the correct level it can be made to expand and re-open the bronchial lumen.
- Laser treatment is a valuable palliative tool. Laser beams can be delivered using a bronchoscope to destroy tumour tissue which is either obstructing the lumen of a bronchus or bleeding. It has the advantage that it can be used after other treatments, such as external beam radiotherapy. The disadvantage is that only superficial tumour is destroyed, and it may not be long before residual tumour grows again.

Sometimes, best results are achieved by the use of more than one of these techniques together. For example, laser treatment may be used to open up a completely blocked bronchus, allowing placement of a catheter for endobronchial brachytherapy which may prolong the period of tumour control.

Superior vena cava compression caused by lung cancer is normally treated with radiotherapy or chemotherapy in the first instance. If this is not effective, or if symptoms later return, it is sometimes possible to restore venous return by enlisting the help of a vascular interventional radiologist who will place an expanding metal stent in the superior vena cava or other compressed veins.

Patients with lung cancer may have a massive haemoptysis as a terminal event. For those dying patients being cared for at home, it is worthwhile prescribing 10–20 mg of diamorphine to be administered immediately in this event by the district nurse or palliative care nurse.

Stomach cancer

In the middle of last century, cancer of the stomach was the leading cause of cancer mortality in Britain. Incidence rates have been falling and the standardised mortality ratio for stomach cancer is now just half of what it was even 20 years ago. Stomach cancer, with fewer than 7,000 deaths per year in England and Wales now accounts for just 5% of cancer mortality. The declining incidence is largely due to changes in diet with a greater consumption of fresh fruit and vegetables, improved food preservation and a reduction in Helicobacter pylori infection. To some extent this fall has been offset by increasing deaths from oesophageal cancer, particularly disease at the gastro-oesophageal junction (Chapter 24). There is an association between gastric cancer and atrophic gastritis, achlorhydria and pernicious anaemia. Patients with hereditary polyposis are also at increased risk of developing stomach cancer.

Stomach cancer is twice as common in men as women. It is rare in people under 40 years of age, and the incidence increases steeply in the over 60s. It is more common among the socially disadvantaged. Screening is of proven value in improving prognosis through earlier diagnosis in Japan where the disease is more common, but has no place in the UK.

PRESENTATION AND DIAGNOSIS

> **SYMPTOMS OF GASTRIC CANCER**
>
> ◆ Dysphagia
> ◆ Indigestion
> ◆ Heartburn or reflux
> ◆ Pain or discomfort in the area of the stomach, chest or upper abdomen
> ◆ Weight loss
> ◆ Anaemia
> ◆ Vomiting

Unfortunately, gastric cancer tends to present with symptoms which are common but non-specific, such as indigestion, heartburn, reflux and pain or discomfort in the area of the stomach, chest or upper abdomen. Such symptoms lead to a large number of general practice consultations, but only about 2% of patients with dyspepsia will have cancer. An average general practitioner (GP) might expect to see one or more patients a week with this type of complaint, but only one patient a year will turn out to have an upper gastro-intestinal tract cancer, of which one in three will be gastric cancer.

> **GUIDELINES FOR URGENT REFERRAL FOR SUSPECTED UPPER GASTRO-INTESTINAL CANCERS**
>
> ◆ Dysphagia – food sticking on swallowing (any age)
> ◆ Dyspepsia at any stage combined with one or more of the following "alarm" symptoms:
>   – weight loss
>   – proven anaemia
>   – vomiting
> ◆ Dyspepsia in a patient aged 55 years or more (age 55 years is considered to be a maximum age threshold; Local Cancer Networks may elect to set a lower age threshold, e.g. 45 years or 50 years) with at least one of the following "high-risk" features:
>   – onset of dyspepsia less than 1 year age
>   – continuous symptoms since onset
> ◆ Dyspepsia combined with at least one of the following known risk factors:
>   – family history of upper gastrointestinal cancer in more than two first degree relatives (FDRs)
>   – Barrett's oesophagus
>   – pernicious anaemia
>   – peptic ulcer surgery over 20 years ago
>   – known dysplasia, atrophic gastritis, intestinal metaplasia
> ◆ Jaundice
> ◆ Upper abdominal mass

When dyspeptic symptoms are combined with weight loss, anaemia or vomiting there is a greater likelihood of cancer being the cause. Recent onset of dyspepsia in older patients, and continuous symptoms, are worrying. Tumours in the region of the cardia may present with dysphagia. Tumours blocking the pylorus will cause vomiting. Jaundice may be caused by metastatic disease.

Criteria for referral for urgent investigation by members of the local upper gastro-intestinal diagnostic team under the "2-week rule" are given in the box.

An upper gastro-intestinal endoscopy, or oesophago-gastro-duodenoscopy will be sufficient to diagnose most cases of oesophageal or gastric cancers. Histological and cytological confirmation of suspected cancers will be achieved by biopsy and brushings. Barium swallows and meals are less useful than endoscopy as the initial investigation of dyspepsia or dysphagia because endoscopy will still be needed to obtain histology from any suspicious lesions identified on the barium examination, and because many suspicious lesions turn out to be benign. However, as it may be possible to get a barium study performed much more quickly than an endoscopy in many places, the former may be preferable as an initial screening investigation. If endoscopy is coupled with an abdominal ultrasound, additional diagnoses which may result in similar symptoms, such as gallstones, liver metastases and pancreatic cancer, will be made.

The majority of patients investigated by this team will not have cancer, but the cause of their symptoms will be found to be a benign disease such as gastritis or peptic ulceration which can then be treated appropriately.

When a diagnosis of stomach cancer is made, the patient will normally be referred on to the specialist oesophago-gastric cancer team, which may be based at a separate hospital serving a number of diagnostic teams. In exceptional cases, patients who are very frail or who have definite metastatic spread precluding a radical approach to treatment may be managed locally without referral to the specialist treatment team. Preoperative staging of the cancer may involve a combination of computed tomography (CT) scans or magnetic resonance imaging (MRI), endoscopic ultrasound and laparoscopy. On the basis of these investigations, patients suitable for an attempt at radical surgery will be selected. Some patients with more advanced disease will be still suitable for surgery with palliative intent.

PATHOLOGY AND STAGING

Most patients with malignant disease arising in the stomach have adenocarcinoma. Macroscopically, this can be categorised into one of four types: fungating or polypoid, ulcerating, superficial spreading or diffusely spreading (linitis plastica). A variety of microscopic patterns are described. Rarely, the tumour may prove to be a lymphoma or a sarcoma, and of course such tumours are managed differently from standard adenocarcinoma.

Gastric cancer can spread locally to involve adjacent structures including the spleen, transverse colon, liver diaphragm, pancreas, abdominal wall, adrenal gland, kidney, small intestine and retroperitoneum. Lymph node spread often occurs early in the course of the disease.

Liver metastases arise as a result of portal vein spread, and involvement of other organs, such as the lungs, occurs by systemic venous metastasis. Spread across the peritoneal cavity to involve the omentum or ovaries is not uncommon.

Gastric cancer is staged postoperatively using a complex TNM system (Chapter 8). The various TNM categories can then be used to assign a stage grouping from Stage I to Stage IV.

RADICAL TREATMENT

Surgery is the only potentially curative treatment for stomach cancer. Often patients have lost a significant amount of weight and are malnourished at the time of diagnosis. A period of total parenteral nutrition may, therefore, be required before and after surgery. Partial gastrectomy is preferable to total gastrectomy where this operation is feasible. It results in a similar chance of cure when either procedure is possible, but with fewer post-operative symptoms and a correspondingly better quality of life. Very extensive operations involving removing many lymph nodes the spleen and pancreas are not usually necessary, and there is no evidence that such radical procedures result in better outcome. If, however, it is necessary to remove the spleen, the patient will require life-long prophylaxis against pneumococcal infection with vaccination and penicillin. In deciding whether or not to undergo surgery, the possibility of cure (about 20%) must be weighed against the risk of peri-operative death (which varies from 5% to about 15% depending on centre).

Side-effects of surgery include "dumping" when the gastric contents flow into the small intestine too quickly, rapid absorption of sugars leads to a surge in insulin followed by hypoglycaemia. Removal of the gastric antrum leads to a loss of intrinsic factor production, and patients will require vitamin B12 supplementation. Normal eating can be compromised by loss of all or part of the stomach, and patients will benefit from the advice and support of a dietician in the postoperative period.

Chemotherapy has been investigated as an adjuvant treatment after potentially curative surgery for gastric carcinoma. Data suggest a very modest benefit, with an absolute survival benefit of only 4% in patients with Stage II and III disease, and just 2% in patients with Stage I disease. It should therefore be discussed with fit patients, although many patients, especially if they are elderly, will decide that the very small likelihood of benefit does not justify the inconvenience and toxicity of chemotherapy.

There is insufficient evidence to support the use of radiotherapy alone or in conjunction with chemotherapy as an adjunct to surgery. Radiotherapy is therefore not recommended as part of the adjuvant treatment of gastric cancer outside clinical trials.

PALLIATIVE TREATMENT

Patients whose cancer is too advanced at the time of diagnosis may still benefit from a palliative resection, or a bypass procedure if the tumour cannot be resected but is causing a gastric outflow obstruction.

Palliative chemotherapy in selected patients may result in improved quality of life and modest prolongation of survival, that is by up to 6 months. The inconvenience and toxicity associated with chemotherapy suggest that it should be avoided in the frail and in those with poor performance status. Widely used agents include anthracyclines, cisplatin and fluorouracil.

The prognosis of patients with stomach cancer is poor. Of those undergoing radical surgery, 20% will be cured. Overall however, only about 5% of patients are alive at 5 years, and for those presenting with advanced disease the median survival is only of the order of 4 months. Due to this, it is wise to involve the community palliative care team early in the patient's illness.

Oesophageal cancer

The incidence of oesophageal cancer varies greatly across the world. In Britain, Europe and North America, it is relatively rare, with an incidence of about 3 per 100,000. It is much more common in South Africa, Iran and China. Men are more often affected than women. The principal risk factors in low-incidence areas seem to be tobacco and alcohol. Carcinogens in food have been postulated to explain the geographical variation in incidence. Genetic factors are not thought to be important. Oesophageal cancer may complicate benign oesophageal conditions. In the cervical oesophagus, as in the postcricoid region, squamous cancer may be associated with iron deficiency (the Plummer Vinson or Paterson Brown Kelly syndrome). Adenocarcinoma may develop in the lower oesophagus in relation to achalasia of the cardia, peptic strictures and glandular metaplasia (Barrett's oesophagus), which are all associated with chronic inflammation.

PREDISPOSING FACTORS AND ASSOCIATED CONDITIONS

- Tobacco
- Alcohol
- Iron deficiency anaemia
- Barrett's oesophagus
- Achalasia of the cardia

The commonest sites are the mid- and lower-thoracic oesophagus. Cancers of the cervical and upper-thoracic oesophagus are rarer. The overwhelming majority are squamous cancers, but about 10% are adenocarcinoma, nearly always at the lower end. Many other histological varieties, for example small cell carcinoma, tumours of salivary gland type and various sarcomas may also occur, but very rarely.

PRESENTATION

Most commonly, oesophageal cancer presents in elderly patients. There is usually gradually progressive difficulty in swallowing, initially for solid foods, especially for chewy things like meat, later for fluids. Occasionally, a sudden difficulty in swallowing, or a choking sensation, due to impaction of food may be the presenting feature. Patients often point to a particular level where they think the food sticks, but this is an unreliable indicator. In most patients, the difficulty in swallowing is associated with weight loss. Sometimes there is pain associated with the swallowing problems. This may be a vague "indigestion" discomfort; occasionally, it may be a more severe continuous pain radiating through to the back. Coughing associated with swallowing or repeated chest infections suggests either aspiration of food due to regurgitation or the development of an oesophago-bronchial or oesophago-tracheal fistula.

INVESTIGATION

Dysphagia always merits investigation. In middle aged or elderly smokers and drinkers, it is especially likely to be due to malignancy. Vigilance should be maintained in patients known to have predisposing conditions, such as achalasia, where a change in symptomatology may herald the development of cancer.

Barium studies and endoscopic examinations can both be useful. A barium swallow is a quick and simple preliminary test, and gives important information about the length and site of a tumour, which may not be gleaned from endoscopy. It is, however, possible for false negatives to occur, especially with tumours of the upper oesophagus. Endoscopy provides opportunities both for biopsy and for palliative procedures, such as intubation and lasering. The general practitioner's choice of initial investigation will depend partly on whether he has access to early endoscopy or whether barium swallow or urgent ENT opinion are more quickly available.

Oesophageal cancer spreads locally, proximal and distal spread may be demonstrated histologically for up to 5 cm from the visible tumour. At least this margin of clearance needs to be taken surgically or radiotherapeutically when potentially curative procedures are undertaken. Laterally, oesophageal cancers spread early into the mediastinum and may invade the bronchial tree, pericardium, great vessels and vertebrae. Lymph node spread also occurs early to nodes in the neck, mediastinum and upper abdomen, depending on the location of the primary tumour. Haematogenous spread occurs less commonly. The liver and lungs are most often involved, bone and brain less frequently. A CT scan of the chest and upper abdomen is the best investigation to judge whether a patient is suitable for radical treatment, as it will show the extent of local spread, nodal involvement and hepatic or pulmonary metastases.

TREATMENT CHOICES

The most important decision to be made in a patient who has been found to have oesophageal cancer is whether there is any possibility for potentially curative treatment. "Potentially" is a key word here, for radical treatment in carefully selected patients, still only yields a 5-year survival rate of around 10–20%. Many patients are deemed unsuitable for radical treatment because of age, frailty and concurrent illness. In younger fitter patients, mediastinal invasion (indicated by, e.g., the presence of a fistula or phrenic or recurrent laryngeal nerve palsy) or lymphatic or distant metastases contraindicate radical treatments. It is important to recognise that some patients are best served by supportive care only, for example analgesia, with no active anti-cancer treatment.

> **TREATMENT CHOICES IN OESOPHAGEAL CANCER**
> - Radical treatment
>   - surgery
>   - radiotherapy
>   - combined modality treatment
> - Palliative treatment
> - Supportive care only

RADICAL TREATMENT

Radical radiotherapy is regarded as the treatment of choice for tumours in the cervical- or upper-thoracic oesophagus.

Surgery is the best treatment for fit patients with a cancer in the middle or lower oesophagus. It is best undertaken by a surgeon with a specific interest in this type of surgery, who might be either a "general" or a cardiothoracic surgeon in different centres. The use of radiotherapy in addition to surgery has been investigated, but has no established value in improving survival rates. Postoperative radiotherapy may, however, diminish the likelihood of local recurrence in some patients. Its use, therefore, may be carefully considered, but it is probably seldom justified. Chemotherapy is also being investigated as an adjunct to surgery, and preliminary data suggest that the use of preoperative cisplatin-based chemotherapy may offer a survival advantage. However, this cannot yet be regarded as standard practice.

Radiotherapy can sometimes be used successfully in patients who have an "operable" tumour, but are not fit for surgery because of intercurrent illness, such as coronary artery disease. For radical radiotherapy to have any reasonable chance of success, the tumour must be localised. The length of the tumour as demonstrated on barium swallow is a useful guide. Tumours longer than about 5 or 6 cm are unlikely to be cured. There is much interest in the use of chemotherapy at the same time as radiotherapy, but the routine use of chemoradiotherapy rather than radiotherapy alone is not yet established.

PALLIATIVE TREATMENTS

For most patients, only palliative treatment is possible. Palliative treatment is also needed for the majority of patients who relapse after initial radical treatment. Surgical resection is not an appropriate palliative treatment for patients whose disease preoperatively is clearly too advanced for an attempt at radical treatment. Some patients are deemed to have had a palliative resection when it is clear at the time of surgery, or on examination of the resected specimen, that not all the cancer has been removed.

Palliative treatment should be aimed at symptom relief. The most common symptom is dysphagia, and the best way of relieving this is by intubation. Tubes are usually placed endoscopically, but occasionally may be inserted peroperatively when tumours are found to be irresectable. Intubation does not restore swallowing to normal and the patient often feels happiest on puréed foods and high-calorie drinks. If the tube does get blocked by food, a fizzy drink is a good way of trying to unblock it. Intubation is not such a good option for tumours in the upper part of the oesophagus. Oesophageal dilatation is not good by itself for dysphagia as there is a risk of perforation and without additional measures the dysphagia usually returns quickly. It may, however, be an essential prerequisite for intubation. Dysphagia can also be relieved by lasering, often in combination with intubation or stenting. It has the advantage of being repeatable, but only deals with disease in the lumen.

Palliative radiotherapy may help dysphagia, but responses are not instant, and so it is often combined with intubation or stenting in the lower oesophagus. Radiotherapy is contraindicated in patients with a fistula, as tumour breakdown may exacerbate rather than relieve symptoms. External beam radiotherapy has the advantage of treating local extension outside the oesophagus and adjacent lymph node masses. It may, therefore, provide good pain relief. High-dose rate afterloading machines have made endoluminal brachytherapy another tool in the treatment of oesophageal cancer. This can deliver a high dose to the centre of the tumour in a single treatment, and can be used to prolong the benefit achieved by lasering. Chemotherapy has no established place in the palliative treatment of oesophageal cancer.

Many patients with advanced oesophageal cancer and their relatives are worried about lack of nutrition. Even when dysphagia is relieved, for example by intubation, many will have a very poor appetite, especially those with metastatic disease. The use of artificial feeding via nasogastric tubes or gastrostomies is not usually to be recommended in the palliative setting. An endoscopically placed percutaneous gastrostomy (PEG) can, however, be valuable supportive care during the time a patient receiving is radical radiotherapy.

OUTCOME

The outcome for patients with cancer of the oesophagus is very poor. For the majority of patients treated palliatively life expectancy is only a few months. Most lose weight and strength and develop chest infections as the terminal event. Occasionally erosion of the tumour into the oesophagus can result in a fatal haematemesis.

For those treated radically, the median survival is perhaps just over a year, less than half can expect to be alive at 2 years, and less than 20% are likely to be cured. Despite this dismal prognosis, it is important to investigate patients who develop dysphagia again after apparently successful initial treatment. In some cases, this will be due to the development of an easily treated benign stricture rather than tumour recurrence.

Pancreatic cancer

Carcinoma of the pancreas remains a major challenge in oncology. It has become more common in recent years, but does not yet feature in the top 10 list of cancers by incidence, accounting for only about 3% of the cancer burden. About 6,000 cases occur in England and Wales each year, so the incidence is similar to that of cancer of the oesophagus. The average general practitioner (GP) may see a new patient with pancreatic cancer every 3 or 4 years. It is predominantly a disease of elderly people: three-quarters of patients are past retirement age. The sex incidence is equal.

This type of cancer is only rarely curable, and it now ranks as the fourth or fifth cause of cancer death in men and women. The causes of pancreatic cancer are poorly understood, but there seems to be an association with cigarette smoking, alcohol intake, chronic pancreatitis and diabetes mellitus.

PRESENTING FEATURES

The classic symptoms are weight loss, pain and jaundice. Obstructive jaundice with pale bowel motions, dark urine and pruritis is a feature in over 80% of cases arising in the head of the pancreas. It is less common when the tumour is in the tail of the organ. The pain may be intermittent at the outset, or related to posture or food, but often becomes severe and unremitting. It may be localised to the epigastric region, be felt as upper lumbar back pain, or both. Weight loss is almost universal, and is often associated with other non-specific symptoms, such as anorexia, nausea, vomiting (due to duodenal compression by tumour), diarrhoea (due to fat malabsorption), fatigue, weakness and anaemia.

PRESENTING SYMPTOMS OF PANCREATIC CANCER

- Obstructive jaundice
- Vomiting and nausea
- Diarrhoea or steatorrhoea
- Weight loss and cachexia
- Upper abdominal or back pain
- Fatigue and anaemia
- Onset of insulin dependent diabetes mellitus
- Hypoglycaemic symptoms
- Depression and psychological symptoms

On examination, the patient will often be icteric, but the absence of jaundice does not preclude the diagnosis. Supraclavicular lymphadenopathy may be present. Abdominal examination may reveal an epigastric mass or tenderness, hepatomegaly, an enlarged gall bladder and less commonly ascites.

Criteria for the early referral under the "2-week rule" of patients with suspected pancreatic (or other upper gastrointestinal tract) cancer have been set out in Chapters 5 and 23.

INVESTIGATION

Liver function tests in a jaundiced patient with pancreatic cancer will show an obstructive picture with elevated bilirubin and alkaline phosphatase, anaemia may be present and clotting may be deranged. The differential diagnosis of the patient with obstructive jaundice will include gallstone disease, hepatitis, cholecystitis and bile duct tumours.

Abdominal ultrasound is the simplest preliminary imaging investigation both for patients with obstructive jaundice and for non-jaundiced patients who have symptoms which may be attributable to pancreatic cancer. Dilated bile ducts and the underlying cause of the jaundice will often be demonstrated. Patients with dilated bile ducts and no evidence of gallstones, and any other patients considered likely to have pancreatic cancer on the basis of symptoms and ultrasound findings, should normally be referred immediately to the specialist pancreatic cancer team at the cancer centre. This may be inappropriate for very frail patients with advanced disease, and following discussion it may be better to move towards symptom control and palliative control.

Following specialist referral, other investigations, such as CT scanning, perhaps with needle biopsy, endoscopic retrograde cholangiopancreatography (ERCP), magnetic resonance cholangiopancreatography (MRCP), or if that fails, percutaneous transhepatic cholangiography (PTC), may be performed. Insertion of a stent to relieve obstructive jaundice may be performed at the same time as ERCP (or PTC).

Where symptoms or imaging clearly show that the disease is metastatic or inoperable, or the patient is unfit for radical treatment by virtue of age, frailty or comorbidity, there may be no advantage in further assessment of the primary tumour. The aim of any treatment offered will be palliative. If radical surgery seems potentially feasible, tumour stage and spread may be assessed by laparoscopy.

PATHOLOGY

The great majority of pancreatic tumours are adenocarcinomas arising from the ducts of the exocrine pancreas. A variety of different histological subtypes are recognised, but these are of little importance.

Tumours may also arise from the endocrine cells of the pancreas, but tumours of this type are less common. They are more likely to be localised and respectable, and the prognosis is likely to be significantly better. They may present with endocrine symptoms, such as episodes of hypoglycaemia rather than with pressure effects, such as obstructive jaundice. Other rare tumours encountered in this location include lymphoma and the childhood tumour, pancreaticoblastoma.

It is always helpful to have histological confirmation of the tumour type before radiotherapy or chemotherapy is embarked upon, but there are risks associated with biopsy, and if the imaging appearances of extensive or metastatic disease are unequivocal, it is reasonable to omit any attempt in obtaining histological confirmation and proceed directly to palliative approach.

STAGING

A TNM classification for pancreatic cancer exists, but it is little used as there is no great virtue in detailed staging beyond designating tumours as being either resectable or unresectable.

A PRACTICAL STAGING SYSTEM FOR PANCREATIC CANCER

- Resectable
- Unresectable

TREATMENT

The only potentially curative treatment for pancreatic cancer is surgical resection (pancreatico-duodenectomy or Whipple's operation). Unfortunately, only 10–15% of patients have apparently localised disease suitable for this procedure. The operation is long, difficult and hazardous. As it is associated with significant morbidity, and a mortality rate of 5–15%, it should not be undertaken lightly or outside specialist centres. The use of octreotide, which diminishes pancreatic sections may reduce the complications of surgery. Cure only occurs if the

tumour is truly localised to the pancreas, and the realistic 5-year survival rate of this procedure is only about 5%, although some specialist centres claim survival rates of up to 20%.

RADICAL TREATMENT FOR PANCREATIC CANCER

- Surgical excision (Whipple's operation)
- Possibly adjuvant chemotherapy

It is not entirely clear whether or to what extent postoperative adjuvant treatment may improve the results offered by surgery alone. This is still an area for clinical trials. It is thought that fluorouracil-based chemotherapy may improve results, but radiotherapy (with or without chemotherapy) is not recommended. There are no data to support the use of neoadjuvant chemotherapy to improve the chances of a successful resection.

Palliative chemotherapy should be considered in fit patients with inoperable or metastatic disease, and in patients whose disease recurs following surgery. A number of trials have suggested that chemotherapy may prolong survival in this group of patients, but only by a matter of weeks or months – others have shown no benefit. An improvement in quality of life has been suggested in some studies, but the inconvenience and toxicity of treatment may outweigh benefits. The decision to receive (or not to receive) palliative chemotherapy should be made by patients, perhaps in conjunction with their relatives, following detailed explanation of the pros and cons. It is not clear what chemotherapy schedule is best. Several regimens, mostly based on fluorouracil with or without an anthracycline drug or platinum compound, are in use. Gemcitabine is a new addition to the chemotherapy options for this disease. The use of chemotherapy with radiotherapy may prolong survival in patients with locally advanced tumour, but it is associated with significant toxicity.

PALLIATIVE TREATMENT FOR UNRESECTABLE PANCREATIC CANCER

- Palliative chemotherapy or chemoradiotherapy in fit patients
- Symptom control and supportive care measures
- Endoscopic or percutaneous stenting or surgical bypass to relieve obstructive jaundice
- Stenting or bypass surgery to relieve duodenal obstruction
- Coeliac plexus nerve block or radiotherapy for pain

The majority of patients with pancreatic cancer are frail and elderly, often with other medical problems, and have locally advanced or metastatic disease. Their untreated life expectancy is only of the order of 3 months. Active anti-cancer treatment is not recommended, and efforts should concentrate on symptom control and supportive care. An early introduction to the specialist palliative care team is advisable. In addition to general palliative care measures, some principal symptoms of pancreatic cancer can be relieved in special ways.

Obstructive jaundice can be relieved by the endoscopic (or less commonly percutaneous) insertion of a stent. Expanding metal wall stents are associated with fewer complications than polythene stents. Stents sometimes block and need to be replaced. Alternatively, a surgical bypass procedure can be performed. This requires more time in hospital and has associated risks. It may be performed at the time of laparotomy done with the aim of resecting the cancer if the disease is found to be inoperable, if a laparotomy is performed for another reason such as to relieve duodenal compression, or if stent insertion is not possible.

Vomiting caused by gastric outflow obstruction as a result of compression of the duodenum by tumour may be overcome by a surgical bypass procedure, such as gastrojejunostomy or sometimes stenting is possible.

Severe pain, not easily relieved by conventional pain control measures, may sometimes be alleviated by a celiac plexus nerve block. Palliative radiotherapy (with or without chemotherapy) may sometimes help pain.

PROGNOSIS

In general, the prognosis for patients with pancreatic cancer is dismal. The median survival of all patients is of the order of 3–6 months, and three-quarters of patients will be dead within a year. Fewer than 5% of patients will be alive at 5 years. Clearly, the specialist palliative care team is very important in the management of this disease.

Cancer of the larynx and pharynx

Cancer arising in the larynx and pharynx is usually a squamous carcinoma. Non-Hodgkin's lymphoma (NHL) may also be seen, usually in the naso- or oropharynx. Tobacco and alcohol consumption are the major causative factors for squamous carcinoma in the larynx and pharynx, and consequently male patients form the majority. Most patients with the rare postcricoid carcinoma are women, which may be due to its association with chronic iron deficiency anaemia. Distant metastasis is unusual, except in nasopharyngeal cancer. Nasopharyngeal cancer is very common in Chinese people and may be due to diet and Epstein–Barr virus (EBV) infection.

THE ANATOMY OF THE LARYNX AND PHARYNX

Anatomy is critical to the presentation, treatment options and prognosis of tumours arising in the upper part of the airway and digestive tract. The anatomy is complex as both the larynx and pharynx are divided into a number of areas, each of which may have several sub-sites with important distinctions between them. To make matters worse, a number of these sub-sites have several names.

The larynx is divided into three parts by the vocal cords (or vocal folds) which constitute the glottis. Below the glottis is the subglottis and above is the supraglottis.

> **DIVISIONS OF THE LARYNX**
>
> ◆ The supraglottis
> ◆ The glottis
> ◆ The subglottis

The supraglottic larynx includes the false cords, the laryngeal ventricles lying between the true and the false cords, the posterior aspect of the epiglottis, the arytenoid region and the mucosal folds which run between the arytenoid cartilages and the epiglottis (the ary-epiglottic folds) which separate the larynx medially from the pyriform fossae of the hypopharynx laterally.

> **DIVISIONS OF THE SUPRAGLOTTIC LARYNX**
>
> ◆ The laryngeal ventricles
> ◆ The false cords
> ◆ The arytenoid area
> ◆ The posterior aspect of the epiglottis
> ◆ The ary-epiglottic folds

The pharynx is also divided into three parts. The upper part is the nasopharynx, the middle part is the oropharynx and the lower part is the hypopharynx. Confusingly, the hypopharynx is sometimes called the laryngopharynx. Sometimes people (incorrectly) use the term laryngopharynx to mean "the larynx and pharynx" rather than to identify a section of the pharynx, and so this term is better avoided.

> **DIVISIONS OF THE PHARYNX**
>
> ◆ The nasopharynx
> ◆ The oropharynx
> ◆ The hypopharynx

The nasopharynx sits underneath the skull base, between the ears (it is connected to the middle ears by the Eustachian tubes) and behind the nasal passages. It is connected to the oropharynx below, the soft palate forming the boundary between the nasopharynx and the oropharynx). The oropharynx contains the tonsils, the posterior third of the tongue, the valleculae and the anterior aspect of the epiglottis.

> **DIVISIONS OF THE OROPHARYNX**
>
> ◆ The underside of the soft palate
> ◆ The tonsils and faucial pillars
> ◆ The posterior third of tongue
> ◆ The valleculae
> ◆ The anterior aspect of the epiglottis

The hypopharynx lies behind the larynx, in continuity with the oropharynx above and the cervical oesophagus below. It is divided into the posterior pharyngeal wall, the pyriform fossae (the pyriform sinuses) and the postcricoid region.

PRESENTING SYMPTOMS OF CANCER IN THE LARYNX AND PHARYNX

Most patients with laryngeal cancer present with hoarseness, often worse at the end of the day. Benign causes such as laryngitis are, however, much more common, but all patients with hoarseness persisting for more than 3 weeks in spite of advice to rest the voice and not to whisper should be assessed in a ears, nose and throat (ENT) clinic to exclude malignancy. This is, particularly, important in middle-aged or elderly male smokers. Laryngeal cancer is not the only malignant cause of persistent hoarseness in smokers as lung cancer invading the mediastinum can cause the left recurrent laryngeal nerve palsy.

The chink between the vocal cords is the narrowest part of the airway and most cancers at this site present early, before the development of lymph node metastases. Other sites in the larynx have a richer lymphatic drainage than the vocal cords, and for this reason also non-vocal cord laryngeal carcinomas, such as supraglottic carcinoma have a much higher incidence of cervical node metastases and often present with a lump in the neck. Full blood count and film can be normal at this stage and an urgent ENT referral should be considered with all neck lumps of more than 2-week duration if no definite site of infection is apparent.

Presentation of pharyngeal cancers is much more variable, although naso-, oro- and hypopharyngeal tumours often present with neck nodes. Presenting symptoms otherwise usually depend on which part of the throat is affected.

Nasopharyngeal tumours may obstruct one or both Eustachian tube orifices and patients may complain of ear pain or deafness because of middle ear effusions. The nasal airway may become obstructed and speech quality may be altered. Erosion of cancer through the skull base may lead to a variety of isolated or multiple cranial nerve palsies.

Oropharyngeal and hypopharyngeal tumours often present with pain referred to the ear. All patients with persistent earache in whom the ear has a normal appearance should have a careful throat examination. This is particularly important if they are smokers and drinkers, and if no abnormality can be found in the ear to explain their pain. Oropharyngeal and hypopharyngeal tumours often cause pain or difficulty in swallowing, and are frequently associated with weight loss. Hoarseness is caused by invasion of the larynx by hypopharyngeal cancers and is a late sign of advanced disease.

General practitioners (GPs) should maintain a high index of suspicion in all patients who develop any of these symptoms and, in particular, older males who drink or smoke, and in people of Chinese origin.

TREATMENT OF LARYNGEAL CANCER

The two most important treatments for laryngeal cancer are radiotherapy and surgery. Chemotherapy is sometimes used, especially in association with radiotherapy, but its value is not yet proven. Across the world treatment policies vary, with surgery being more greatly favoured in the US than in Britain. Not surprisingly, surgeons are more likely to advocate surgery than oncologists.

In early laryngeal cancer, whether glottic or supraglottic, both surgery and radiotherapy can produce excellent cure rates. What distinguishes the choice of treatment is the side-effects. Radiotherapy for early laryngeal cancer is well tolerated with a minimal long-term complication rate. Clearly laryngectomy, depriving the patient the power of normal speech and resulting in the need for a tracheostomy, would be unnecessary interference in this situation. More limited surgery, such as laser cordectomy for an early vocal cord carcinoma, or a horizontal partial laryngectomy for a supraglottic carcinoma may be as effective, but voice quality and swallowing may not be as good as after radiotherapy.

In more advanced laryngeal cancer, surgery might produce slightly better results in terms of local control and survival, but radical radiotherapy can still cure a significant proportion without the need for loss of normal speech and a tracheostomy. If radical radiotherapy fails to control the disease, or results in laryngeal necrosis, salvage surgery is still usually possible. The principal indications for primary surgery are stridor, when a tracheostomy is needed; cartilage invasion; and the presence of bulky lymph nodes which are not likely to be sterilised by radiotherapy.

Even so these indications are not absolute, as stridor may sometimes be improved by lasering, avoiding the need for tracheostomy and allowing radical radiotherapy to be safely given. Similarly, initial chemotherapy may shrink down enlarged nodes, allowing radiotherapy to have a better chance of achieving a cure. Conversely, radiotherapy is often needed after surgery, especially if resection margins are close or if there is lymph node involvement.

SPEECH AFTER LARYNGECTOMY

Oesophageal speech is the best form of speech in patients without a larynx. It entails the controlled regurgitation of swallowed air which causes pharyngeal vibrations to emulate normal phonation. This sound is then articulated as normal by the tongue and mouth to produce words. The voice quality it produces is gruff, and is more suited to men than women. It is a difficult technique to learn well, and requires patience, motivation and intensive speech therapy. Younger patients with good family support are more likely to get good oesophageal speech. Factors such as post-operative scarring and a hiatus hernia may prevent the successful development of oesophageal speech. Only about one-third of patients develop good oesophageal speech.

Fortunately, in recent years the introduction of speaking valves (or neo-glottises) has provided a satisfactory alternative of semi-normal speech. Either at the time of laryngectomy, or subsequently as a secondary procedure, the surgeon creates a tracheo-oesophageal fistula at the top of the trachea, behind the tracheostomy. Various types of plastic valves, such as the Blom–Singer valve, can then be inserted into this fistula. If the patient then covers the opening of the tracheostomy with a finger and tries to breathe out, air passes through the valve from the trachea into the oesophagus and up into the pharynx. The vibrations produced in the valve form the basic sound which is then articulated into words.

Until a patient has developed oesophageal speech or has become able to use his speaking valve, one of several types of electromechanical vibrators can be used. Vibrators can also be used as a permanent solution. These external devices are usually held against the patient's throat and produce a constant buzzing sound. This noise is modified by articulation and hopefully produces intelligible speech. At best this speech is artificial, monotone, difficult to listen to, and is like that produced by Dr Who's ancient enemy, the Daleks.

TREATMENT OF PHARYNGEAL CANCER

Malignant tumours of the nasopharynx are always inoperable, and are always treated with radiotherapy, often in conjunction with chemotherapy which is thought to improve the generally poor results.

Early tumours of the oropharynx are usually best treated with radiotherapy. Surgery is often recommended for moderately advanced cancers of the lateral wall of the oropharynx, especially in the presence of lymph node involvement. This may entail splitting of the mandible, a flap reconstruction of the pharyngeal defect and a radical neck dissection. Postoperative radiotherapy is often needed if there are close or positive margins, multiple involved lymph nodes or extracapsular spread of tumour from lymph nodes. Cancers of the posterior third of tongue are usually too advanced for surgery. Anyway, as surgery would entail removal of both the whole tongue and the larynx (a total glossolaryngectomy), radiotherapy is the preferred option. Such cancers often have advanced lymph node involvement which may be bilateral. As bulky lymph nodes are difficult to cure with radiotherapy alone, a radical neck dissection with radiotherapy to the primary tumour is sometimes advocated, thereby avoiding particularly unpleasant surgery with the associated functional loss.

Lymphoma arising in the pharynx is treated with chemotherapy and radiotherapy in the same way as lymphoma at other sites. Surgery is not required except for biopsy.

The majority of hypopharyngeal carcinomas are advanced at presentation, and often have involved nodes. In fit patients, radical surgery followed by radiotherapy probably offers the best chance of cure. Surgery is usually a laryngopharyngectomy often in association with a neck dissection. The missing part of the pharynx is replaced either by a bit of jejunum which is transplanted from the abdomen, or by pulling up the stomach through the thorax. Many patients are unwilling for, or are too frail for, or are anaesthetically unfit for, such extensive surgery, and radiotherapy is used.

Radiotherapy for advanced laryngeal and pharyngeal cancers is, however, not without problems. It can produce a very considerable mucosal reaction that makes eating difficult for many weeks. This reaction can be made more severe and more prolonged by the prior or concomitant use of chemotherapy. In addition to the deleterious effects of malnutrition itself, these patients are very susceptible to the development of life-threatening chest infections because of the aspiration of food into airways possibly already compromised by smoking. The advent of endoscopic technology has made management of nutritional difficulties during and after treatment much easier to manage than previously. The percutaneous endoscopic gastrostomy (PEG) placement of gastrostomy tubes is now commonplace, if not routine, in the management of patients undergoing treatment for pharyngeal cancer.

OUTCOME

Early laryngeal cancer, for example a cancer confined to the vocal cords, can be cured in 90% of cases. The small number of patients whose disease is not cured by radiotherapy alone can usually be salvaged by laryngectomy. More advanced laryngeal cancers are more difficult to treat, but a patient with a laryngeal cancer causing vocal cord fixation which has not spread to the lymph nodes has a two-thirds chance of being cured – half of such patients will retain their larynx if treated with radiotherapy. The outcome for supraglottic cancers is less good than that of glottic ones. They tend to be more advanced locally, and there is a much greater incidence of lymph node involvement at the time of presentation.

Nasopharyngeal and hypopharyngeal cancers are often advanced at presentation, when the likelihood of cure is small. Early oropharyngeal cancers have a reasonable prospect of cure.

For patients with laryngeal and pharyngeal cancer, the cure of the cancer is not necessarily the same as long-term survival. As a group, they have a high incidence of other alcohol- and tobacco-related problems, such as malnutrition, vascular disease and cirrhosis, in addition to socio-economic problems.

Second primary tumours related to tobacco and alcohol, either elsewhere in the head and neck or in the lung, may affect up to one-third of those cured of their original primary tumour.

Cancer of the lip and mouth

ANATOMICAL SUB-SITES OF THE LIP AND ORAL CAVITY WHERE CANCER MAY OCCUR

- External lip (vermilion border)
- Buccal mucosa
- Upper alveolus and gingiva
- Lower alveolus and gingiva
- Hard palate
- Anterior two-thirds of the tongue
- Floor of mouth

CANCER OF THE EXTERNAL LIPS

The lips are the most common location for mouth cancer. The lower lip is affected in over 90% of cases. Men are affected very much more commonly than women. Patients are usually elderly. Sun exposure is an important aetiological factor, and so it is more common in those with an outdoor occupation, and in those who have lived in or frequently visited sunny countries. White people are more susceptible than those with pigmented skin. Other aetiological factors include cigarette and pipe smoking, alcohol and chronic erosive skin disease, such as lichen planus. The histology is almost always squamous carcinoma.

Clinical presentation

Most commonly, the tumour arises on the vermilion border of the lower lip, just outside the line of contact with the upper lip. Most commonly, the tumours are exophytic. When the tumour is greater than 1 cm in diameter, necrosis and ulceration may develop. There is often a history of intermittent crusting with bleeding on removal of the crust. Less commonly, the tumour may present as a non-healing fissure in the lip or as an ulcer with minimal elevation. Lymph node metastases occur at presentation or, subsequently, in about 10% of patients. Enlarged lymph nodes may be present which do not contain secondary spread: infection of the tumour or poor oral hygiene may cause reactive lymphadenopathy.

Staging

Cancers of the lip and other sub-sites in the oral cavity, are staged by the TNM system (Chapter 8). This is important for guiding treatment choices and for predicting outcome. As with other squamous cancers of the head and neck, it is the T- and the N-categories which are most important; distant metastases are exceptionally rare.

Treatment

Early cancer of the lip can be managed equally well by either radiotherapy or surgery. Surgery is preferable for small lesions, wedge excision biopsy will provide tissue for diagnosis, and will be the adequate treatment. Surgery is also preferable in younger patients as they will be spared the late effects of radiotherapy which include thinning of the substance of the lip, altered pigmentation of the skin and telangiectasia. Radiotherapy may be preferred for more advanced but still localised tumours; alternatively, a more major resection with reconstruction may be appropriate. Postoperative radiotherapy may be required, especially, if there is lymph node involvement.

Prognosis

Localised tumours less than 2 cm in diameter will be cured by either surgery or radiotherapy in between 80% and 90% of cases. Well-differentiated tumours have a better outlook than moderately or poorly differentiated cancers. With larger tumours, or if there is lymph node spread, the prognosis is worse and only about half in this category will be cured.

ORAL CAVITY CANCER

Oral cavity cancer is a disease of the middle aged and elderly. Men are more commonly affected than women. The overwhelming majority (i.e. 85%) of oral cavity cancers are squamous cell carcinoma. Minor salivary gland carcinomas (Chapter 28) comprise 5%, the remainder are a variety of rare tumour types. The most common location of cancers within the oral cavity is on the anterior two-thirds of the tongue (35%) and the floor of mouth (30%). The primary is on the gums in 20%, and the remaining 15% occur on the buccal mucosa, the hard palate or in the retromolar region.

There are many predisposing factors in the development of oral cancer, but, as at so many other sites, alcohol and tobacco (smoked or chewed) are the principal culprits in Western society. Leucoplakia is a pre-malignant lesion. It appears as a white plaque in the mouth which, unlike a patch of candidiasis, cannot be wiped off. There is a spectrum of change from moderate dysplasia, through severe dysplasia and carcinoma *in situ,* to invasive squamous cancer. The variant, erythroleucoplakia, appears as a velvety red patch, and is more likely to become malignant than a simple white patch. Investigations may reveal a "field change" within the oral cavity where the area of dysplasia and potential malignant change is much larger than is apparent. Tumours may be multifocal in origin in such cases.

Presenting features

Most oral cavity cancers present as a progressive swelling or as a non-healing ulcer. Early on, they may be relatively asymptomatic, although pain can be a prominent feature. Referred pain affecting the ear can lead to a delayed diagnosis. All older smokers and drinkers presenting with earache should have their mouths carefully examined. Presentation is often to the dentist rather than the doctor, and routine dental examination should include careful inspection of all parts of the mouth for lesions which might be malignant. Sometimes, the presence of a tumour may lead to loosening of a tooth, or to dentures becoming ill fitting. Fungating tumours are associated with an offensive odour. Functional disturbances, such as difficulty in eating or speaking, are features of advanced disease. Lymph node metastases are present in about half the cases.

Investigation

All patients with a suspicious oral cavity lesion should be referred to a head and neck clinic urgently for assessment. An initial examination in the outpatient setting will provide a lot of information about the site and the extent of the tumour, but an examination under anaesthetic (EUA) is usually necessary to allow biopsy and to examine less easily accessible areas of the upper aerodigestive tract which may be harbouring a synchronous neoplasm. Dental assessment is important as the state of the teeth may be relevant to the treatment chosen, and care of any teeth will be important during the follow-up period. Radiological investigations including an orthopantomogram (OPG), computed tomography (CT) or magnetic resonance imaging (MRI) scan and chest radiography are often indicated to evaluate the state of the teeth, to confirm the extent of local disease, especially, if there is any possibility of local bone erosion and to identify pulmonary metastases or an associated lung cancer.

Following this evaluation, the histological type of the tumour will be confirmed, and the stage of the disease will have been determined. More information is, however, required before a treatment plan can be formulated in the combined head and neck clinic by the surgeon and the oncologist in conjunction with the patient and family members.

It is also important to assess the patient from a general medical point of view, as co-morbidity is common and may influence treatment choices. Similarly, the patient cannot be treated without reference to his or her social background, as many patients with head and neck cancer come from a disadvantaged setting which may influence the feasibility and suitability of different treatment approaches.

Treatment

> **TREATMENT OPTIONS FOR SMALL LOCALISED ORAL CAVITY TUMOURS**
>
> ◆ Surgery alone
> ◆ Radiotherapy alone

Small, localised tumours can be treated with either surgery or radiotherapy alone, with little morbidity and equal survival rates at about 80%. The advantages of surgery are that in the case of a small accessible lesion, surgical treatment is quick and efficient with little need for reconstruction and it also permits complete histological assessment of the lesion which may guide the need for prophylactic treatment of neck nodes which may harbour occult metastatic disease. Radiotherapy, for example for a carcinoma of the lateral border of the anterior two-thirds of the tongue, may avoid the loss of normal tissue and function which may accompany surgery. It can be given in the form of an interstitial implant (Chapter 12) or external beam radiotherapy. The former has the advantage of being quicker to deliver and having fewer adverse effects (e.g. xerostomia) on normal tissue.

> **TREATMENT OPTIONS FOR ADVANCED ORAL CAVITY CANCERS**
>
> ◆ Excisional surgery (with or without reconstruction) and postoperative radiotherapy
> ◆ Radical radiotherapy or chemoradiotherapy alone
> ◆ Transoral laser resection and postoperative radiotherapy
> ◆ Symptom control and palliative care only

Radiotherapy alone is less likely to be successful for more advanced tumours, and even there is no clinically detectable lymph node involvement the likelihood of occult involvement rises with increasing primary tumour size. Surgery is, therefore, preferable as the initial treatment. Resection of the primary tumour can be accompanied by a therapeutic neck dissection if there is lymph node involvement, or by a selective sampling of nodes in the relevant part of the neck for histological assessment if clinically the neck is free of disease.

Operations of this type are major procedures, often a temporary tracheostomy is needed, and the patient may be left with significant functional or cosmetic impairment. Nutritional support, for example via a gastrostomy, may be required. It is often very helpful for patients and their families to have detailed discussions with a head and neck clinical nurse specialist as well as the head and neck surgeon prior to a final decision being made about treatment.

Following surgery for locally advanced disease, or if there was lymph node involvement, postoperative radiotherapy or chemoradiotherapy to the primary site and lymphatic drainage areas in the neck will, usually, be required.

Perhaps the greatest advance in the management of oral cavity cancer in recent years has been an improvement in reconstructive techniques. Often a plastic surgeon will be part of the team performing the operation. There are many techniques available to assist in functional and cosmetic reconstruction.

SOME TECHNIQUES USED IN RECONSTRUCTION

- Spit skin grafts
- Full thickness skin grafts
- Local pedicled skin flaps
- Pedicled myocutaneous or muscle only flaps
- Fascial flaps
- Bone, muscle and skin-free tissue transfer, for example radial free forearm flap, fibula flap

---

Alternative approaches to advanced disease include radiotherapy or chemoradiotherapy alone. This, in selected cases, may result in less functional morbidity, and may be the chosen method of treatment in other cases if the patient refuses, or is not fit for, a major surgical procedure. Generally, however, the results of radiotherapy alone for advanced disease are not as good as those of combined modality treatment.

A new approach, which is presently being evaluated, is transoral laser resection of the tumour followed by radiotherapy. Laser resection is an effective way of substantially

---

PRINCIPLES OF RECONSTRUCTIVE SURGERY

- The reconstruction technique should not interfere with or limit any excisional surgery
- Form and function should be restored as quickly as possible
- Operative morbidity and mortality should not be increased unnecessarily by the reconstruction method chosen
- As a general rule, resection and reconstruction should take place as a one-stage procedure
- Procedures that involve soft tissue and bone reconstruction should not be used where a prosthesis would provide a better alternative

---

debulking the tumour and often removing all macroscopic disease. It is not, however, a classical "oncological operation" in that it does not remove the tumour in its entirety in one piece with clear margins. Viable cells will almost always be left in the tumour bed, hence the need for radiotherapy. It has the advantages of producing less functional morbidity than a classical resection, and often avoids the need for a major reconstructive procedure. Results may, however, be better than for radiotherapy alone, as the principal tumour bulk is removed.

Finally, it should not be forgotten that sometimes, due to the extent of the tumour or the frailty or comorbidity of the patient, active anti-cancer treatment with either curative or palliative intent is not appropriate. For these patients, specialist palliative care input, preferably in the community with access to a hospice if necessary, is essential.

Prognosis

The outcome for treatment of early oral cavity cancer is good. Perhaps four out of five patients may expect to be cured, so many live to develop second primary cancers at other sites in the oral cavity or other parts of the aerodigestive tract, or may succumb to other smoking- and drinking-related diseases.

With more advanced disease, the outlook is less good, with cause specific 5-year survival rates generally between one-third and two-thirds, depending on stage and grade of the tumour, and whether medical or social factors have compromised treatment. Again, social deprivation, the high level of other smoking- and drinking-related diseases, and second malignancies often lead to a poor survival overall, even when the initial cancer is successfully controlled.

Salivary gland cancer

Salivary gland tumours are not uncommon and, although the majority are benign, they need to be approached with great care in order to detect cancers, while there is still a chance of cure without undue complications. They may arise in either of the two pairs of major salivary glands, the parotid and the submandibular glands, or in any of the hundreds of minor salivary glands, which occur in the mucosa of the upper aerodigestive tract, especially the hard palate and oropharynx.

> **LOCATION OF SALIVARY GLAND TUMOURS AND RISK OF MALIGNANCY**
>
> ◆ Parotid glands – 1:6 malignant
> ◆ Submandibular glands – 1:3 malignant
> ◆ Minor salivary glands – 1:2 malignant

BENIGN CONDITIONS

A variety of benign conditions can cause a transient or permanent swelling in the salivary glands, in addition to a true neoplasm, whether benign or malignant. These include mumps, acute bacterial infections, salivary calculi, the granulomatous diseases, sarcoidosis and tuberculosis, and cysts, which may be a manifestation of HIV disease. In addition, as there are lymph nodes within the substance of the parotid gland, any cause of lymph node enlargement (benign or malignant) can cause a swelling at this site.

Benign tumours are fairly clearly circumscribed and are usually solitary, although bilateral cases may occur. They do not infiltrate the overlying skin or give rise to facial nerve paralysis: these are clear signs of malignancy. However, as with breast lumps, the absence of definite indicators of malignancy does not mean that a lesion is benign, and so all patients with a persistent discrete swelling in the parotid or submandibular regions, or in the oral cavity or throat, should be referred to a head and neck surgeon without delay.

> **BENIGN SALIVARY GLAND TUMOURS**
>
> ◆ Pleomorphic adenoma
> ◆ Monomorphic adenomas
>   – Warthin's tumour (or adenolymphoma)
>   – Oncocytoma (or oxyphil cell adenoma)

Pleomorphic adenoma is the commonest benign tumour, accounting for three-quarters of all parotid gland and half of all submandibular gland tumours. Apart from some occasional discomfort, and, of course, the presence of the lump itself, they are usually asymptomatic. The sex ratio is equal, and the average age at presentation is 40 years. Fine needle aspiration cytology may be helpful in giving a preoperative diagnosis, and imaging of parotid tumours with CT or MRI will usually show that the tumour is confined to the superficial lobe. The initial treatment should be wide local excision, which usually means removal of the whole submandibular gland or a superficial parotidectomy sparing the facial nerve or an equivalent surgical procedure, if the tumour is located in a minor gland. Lesser procedures are accompanied by an unacceptable risk of local recurrence. In the past, radiotherapy was given after the limited surgical procedure of "enucleation", but nowadays an adequate surgical excision is preferred initially to minimise risks of recurrence, as with repeated excisions, the likelihood of damage to the facial nerve or of malignant transformation becomes greater. Even with complete excision, pleomorphic adenomas may recur, sometimes after an interval of many years, and postoperative radiotherapy can be called for following surgery for recurrence, even though the tumour remains histologically benign.

There are several types of monomorphic adenoma, the commonest being Warthin's tumour, also called adenolymphoma, a benign tumour occurring most often in the parotid gland in elderly men. Surgery alone is sufficient. Oncocytoma or oxyphil adenoma is less common. It tends to be cystic and occurs in older men and women.

MALIGNANT SALIVARY GLAND TUMOURS

> **MALIGNANT SALIVARY GLAND TUMOURS**
>
> ◆ Acinic cell carcinoma
> ◆ Adenocarcinoma
> ◆ Adenoid cystic carcinoma
> ◆ Carcinoma arising in a pre-existing pleomorphic adenoma
> ◆ Lymphoma
> ◆ Mucoepidermoid carcinoma
> ◆ Squamous cell carcinoma

There are many different types of salivary gland cancers and they vary significantly in histological grade and clinical behaviour.

Acinic cell tumours

They are at the better end of the spectrum. They tend to behave like a pleomorphic adenoma, although some may have an aggressive malignant course. The sex incidence is equal and they may occur at any age from childhood onwards with a peak incidence in people in their 40s. The likelihood of survival at 5 years is excellent, but there is a tendency for late local nodal or metastatic recurrence, sometimes after an interval of decades, which reduces the 20-year survival rate significantly.

Adenocarcinoma

Adenocarcinoma can arise at any site, at any age and in both sexes. It is often advanced at presentation having grown rapidly, caused facial nerve paralysis and perhaps infiltrated the skin. It behaves in a highly malignant fashion and survival rates are poor.

Adenoid cystic carcinoma

This is the most common malignant tumour type, accounting for 40% of all cases. It is most common in the minor glands, tends to affect women more than men and is more common in older people. It is only slowly growing, and the natural history often extends over many years. There is a marked tendency for spread of the tumour along nerves, and parotid adenoid cystic carcinomas may well recur in the brain, the tumour having tracked along the course of the facial nerve through the temporal bone to gain access to the cranial cavity. Distant metastases, especially in the lungs, are not uncommon, but patients may live with metastases for many years.

Carcinoma arising in a pleomorphic adenoma

This is not common, and is most likely to be found in patients who have had treatment on many occasions over the years for recurrent pleomorphic adenomas.

Lymphoma

Any type of lymphoma may arise in the pre-auricular lymph nodes, which are situated in the substance of the parotid glands anterior to the ear. It is classified, staged and treated as lymphoma arising at any other site.

Mucoepidermoid carcinoma

This arises more commonly in minor glands. The sex ratio is equal, and it can occur at any age from childhood to old age. Most commonly, it behaves in a low-grade fashion, rather like a pleomorphic adenoma. In some cases, however, it can be highly malignant, with the early development of lymph node involvement in the neck and distant metastases.

Squamous cell carcinoma

This is not common, but it is important to differentiate a true primary parotid salivary gland squamous carcinoma from a metastasis in a lymph node due to a primary tumour at another site, such as on the scalp. Such a primary tumour might have been small and have been excised some time previously and forgotten about by the patient. Mention of past malignancies in a general practitioner's referral letter can be enormously helpful to the head and neck surgeon. Genuine primary salivary gland squamous cell cancers tend to occur in elderly men. They are often rapidly growing and cause pain, facial nerve palsy and skin fixation with ulceration. Neck node metastases are likely to be present at the time of diagnosis, and the prognosis is very poor.

INVESTIGATION AND TREATMENT

In the majority of cases, the surgeon in the head and neck clinic will not be able to determine whether a salivary gland swelling is benign or malignant just by clinical examination, although findings on examination are of great importance. Fine needle aspiration for cytology, coupled with imaging investigations may yield a diagnosis preoperatively in many patients, but for some, the fact that they have cancer will only be revealed by the definitive surgical histology report. Complete conservative surgery is often adequate for many low-grade cancers. Cancers that are more advanced at presentation will often require more extensive operations, involving, for example, sacrifice of the facial nerve, coupled with postoperative radiotherapy. Some malignant tumours, usually adenocarcinoma or squamous carcinoma, are too advanced at presentation for potentially curative surgery to be performed. In these cases, radiotherapy may provide good palliation of pain, swelling and ulceration, but cure is not a likely outcome.

In summary, therefore, all patients presenting with swellings in the salivary gland area, which persist for more than 2 weeks, should be referred to a head and neck surgeon for investigation.

CHAPTER 29
Thyroid cancer

There are different types of thyroid cancer, which vary from the highly malignant to exceptionally indolent. This spectrum of natural history extends from anaplastic cancer (a disease which often proves fatal within a few weeks) to papillary cancer (a condition which may, if it is not cured, recur over many decades). Patients of almost any age may be affected, but the disease is most common in younger adults. Papillary cancer is the most common type in children and younger adults, and anaplastic cancer is usually confined to the elderly. As with other thyroid conditions, it is much more common in females: the female to male ratio is 3 : 1. Thyroid cancer is not common, but it is important to minimise delay in diagnosis both for eventual outcome and for decreasing adverse effects of treatment.

TYPES OF THYROID CANCER

The main cell types in the normal thyroid gland are the follicular cells, which produce the protein thyroglobulin from which the thyroid hormone thyroxine is derived, and the parafollicular or C-cells, which produce the orphan hormone calcitonin.

> **NORMAL THYROID CELL TYPES**
> - Follicular cells: produce thyroglobulin
> - Parafollicular cells: produce calcitonin

The majority of thyroid carcinomas – about 95% – are derived from the follicular cells. These may be differentiated tumours, which are described as either papillary or follicular or mixed. Undifferentiated or anaplastic thyroid cancers also arise from follicular cells. Papillary cancers and mixed cancers, which are treated in the same way as papillary cancers, account for about half of all cases, pure follicular cancers account for about one-quarter of all cases, and about one in five is an anaplastic cancer. Medullary carcinoma of the thyroid arises from the parafollicular cells and accounts for only about 1 in 20 cases. Other tumours can also occur in the thyroid gland, but only lymphoma is seen with any frequency. This is almost always a high-grade non-Hodgkin's lymphoma.

> **HISTOLOGICAL TYPES OF THYROID CANCER**
> - Follicular cell origin
>   - papillary carcinoma
>   - follicular carcinoma
>   - anaplastic carcinoma
> - Parafollicular cell origin
>   - medullary carcinoma
> - Non-thyroid cell origin
>   - non-Hodgkin's lymphoma

PRESENTATION

Most commonly, thyroid cancers present as a swelling in the neck. These are usually solitary, slowly growing nodules, which are clearly within the thyroid gland because they move with the larynx on swallowing. When examining the neck, it should be inspected from the front and palpated from behind the patient. The differential diagnosis includes common benign thyroid nodules, but patients with solitary nodules should always be referred for investigation. If malignant, they are most likely to be well-differentiated papillary cancers. Occasionally, thyroid cancers may present with cervical lymphadenopathy without a clinically detectable thyroid abnormality. Rapidly enlarging diffuse anterior neck masses rarely move with swallowing because they have become fixed to other structures. They are almost always malignant and may be either anaplastic cancers or lymphoma. Hoarseness may be a feature.

INVESTIGATION

While patients with a small, smooth symmetrical goitre may be observed in the community, all patients presenting with a distinct palpable thyroid nodule, with or without an underlying goitre, should be referred for urgent investigation. This is especially important with larger nodules or if there is a rapid change in size. Likely investigations will include radionuclide scanning, ultrasound and fine needle aspirate for cytology. Patients whose initial investigations yield suspicious or positive results will require surgical exploration. In patients with a suspicious nodule (not yet proven to be malignant), a thyroid lobectomy will be performed.

INITIAL TREATMENT OF PAPILLARY AND FOLLICULAR CANCER

Surgery is necessary for all patients with operable differentiated cancers of follicular cell origin. When cancer is confirmed following lobectomy for a suspicious lump, the question of further surgery arises. In most cases, a complete thyroidectomy will be performed. Occasionally, if the lump is small (say, less than 1 cm diameter) and the margins are clear, a surgeon may be content to follow up the patient carefully rather than re-operate immediately. If initial investigations have confirmed the lump to be malignant, a near total thyroidectomy will be performed in most cases as the definitive surgical procedure. This involves removal of almost all the thyroid gland, leaving only a sliver of tissue containing at least one parathyroid gland. If there are enlarged nodes, these should be removed at the time of thyroidectomy. There is no need to perform a block dissection as is often the case in squamous cancer of the head and neck, but occasionally, it may be necessary to remove nodes from the superior mediastinum. Complications of thyroid surgery include transient or permanent hypocalcaemia due to removal of parathyroid tissue and transient or permanent hoarseness due to recurrent laryngeal nerve damage. Many patients will complain that their voice sounds abnormal for up to 3 months postoperatively, even in the absence of any nerve damage.

> ### TREATMENT OF PAPILLARY AND FOLLICULAR THYROID CANCER
>
> ◆ Surgery – usually near total thyroidectomy
> ◆ Radioactive iodine – to ablate thyroid remnant
> ◆ External beam radiotherapy – rarely if residual disease in the neck
> ◆ Radioactive iodine – rarely for metastatic disease
> ◆ Thyroxine replacement – suppressive doses

Following thyroidectomy, patients will become hypothyroid unless they receive thyroid hormone-replacement therapy. Patients may sometimes be started on thyroid hormones immediately after surgery, or they may be left without replacement pending further treatment.

After surgery has removed all macroscopic disease from the neck, any residual thyroid tissue should be ablated by treatment with radioactive iodine, except in the rare case of a patient with a very good prognosis small tumour,

who has been treated with partial thyroidectomy only. This may be done 3 weeks to 3 months after surgery. Patients need to be off thyroid hormone replacement (if they have started it) long enough for endogenous thyroid-stimulating hormone (TSH) levels to rise. Unless TSH levels are high, uptake of the radioiodine by residual thyroid tissue will be poor and ineffective. If a patient has been started on thyroxine (T4) after surgery, they should be changed to the shorter-acting analogue liothyronine (T3) 20 micrograms three times a day, 4 weeks prior to the planned radioiodine treatment. Liothyronine should then be stopped 10 days prior to the radioiodine.

Radioactive iodine is administered orally, usually as a capsule, although liquid preparations are available. The patient will require hospitalisation for about 3–4 days following the radioiodine for radiation protection purposes. A scan will be performed before discharge, but this is only likely to show uptake into residual normal thyroid tissue in the neck, even if distant metastases are present. Following return home, the patient will still be radioactive for some time, and should not have contact with children or pregnant women, and use of a separate toilet may be advisable.

External beam irradiation of the neck (and sometimes the upper mediastinum as well) is only rarely necessary. It is indicated if there is residual inoperable disease in the neck, especially if the uptake of radioactive iodine is poor, or if pathological findings such as positive margins or extracapsular nodal spread indicate a high likelihood of microscopic residual disease. This will be a radical course of treatment, and is likely to be complicated by an acute skin reaction and dysphagia due to mucositis. Permanent xerostomia may result if extensive nodal spread means that the whole neck and salivary glands require treatment.

TREATMENT OF METASTATIC DISEASE

About 3 months after initial treatment, it is wise to perform a diagnostic radioiodine scan. Again this requires a changeover from thyroxine to liothyronine, which should be stopped 10 days prior to the scan. On this occasion, only a small tracer dose is given and hospitalisation is not required. This scan should confirm successful ablation of the thyroid remnant, and hopefully the absence of metastatic disease in the lungs or elsewhere. If the thyroid remnant has not been ablated, a further ablative dose of radioiodine is needed. If metastatic disease has been demonstrated, then one or more therapy doses of radioiodine will be required. Bone metastases are unusual and carry a poorer prognosis than lung metastases. External beam radiotherapy may be needed. Chemotherapy is very little use in thyroid cancer.

FOLLOW-UP

When treatment is complete, the patient should be on supraphysiological-replacement doses of thyroxine (often 200–300 micrograms daily) to keep the TSH level completely suppressed. The dose should be as low as possible, consistent with good TSH suppression. When the TSH level is well suppressed, regular monitoring of the tumour marker thyroglobulin is performed. If there is a rise in thyroglobulin levels, a further radioiodine scan can be performed to identify the site of relapse.

PROGNOSIS OF PAPILLARY AND FOLLICULAR CANCERS

The majority of patients with well-differentiated thyroid cancer of follicular cell origin will be cured. Even those who are destined ultimately to die from their disease may live for decades. The most important intrinsic prognostic factor is age: patients over the age of 40 fare significantly worse. Patients with only moderately-well differentiated tumours have an increased mortality. Tumour size and extent are also of independent prognostic significance. Patients with small tumours do well, but those with large cancers, especially if there is local extension into surrounding organs, such as the larynx or oesophagus, or with nodal metastases are more likely to develop local recurrence or distant metastases. The most important treatment-related factor affecting prognosis is adequate TSH suppression.

Distant metastases are present in 5–10% of patients at the time of diagnosis, and may subsequently develop in a similar proportion of patients whose disease is initially localised. With radioiodine treatment, a significant proportion may be cured, or at least live for many years. Patients whose tumours do not take up iodine fare worse. Patients with large pulmonary metastases, or with bone disease fare worse than those with very small pulmonary nodules.

ADVERSE PROGNOSTIC FACTORS FOR PAPILLARY AND FOLLICULAR CANCERS

- Age over 40 years
- Less well-differentiated histology
- Larger primary tumours
- Extensive local or distant disease

TREATMENT OF ANAPLASTIC THYROID CANCER

Anaplastic cancers usually present in elderly women as rapidly growing hard diffuse swellings in the neck, which infiltrate surrounding tissues and often lead to stridor. They are usually inoperable, but surgery is necessary to obtain histological confirmation of the diagnosis as lymphoma can present in a very similar way, but has a very different prognosis, if treated appropriately. Tracheostomy is sometimes necessary. Palliative radiotherapy and corticosteroids may produce improvement, but this is usually transient. Results of chemotherapy are disappointing and it is not used routinely. The median survival is only a few months, exceptionally patients may live up to a year.

TREATMENT OF MEDULLARY THYROID CANCER

Medullary cancers do not take up radioiodine. Treatment is, therefore, with surgery either alone or combined with external beam irradiation, if there is residual disease. As growth of medullary cancers is not promoted by TSH, TSH levels do not need to be suppressed and normal-replacement doses of thyroxine are adequate. Calcitonin, together with carcino-embryonic antigen (CEA) rather than thyroglobulin is used as a tumour marker. Patients with medullary carcinoma of the thyroid may have a family history, and the disease is rarely part of a multiple endocrine neoplasia syndrome.

TREATMENT OF THYROID LYMPHOMA

Thyroid lymphoma is most often seen as a rapidly progressing neck swelling in elderly women. Clinically, it may be indistinguishable from anaplastic cancer, and so accurate histological assessment is essential. It often arises on a background of auto-immune thyroiditis (Hashimoto's disease). Most commonly, it is a high-grade B-cell non-Hodgkin's lymphoma. Separate cervical lymph nodes may or may not be palpable. It is staged in the same way as any other lymphoma, but usually proves to be localised. Treatment is usually with radiotherapy to the neck, which brings about resolution of the often massive swelling within a few days, followed by chemotherapy. Chemotherapy alone may be used.

Other head and neck cancers

This chapter deals with rarer tumours of the head and neck region: cancers arising in the nose and paranasal sinuses and the ear; paragangliomas or glomus tumours; and finally, but by no means the least important, the management of patients presenting with metastatic squamous cancer in cervical lymph nodes when no primary tumour is apparent.

The management of the more common cancers of the head and neck is described in other chapters. Squamous cell carcinomas, the larynx and the pharynx have been covered in Chapter 26. The lips and oral cavity have been dealt with in Chapter 27. The classification and management of tumours of the major and minor salivary glands are set out in Chapter 28. Thyroid cancers have been covered in Chapter 30. The management of skin cancer arising on the head and neck, and mucosal melanoma, is included in Chapter 34. The classification and treatment of lymphomas and soft tissue sarcomas arising in the head and neck region are dealt with in Chapters 41 and 44.

TUMOURS OF THE NOSE AND PARANASAL SINUSES

The nose and paranasal sinuses represent not only two of the rarest sites of origin of head and neck cancer, but also give rise to a great variety of histological types. They are characterised clinically by a tendency to late presentation with locally extensive disease and late nodal metastasis.

SITE OF ORIGIN OF SINO-NASAL TUMOURS

◆ Nasal fossa	45%
◆ Maxillary antrum	30%
◆ Ethmoid sinus	5%
◆ Uncertain due to disease extent	20%

Nose and sinus tumours are more commonly due to industrial carcinogens than many other tumour types. These include hardwood dust in the furniture industry, which is especially associated with ethmoid adenocarcinoma. There is also an increased incidence in boot and shoe industry workers. Those working in the nickel and chromium industries tend to develop squamous cancers.

Men are more commonly affected than women, and average patients are in their 50s. Sino-nasal tumours may present with a variety of symptoms.

PRESENTING FEATURES OF NOSE AND PARANASAL SINUS TUMOURS

- ◆ Nasal obstruction, discharge or bleeding
- ◆ Facial pain or swelling
- ◆ Loose dentition in the upper jaw or a palatal mass or ulcer due to inferior extension of tumour
- ◆ Trismus as a result of posterior extension of tumour
- ◆ Diplopia or proptosis as a result of orbital invasion

Nose and paranasal sinus tumours are usually localised at presentation. Even if locally advanced, lymph node metastases are unusual, occurring in only about 10% of patients at some point during their illness. Distant metastases are unusual.

Following a biopsy to identify the histological type, and imaging investigations to determine the local extent of disease, a treatment plan can be formulated in the combined consultation clinic by the head and neck surgeon and the oncologist.

If the disease is localised and the patient's condition permits it, radical surgery is the treatment of choice. Nowadays, new techniques enable radical removal of even advanced sino-nasal tumours with minimal morbidity or disfigurement. Craniofacial resection enables removal of the whole ethmoid complex and central skull base leaving no external sign of interference. Mid-facial degloving provides the surgeon with access to allow resection of even very extensive tumours with no visible scars.

Sometimes, however, it is necessary to remove the eye if there is orbital involvement, or part of the upper jaw in the case of tumours in this region. Carefully planned reconstructive surgery and improvements in prosthetics including osseo-integrated implants have significantly improved the cosmetic and functional outcome for patients requiring such major surgery. Usually, postoperative radiotherapy is required following surgery for sino-nasal tumours.

TUMOURS OF THE EAR

Tumours of the pinna are most commonly squamous cell cancers or sometimes basal cell carcinomas. These relatively common tumours are essentially skin cancers, and their management is covered in Chapter 34. The general practitioner can sometimes be the first person to notice a tumour of the pinna coincidentally during a routine consultation.

Tumours of the external auditory meatus and of the middle ear and mastoid are rarer. Cholesteatoma is the most common benign tumour at this site. Again, squamous carcinoma is the most frequently seen malignant tumour, but other histological entities, such as mucoepidermoid carcinoma, adenoid cystic carcinoma and adenocarcinoma, may occur.

These tumours may present with aural discharge or bleeding, an exophytic growth from the ear canal, deafness, pain and sometimes facial nerve palsy. As these tumours can arise against a background of chronic middle ear infection, the clinician must be alert to the potential significance of a change in the pattern of symptoms, or to the unexpected persistence of symptoms.

These tumours can often be very extensive at presentation with involvement deep into the temporal bone. Treatment is principally surgical in the first instance, usually, with postoperative radiotherapy. The prognosis is not good, and less than one-half will be cured.

PARAGANGLIOMAS

Paragangliomas are rare tumours, which are thought to arise from chemoreceptor cells; hence, the alternative name of chemodectoma. They are also called glomus tumours. They are usually benign, but about 5% have malignant potential and bone and lung metastases may develop. Paragangliomas in the head and neck arise at four sites.

Carotid body tumours and glomus vagale present as lumps in the neck, while glomus tympanicum and glomus jugulare most commonly present with deafness, sometimes associated with tinnitus, vertigo, pain and cranial nerve palsies. Progression is slow, and the natural history is correspondingly long.

> ### NAME AND LOCATION OF HEAD AND NECK PARAGANGLIOMAS
> - Carotid body tumour: medial aspect of carotid bulb
> - Glomus vagale: nodose ganglion of the vagus nerve
> - Glomus tympanicum: middle ear
> - Glomus jugulare: the jugular bulb

Treatment of these tumours is principally surgical, but radiotherapy may be used in patients who are unsuitable for surgery by virtue of frailty or extent of disease, who refuse operation, or who develop recurrence after initial surgery.

METASTATIC CANCER IN NECK NODES WITH NO IDENTIFIABLE PRIMARY TUMOUR

> ### LYMPH NODE LEVELS IN THE NECK
> - *Level I*: Mental and submandibular nodes found in the upper part of the anterior triangle of the neck. Primary sites include the lower lip, oral cavity, face, nose and paranasal sinuses.
> - *Level II*: The upper jugular, or upper deep cervical, group of nodes lies behind the upper one-third of the sternomastoid muscle. Primary sites include the oral cavity, oropharynx, nasopharynx, hypopharynx and supraglottic larynx.
> - *Level III*: The middle jugular group lies behind the central part of the sternomastoid muscle. Primary sites include the thyroid, larynx, hypopharynx and cervical oesophagus.
> - *Level IV*: The lower jugular group of nodes lies behind the lower third of the sternomastoid muscle. Primary sites include abdominal organs, breast and lung as well as thyroid and oesophagus.
> - *Level V*: The posterior triangle group of nodes includes nodes in the supraclavicular fossa. Primary sites include nasopharynx and those sites listed for Level IV.
> - *Level VI*: The anterior compartment group contains those nodes in the centre of the neck anteriorly from the level of the hyoid bone down to the suprasternal notch. Primary sites include the thyroid gland, the larynx and the hypopharynx.
> - *Level VII*: These nodes are in the anterior mediastinum, not in the neck.

While head and neck cancer usually presents with symptoms due directly to the primary tumour, it is not uncommon for the patient to present with a lump in the neck due to an enlarged lymph node or group of nodes with no primary tumour detectable even on detailed clinical examination. This situation is not always clear-cut, as neck swellings may be due to things other than cervical lymphadenopathy, and cervical lymphadenopathy will be due to a benign condition. It can be helpful to get a full blood count, film and a Paul Bunnell or monospot test, if there is a persistent lymph node or neck lump, especially in a younger patient, as this may point to an inflammatory cause, such as infectious mononucleosis.

Patients should be referred to a head and neck clinic for urgent investigation under the 2-week rule (Chapter 5), if they have an unresolved neck mass for 3 weeks. The index of suspicion rises, if there are other symptoms, such as hoarseness or dysphagia, and in smokers and drinkers over the age of 45, especially if they are male.

The initial history taken in the head and neck clinic will identify the risk factors for malignancy and any additional symptoms, which might point to the underlying diagnosis. Physical examination will define whether the swelling is solitary or if additional swellings are present; whether it arises from a lymph node or another structure; and if there is a detectable primary tumour in the oral cavity, pharynx, larynx or at another site, such as the scalp or in the thyroid gland.

The location of lymph nodes in the neck may give a clue as to the likely primary site. The lymphatic drainage sites of head and neck cancers are classified into a number of "levels" for the purposes of description, and for neck dissection purposes, as described in the box below.

Following history and examination, one of the most important initial investigations will be fine needle aspiration of the lump for cytology (Chapter 7). This will, usually, indicate reliably whether or not the lump is malignant, and if so, the histological type. If it is a squamous cancer, the head and neck surgeon will undertake an examination under anaesthesia including bronchoscopy and oesophagoscopy. If no abnormality is visible, blind biopsies of the post-nasal space and the tongue base will be performed, and an ipsilateral tonsillectomy undertaken, as these are the most common sites for an occult primary tumour. Imaging investigations will include a chest X-ray and, usually, a CT scan. Open biopsy of the lymph node should not be undertaken unless no primary tumour can be found.

Often, by this stage, a definite diagnosis will be possible. For example, it may be a nasopharyngeal carcinoma or a squamous cancer of the tonsil with neck node spread, or a lymphoma. If, after full investigation, it turns out to be metastatic squamous carcinoma with no detectable primary tumour, then one of two approaches is possible. Radical radiotherapy to the whole neck including potential primary sites in the pharynx used to be the preferred option, and often resulted in no recurrence of the cancer. It is, however, associated with significant morbidity, and may be overtreatment. Nowadays, a radical neck dissection with postoperative radiotherapy limited to the affected side of the neck tends to be preferred. It provides good local control and results in fewer long-term sequelae than extensive radiotherapy. With careful follow-up, there may be no further problems. If a previously occult primary tumour becomes manifest, it can be dealt with on its own merits.

Cervical cancer

Cervical carcinoma is not the most common gynaeco-logical cancer, yet it has a higher public profile than, say, ovarian cancer, because it affects younger women and because of well-publicised failings in the cervical smear-screening system. However, deaths from carcinoma of the uterine cervix are thankfully becoming less common, largely due to the genuine efficacy of the screening programme. This aims to detect pre-malignant change which can be successfully treated before invasive squa-mous cancer develops (Chapter 6). However, screening does not detect all cases, and is not designed to detect adenocarcinoma. The recent introduction of chemoradio-therapy for advanced disease may have some further impact on survival figures.

Relative frequency of gynaecological cancers
(England and Wales)

Site	Number of cases	Incidence per 100,000 women	Number of deaths	Mortality per 100,000 women
Ovary	5,388	20.3	3,985	15.0
Endometrium	3,912	13.8	774	2.9
Cervix	3,400	10.4	1,225	4.6
Vulva	803	3.1	346	1.3
Vagina	209	0.8	89	0.3

Cervical cancer is a relatively rare cancer, account-ing for only about 6% of all malignancies in women in the Western world (although about 12% worldwide). In England and Wales in 1992, about 3,400 new cases were confirmed. Compare this with about 25,000 new cases of breast cancer. This means that the average general prac-titioner (GP) may expect to see a new case only every 9 years or so, but thousands of cervical smears will have been performed during this time.

Risk factors for the development of cervical carcinoma include early age at first intercourse, multiple sexual part-ners, smoking and lower socio-economic class.

As cervical and other gynaecological cancers are rela-tively rare, it is important that there are clearly identi-fied specialist gynaecological oncology services where expertise can be centralised. A district general hospital cancer unit should have a dedicated diagnostic and assess-ment service for women with symptoms suspicious of a gynaecological cancer, and for the investigation of asymp-tomatic women who present with abnormal smear tests. Cancer centres will have specialised multiprofessional gynaecological oncology teams responsible for the treat-ment of women referred with a definite diagnosis of female genital tract malignancy from a number of cancer unit diagnostic services.

REFERRAL OF SYMPTOMATIC PATIENTS FOR URGENT INVESTIGATION

> A recent normal cervical smear does not exclude the diagnosis of cervical cancer

Cervical cancer has a fairly constant rate of incidence in women over the age of 30 years, unlike ovarian and endometrial cancer, which are predominantly conditions of older women. The usual symptomatic presentation of cervical cancer is with vaginal bleeding, which may be intermenstrual, post-coital or post-menopausal. Abnor-mal bleeding must be taken seriously in women of any age. A recent normal cervical smear does not exclude the diagnosis of cervical cancer. National guidelines suggest that patients should be referred to a gynaecologist for urgent investigation under the "2-week rule" (Chapter 5), if there is any clinical suspicion of cervical cancer, particularly

- if there is a suspicious lesion seen on speculum examination,
- if there is more than one, or a single heavy, episode of post-menopausal bleeding in women aged for more than 55 years, who are not on hormone-replacement therapy (HRT),
- post-coital bleeding lasting for more than 4 weeks in a woman aged over 35 years.

Some GPs, however, will follow a more cautious approach and refer after one episode of post-coital or post-menopausal bleeding.

DIAGNOSIS

If cervical cytology is suspicious but the cervix appears to be relatively normal on speculum examination, colposcopy and biopsy is indicated. Sometimes, cone biopsy may be necessary in the presence of cervical intra-epithelial neoplasia to exclude the presence of invasive cancer. If the cervix appears abnormal, examination under anaesthesia (EUA) for biopsy and staging purposes may be the first investigation. An EUA and cystoscopy is always required for staging purposes when invasive cancer is confirmed.

PATHOLOGY

For all practical purposes, cervical cancer is either squamous cell (90%) or adenocarcinoma (10%). Other types, such as adenosquamous carcinoma, small cell carcinoma, lymphoma and sarcoma are all very rare. Both squamous carcinoma and adenocarcinoma are treated similarly. The difference lies in the aetiology and, therefore, the possibility of detection by screening. Squamous carcinoma is now thought to be caused principally by infection with various subtypes of human papilloma virus (HPV), which is sexually transmitted. The changes usually commence at the transition zone, where the squamous epithelium of the ectocervix meets the cuboidal epithelium of the endocervix. Abnormal cells in this area are readily detected by exfoliative cytology. Adenocarcinoma, which may occur in women who have never been sexually active, usually arises from glandular tissue in the cervical canal. Malignant cells arising in this area are not reliably picked up by cytological testing.

HISTOLOGY OF CERVICAL CARCINOMA

- Squamous cell carcinoma   90%
- Adenocarcinoma   10%

STAGING

Cervical cancer was one of the earliest tumour sites to be given a staging classification. The original "League of Nations" staging classification, sometimes called the FIGO (Fédération Internationale de Gynécologie et d'Obstétrique) classification, has been in place for more than half a century with only minor modifications. It has been adopted as the basis for the more modern TNM classification. The principal staging categories (but not all the details) are shown in the boxes.

BASIC TNM AND FIGO CLASSIFICATION OF CERVICAL CARCINOMA

TNM categories	FIGO stages	
TX		Primary tumour cannot be assessed
T0		No evidence of primary tumour
Tis	0	Carcinoma *in situ* (pre-invasive carcinoma, CIN III)
T1	I	Cervical carcinoma confined to uterus (extension to corpus should be disregarded)
T2	II	Cervical carcinoma invades beyond uterus but not to pelvic wall or to the lower third of the vagina
T3	III	Tumour extends to the pelvic wall and/or involves the lower third of the vagina, and/or causes hydronephrosis or non-functioning kidney
T4	IV	Tumour invades mucosa of the bladder or rectum, and/or extends beyond true pelvis

TNM T1 AND FIGO STAGE I

TNM categories	FIGO stages	
T1	I	Cervical carcinoma confined to uterus (extension to corpus should be disregarded)
T1a	IA	Invasive carcinoma diagnosed only by microscopy. All macroscopically visible lesions – even with superficial invasion – are T1b/IB
T1a1	IA1	Stromal invasion no greater than 3 mm in depth and 7 mm or less in horizontal spread
T1a2	IA2	Stromal invasion more than 3 mm and not more than 5 mm with a horizontal spread 7 mm or less
T1b	IB	Clinically visible lesion confined to the cervix or microscopic lesion greater than T1a2/IA2
T1b1	IB1	Clinically visible lesion 4 cm or less in greatest dimension
T1b2	IB2	Clinically visible lesion more than 4 cm in greatest dimension

TNM T2 AND FIGO STAGE II

TNM categories	FIGO stages	
T2	II	Cervical carcinoma invades beyond uterus, but not to pelvic wall or to the lower third of the vagina
T2a	II	Without parametrial involvement
T2b	IIb	With parametrial involvement

TNM T3 AND FIGO STAGE III

TNM categories	FIGO stages	
T3	III	Tumour extends to the pelvic wall and/or involves the lower third of the vagina, and/or causes hydronephrosis or non-functioning kidney
T3a	IIIA	Tumour involves lower third of the vagina, no extension to pelvic wall
T3b	IIIB	Tumour extends to pelvic wall and/or causes hydronephrosis or non-functioning kidney

FIGO STAGE IV CERVICAL CARCINOMA

Stage

IVA	T4a, any N, M0 in TNM system Tumour invades mucosa of the bladder or rectum, and/or extends beyond true pelvis
IVB	Any T, any N, M1 in TNM system Distant metastasis

N AND M STAGE IN TNM CLASSIFICATION

Stage

Regional lymph nodes (N)
NX Regional lymph nodes cannot be assessed
N0 No regional lymph node metastasis
N1 Regional lymph node metastasis

Distant metastasis (M)
MX Distant metastasis cannot be assessed
M0 No distant metastasis
M1 Distant metastasis

TREATMENT OF PRE-INVASIVE DISEASE

The precursor lesion of invasive squamous carcinoma of the cervix is dysplasia or carcinoma *in situ* (cervical intra-epithelial neoplasia – CIN). This development of invasive cancer from carcinoma *in situ* can be quite slow. In untreated patients with *in situ* cervical cancer, only 30–70% will develop invasive carcinoma over a period of 10–12 years. However, in about 10% of patients, lesions can progress from *in situ* to invasive in less than a year.

Properly treated, control of truly *in situ* disease should be nearly 100%. Failure to detect invasive disease may be the most common cause of failure, so careful assessment to exclude invasive disease is mandatory before therapy for carcinoma *in situ* is undertaken. Treatment options include loop electrosurgical excision procedure, laser therapy, cone biopsy and cryotherapy. In pre-menopausal women, especially when the endocervical canal is involved, laser or cold-knife conisation may be used for selected patients to preserve the uterus and fertility. Hysterectomy is an accepted therapy for the post-reproductive age group and is particularly indicated when the neoplastic process extends to the inner cone margin.

During pregnancy, no therapy is warranted for pre-invasive lesions of the cervix, including carcinoma *in situ*, although expert colposcopy is recommended to exclude invasive cancer.

TREATMENT OF EARLY INVASIVE (STAGE IA) CERVICAL CARCINOMA

Various treatment options are available, and the outcomes should be equivalent.

TREATMENT OF STAGE IA CERVICAL CARCINOMA

◆ Cone biopsy
◆ Simple hysterectomy
◆ Radical hysterectomy
◆ Intracavitary radiotherapy

In patients wishing to preserve fertility, cone biopsy alone may be adequate treatment, if the depth of invasion is less than 3 mm, no vascular or lymphatic channel invasion is noted, and the margins of the cone are negative.

If fertility is not an issue, simple hysterectomy is an alternative for the same group of patients. Ovarian preservation should be considered in younger women. Radical hysterectomy should be considered, if there is pathological evidence of more advanced disease, for example positive margins after cone biopsy or lymphovascular invasion.

Intracavitary radiation alone is an alternative for women who are not candidates for surgery.

TREATMENT OF STAGES IB AND IIA CERVICAL CARCINOMA

The basic choice in this patient group lies between primary surgery (with or without postoperative radiotherapy depending on histological findings) or radical radiotherapy (with or without chemotherapy). While for the same stages of disease, both approaches yield similar outcomes in terms of tumour control, surgery, where feasible, is preferred as it is less likely to affect bladder or bowel function and sexual enjoyment.

Primary surgery, which usually entails total abdominal hysterectomy including a cuff of vagina, bilateral salpingo-oophorectomy and pelvic lymph node dissection (Wertheim's procedure) is usually the treatment of choice in younger, fitter patients, especially those with small volume disease. Ovarian preservation is sometimes possible. This type of surgery should be performed only by specialist gynaecological oncology surgeons working in cancer centres. If there is pathological evidence of lymph node involvement, positive resection margins or residual parametrial disease, postoperative external beam radiotherapy is advisable. Careful preoperative assessment and selection of patients with more advanced disease for initial radiotherapy should mean that only a minority of patients require both surgery and radiotherapy. There is evidence that use of cisplatin-based chemotherapy along with radiotherapy improves outcome significantly.

In other patients, those who are older, less fit or who have more advanced disease, radiotherapy is usually the preferred option. This usually involves a combination of external beam radiotherapy to the pelvis and one or more intracavitary caesium insertions. Again, use of concomitant cisplatin chemotherapy is recommended in those who are fit enough.

TREATMENT OF ADVANCED (STAGES IIB, IIIA, IIIB AND IVA) CERVICAL CARCINOMA

Advanced disease is not usually suitable for primary surgery, and chemoradiotherapy is the standard treatment. There is good evidence that the addition of cisplatin (with or without other drugs, such as fluorouracil) gives better results than radiotherapy alone. However, not every patient will be considered fit enough for concomitant radiotherapy, and the frail and elderly, and those with impaired organ function (such as renal failure) may be better treated by radiotherapy alone. Radiotherapy will involve a combination of external beam and intracavitary irradiation. Ureteric obstruction, although it is a sign of advanced disease, does not by itself preclude attempts at curative treatment. Nephrostomies and/or ureteric stenting will be required prior to definitive treatment.

Exceptionally, carefully selected patients with extensive central pelvic disease may be suitable for radical pelvic surgery involving urinary or faecal diversion. It should go without saying that this type of pelvic excenteration should be performed only by very experienced surgeons.

TREATMENT OF METASTATIC (STAGE IVB) CERVICAL CANCER

There are no reliably curative approaches for the small group of patients who present with haematogenous metastases. Treatment will be essentially palliative in intent, although there may be a case in carefully selected patients for attempting to maximise the duration of disease control by giving "radical" treatment with chemoradiotherapy.

TREATMENT OF RECURRENT CANCER

Patients with recurrent cancer require careful assessment. Radiotherapy or chemoradiotherapy may be curative in women who have a localised pelvic recurrence after initial treatment with surgery alone. Exceptionally, surgery may be used to salvage a patient with recurrent disease in the pelvis following initial treatment with radiotherapy. For many patients, however, especially those who have developed distant metastases, only palliative care may be possible. If untreatable pelvic recurrence develops and causes ureteric obstruction, urinary diversion is not usually appropriate.

INVASIVE CERVICAL CANCER IN PREGNANCY

Treatment of invasive cervical cancer during pregnancy depends on the stage of the cancer and the maturity of the foetus when the cancer is detected. Immediate therapy, appropriate for the disease stage, is usually recommended when the cancer is diagnosed early in pregnancy. Therapy is delayed until after delivery of the baby only if the cancer is detected in the third trimester. In selected patients with Stages IA and early IB cervical cancer diagnosed in early or mid pregnancy, however, may be reasonable to wait for foetal maturity before initiating treatment. Naturally, pregnant patients require very careful counselling before any decisions are made.

OUTCOME

The prognosis of patients with cervical cancer depends on a number of factors, but the stage of the disease is important. Whatever the stage, the outcome is likely to

APPROXIMATE 5-YEAR SURVIVAL BY FIGO STAGE	
◆ I	80%
◆ II	60%
◆ III	30%
◆ IV	10%

be worse if the disease is bulky. In "operable" disease, the outcome will be worse if there is pelvic lymph node involvement, and this in turn is more likely with less well-differentiated tumours and when there is histological evidence of lymphatic or vascular invasion.

COMPLICATIONS OF TREATMENT

Successful treatment for cervical carcinoma comes at the price of significant morbidity. Most patients treated with either surgery or radiotherapy will lose their fertility, the exception being those treated by cone biopsy for Stage IA disease. Ovarian function will be lost in premenopausal women treated either by surgery involving oophorectomy or by radiotherapy. Fortunately, cervical carcinoma is not hormone sensitive malignancy, and so HRT is not associated with any problems. HRT is, therefore, recommended for younger women, say under the age of 45 or 50 years, who undergo oophorectomy or lose their ovarian function as a result of cervical cancer treatment, both to prevent osteoporosis and to improve their quality of life.

Patients who have a radical hysterectomy without radiotherapy will have a shortened vagina, which may affect sexual function. Patients treated with postoperative radiotherapy or radiotherapy alone may develop vaginal adhesions or vaginal stenosis, which may significantly affect sexual function. They should be provided with lubricants and vaginal dilators and encouraged to use these daily to minimise the scarring, which may take place. Regular sexual intercourse will help to maintain the vaginal cavity, but dryness after radiotherapy means that adequate lubrication is essential. Division of adhesions during sex, or trauma to the vaginal mucosa may lead to post-coital bleeding, and careful investigation will be necessary to exclude recurrent disease. Radiation changes in the bladder may lead to a smaller bladder capacity and intermittent haematuria. Clearly, haematuria will need to be investigated to rule out a more sinister cause than radiation damage. Radiation proctitis may lead to rectal bleeding. Discussion about these possible effects with the oncologist, GP or clinical nurse specialist before they occur will be helpful for patients, who may otherwise feel that all attention is given to the tumour, but that the patient herself is neglected.

Ovarian cancer

Ovarian cancer is the most common gynaecological malignancy. There are over 5,000 new cases per year in the UK, so a general practitioner (GP) with a list size of 2,000 patients might expect a new patient every 5 years or so. The mortality of ovarian cancer is high, with a 5-year survival rate of only about 35%, so deaths from ovarian cancer outnumber those from cervix and endometrium combined. Ovarian cancer is most common in nulliparous women, and the risk is proportional to the number of years of ovulation, so there is also an association with an early menarche and a late menopause. Suppression of ovulation by the oral contraceptive pill may be protective. Most cases of ovarian cancer are sporadic, but in about 5% there may be a genetic predisposition such as BRCA-1 or less commonly BRCA-2 mutation. The familial cancer predisposition syndromes and their management are discussed in Chapters 1 and 4.

PATHOLOGY

> **PRINCIPAL PATHOLOGICAL TYPES OF OVARIAN TUMOURS (WHO)**
>
> *Common epithelial tumours* (benign, borderline or malignant)
> - Serous tumour
> - Mucinous tumour
> - Mixed epithelial tumour
> - Undifferentiated carcinomas
>
> *Sex cord stromal tumours*
> - Granulosa cell tumour
> - Androblastoma: Sertoli–leydig cell tumour
>
> *Germ cell tumours*
> - Dysgerminoma
> - Endodermal sinus tumour (yolk sac tumour)
> - Choriocarcinoma
> - Teratoma
>
> *Others*

The pathology of primary ovarian neoplasms is very diverse. There is a broad spectrum of malignancy from definitely benign, through borderline tumours which have low metastatic potential, to frankly malignant tumours which may be well, moderately or poorly differentiated. A number of classifications are available, of which the World Health Organisation (WHO) system is the most widely used. The majority of cancers, about 85%, arise from the surface epithelium of the ovary and the peak age incidence is in women aged from 50 to 70. Among the various sorts of epithelial cancers, histological grade is of greater prognostic importance than the subtype. Rarer tumours arise from ovarian germ cells, from endocrine cells (sex cord stromal tumours) and other cell types and are more commonly seen in younger women. Metastases from other cancers can be found in the ovaries, but this is not a common presenting feature. More often they arise on the background of, for example, previously treated lobular breast cancer, or stomach cancer, when they are known as Krukenberg tumours.

PRESENTATION

There is no clear evidence that population screening is effective in reducing death from ovarian cancer, and so there is no national programme. Screening of selected groups of women at high risk, for example those known to carry a mutation of BRCA-1, may be different, and there are ongoing clinical studies in this area. Screening has been discussed further in Chapter 6.

The majority of patients with ovarian cancer have a symptomatic presentation. As the disease has usually spread beyond the pelvis at the time of diagnosis, non-specific symptoms such as bloating, swelling of the abdomen, vague abdominal discomfort, backache, fluid retention, "indigestion", altered bowel habit and weight loss predominate. Local symptoms such as a feeling of pressure in the pelvis and urinary frequency may also occur. Symptoms from distant metastases at presentation are very rare. Many patients with ovarian cancer initially have such vague symptoms that the GP is not consulted for some time. When a previously fit woman with these non-specific symptoms does eventually come for a consultation, a high index of suspicion for ovarian cancer is necessary.

On abdominal examination, a mass arising from the pelvis is often palpable, and ascites is often present. On pelvic examination, it is usually possible to feel a mass *per vagina* (PV) and *per rectum* (PR), even if abdominal examination is normal. Occasionally, enlarged lymph nodes are palpable.

The first line of investigation is usually an abdominal and pelvic ultrasound which may show a pelvic mass, often partly solid, partly cystic, lymphadenopathy, ascites and tumour nodules within the abdomen. In women with a pelvic mass, the ultrasound, combined with the blood tests CA 125, and taking the age of the patient into account may well point strongly to a diagnosis of ovarian cancer. These three parameters together can be used to define a risk of malignancy with 80–90% sensitivity and specificity. The GP will refer the patient to a gynaecologist who will arrange for further investigation and management by a multidisciplinary gynaecological cancer team, including a specialist gynaecological oncologist. A computed tomography (CT) scan will usually be requested to demonstrate the extent of the disease more fully. If symptoms are more vague, the initial referral may be to another specialist such as a gastro-enterologist or a general abdominal surgeon. As soon as a diagnosis of ovarian cancer seems likely, the patient should be referred on to the specialist multidisciplinary team.

STAGING

SIMPLIFIED FIGO STAGING SYSTEM FOR OVARIAN CANCER

Stage I Limited to the ovaries
    IA   One ovary, capsule intact
    IB   Both ovaries, capsule intact
    IC   Capsule ruptured, tumour on surface, malignant cells in ascites or peritoneal washings
Stage II Pelvic extension
    IIA   Uterus, tubes
    IIB   Other pelvic tissues
    IIC   Malignant cells in ascites or peritoneal washings
Stage III Peritoneal metastasis beyond pelvis and/or regional lymph node metastasis
    IIIA Microscopic peritoneal metastasis
    IIIB Macroscopic peritoneal metastasis $\leqslant 2$ cm
    IIIB Macroscopic peritoneal metastasis > 2 cm and/or regional lymph node metastasis
Stage IV Distant metastasis, excluding peritoneal metastasis
    Note: Liver capsule metastasis is Stage III, liver parenchymal metastasis is Stage IV. Pleural effusion must have positive cytology for Stage IV.

The principles of cancer staging have been discussed in Chapter 8. The staging of ovarian cancer is important in determining the correct treatment and in predicting prognosis. Ovarian cancer is staged most commonly according to the International Federation of Obstetrics and Gynaecology (FIGO) system. A separate TNM classification exists which parallels the FIGO system. Although the stage can be guessed at preoperatively, the definitive diagnosis and staging cannot usually be stated before surgery. There is evidence that staging is more accurate and reliable when performed by specialist gynaecological oncologists.

SURGERY

An operation is usually undertaken shortly after diagnosis in patients with ovarian cancer. There is evidence of better outcome if it is performed by a gynaecologist rather than a general surgeon, and even better if performed by a specialist gynaecological oncologist rather than a general gynaecologist. The specialist multidisciplinary team, therefore, plays a crucial role in the management of patients with ovarian cancer. Patients should be advised by their GP that it is in their interests to be assessed and treated in a specialist centre, even if that does involve some travelling away from home.

In addition to obtaining tissue to confirm the diagnosis, surgery enables accurate staging of the disease and is an important part of treatment. Surgery is potentially curative in Stage I and II disease. Usually, surgery will comprise a total abdominal hysterectomy and bilateral salpingo-oophorectomy (BSO) along with removal of the omentum. If there is no ascites or other obvious disease beyond the confines of the pelvis, peritoneal washings and retroperitoneal lymph node biopsies may show that the disease is more advanced than was initially apparent. For the small number of pre-menopausal women with early, unilateral invasive cancer or with borderline tumours, unilateral salpingo-oophorectomy (USO) can be offered in an attempt to preserve fertility with only a small chance of recurrence.

The majority of patients, however, have more advanced disease. Although it is never possible to remove all tumour in Stage III disease it is clear that maximum debulking surgery in epithelial ovarian cancer makes chemotherapy more likely to be successful and extends survival. In the rare case of an ovarian germ cell tumour, chemotherapy alone should be curative without the need for such radical surgery, and fertility may often be preserved. The operation ideally will include total abdominal hysterectomy, bilateral salpingo-oophorectomy, omentectomy and removal of as many tumour deposits as possible. The ideal is to remove all macroscopic tumour. As this is only rarely possible, surgery should aim to ensure that the volume of residual disease is as small as can reasonably be achieved, hopefully with no tumour deposits greater than 2 cm diameter remaining. In many patients with advanced disease, maximum cytoreductive surgery is not possible at presentation. In these patients, consideration should be given to interval surgery (sometimes called "second-look laparotomy") after chemotherapy, if there has been a good response, as previously inoperable disease may have been rendered resectable. This is probably especially important if the first operation was not performed by an experienced gynaecological oncologist.

The role of further surgery in patients whose disease relapses after good quality initial surgery and chemotherapy is less clear-cut. There is no evidence that this practice contributes to a better outcome, but it may be justified in patients who are fit when a long interval has elapsed since the original treatment.

CHEMOTHERAPY

Chemotherapy is indicated for all women with epithelial ovarian cancer other than those with well- or moderately well-differentiated Stage IA and IB cancers. Over the years, the type of chemotherapy used has changed from older alkylating agents, such as chlorambucil and cyclophosphamide, as the platinum drugs cisplatin and carboplatin became available. Over the last decade the value of the taxane, paclitaxel has become apparent.

Chemotherapy for ovarian cancer has been a very controversial area, not least because of the expense of the drugs, but also because although undoubtedly effective at relieving symptoms and prolonging life, most patients with advanced ovarian cancer will still die from their disease. As a result of this controversy, many large-scale randomised trials have been performed and the evidence base for the use of chemotherapy, and for favouring one drug or combination over another is now much firmer. The use of platinum drugs has consistently been found to be beneficial in comparison with older schedules. The 5-year-survival rates are increased by about 5% from 25% to 30%. No difference in efficacy has been found between carboplatin and cisplatin, but carboplatin use is associated with a better quality of life. The addition of paclitaxel to platinum based, chemotherapy has improved the outcome in terms of median survival by approximately 1 year from about 2–3 years. The standard treatment schedule is six courses, and no convincing benefit has yet been shown for more protracted schedules. Similarly, dose intensification has not been shown to be beneficial.

Cost-based differences in prescribing practice of chemotherapy for ovarian cancer have had a high public and political profile. The so-called postcode lottery has meant that paclitaxel was available even in the same cancer centre for some women but not for others depending on their health authority of residence. As a result, assessment of the value of paclitaxel was one of the first priorities for NICE, the newly formed National Institute for Clinical Excellence. The guidance from NICE in May 2000 stated that "paclitaxel in combination with platinum therapy (cisplatin or carboplatin) should be the standard initial therapy for patients with ovarian cancer following surgery. The use of paclitaxel/platinum-combination therapy in the treatment of recurrent or resistant ovarian cancer is recommended, if the patient has not previously received this drug combination." The situation remains a dynamic one, however. Preliminary results from another large randomised trial, ICON 3 do not appear to substantiate the routine use of paclitaxel, but the data are as yet too immature to influence policy or practice. NICE will update its guidance periodically taking into account any new evidence.

The other available taxane, docetaxel, has been shown to have useful activity in ovarian cancer, but large-scale clinical studies have not yet been conducted and the drug is not licensed for this indication. Similarly, other relatively new drugs are being studied in early phase clinical trials and may in time assume an important role.

Women who relapse after chemotherapy for epithelial ovarian cancer are incurable, and the prognosis is poor, with a median survival of only about 9 months. Nonetheless, some do respond to further treatment, especially if their disease-free interval has been longer than a year. Those responding to second-line chemotherapy will experience a survival benefit.

RADIOTHERAPY

Although radiotherapy historically had some benefit in patients with ovarian cancer, its use has now been almost completely superseded by chemotherapy. Radiotherapy now plays only a minor role in the palliative treatment of chemorefractory advanced disease, such as for pain from pelvic recurrence or for bleeding from deposits at the vaginal vault.

PALLIATIVE CARE

The palliative care of women with ovarian cancer is challenging, not just quantitatively as over 4,000 women die each year in the UK from this disease, but qualitatively as they commonly experience difficult to manage problems such as ascites and intestinal obstruction.

Simple ascites can be managed by abdominal paracentesis, but this is uncomfortable and will lead to protein depletion and dependent oedema. The use of intraperitoneal sclerosants to diminish the likelihood of reaccumulation of ascites is not beneficial and can lead to complications. Sometimes, surgery to insert a Le Veen peritoneal venous shunt can be considered, but this is not always successful and can also be accompanied by complications.

Subacute intestinal obstruction will usually settle with conservative management, but often recurs. Surgery is sometimes appropriate, especially if there is no known intra-abdominal tumour as it may be due, for example, to adhesions which may be divided successfully. More often, the small bowel is obstructed by tumour masses at multiple levels which would not easily be relieved surgically. In these cases, other measures such as high-dose parenteral steroids or octreotide infusions may be helpful.

Pain is a common feature of end-stage ovarian cancer, and can be managed in the usual ways (Chapter 50). Care has to be taken, of course, to ensure that it is not due to a relatively easily remediable cause such as constipation, and conversely that treatments such as opioid analgesia do not lead to other problems such as constipation.

RARE OVARIAN TUMOURS

Ovarian tumours other than the common epithelial cancers are all rare. The different types listed earlier in this chapter together account for fewer than 15% of cases, and so a GP is unlikely to see most of these. Nonetheless, it may be helpful to outline the salient features of each tumour type in case they are encountered.

Ovarian fibroma, sometimes called a Brenner tumour is benign and usually cured with surgery alone.

Borderline ovarian tumours have low metastatic potential, but it is unwise to think of them as benign. The 5-year survival rates are good at over 90%, but late relapse and metastasis occur and 5-year survival does not equate with cure. Fifteen-year survival rates are only of the order of 70–80%.

Ovarian germ cell tumours are similar in many ways to testicular germ cell tumours. They may occur in childhood and are most common in young adults. The most common sort is the benign ovarian teratoma or dermoid cyst which is cured by surgery alone. Dysgerminoma is the most common malignant type, and is similar histologically to testicular seminoma. There is a tendency for the disease to be bilateral. A high proportion of patients were cured by surgery and radiotherapy, in past eras; nowadays, chemotherapy following surgery is preferred. The prognosis is extremely good, and fertility may be preserved after limited surgery and chemotherapy. Several varieties of non-germinomatous ovarian germ cell tumours may be encountered. Unlike dysgerminomas, these usually produce tumour markers, for example alpha-fetoprotein (AFP) in the case of endodermal sinus (yolk sac) tumours and beta human chorionic gonadotrophin (bhCG) in the case of choriocarcinoma. The advent of modern chemotherapy has transformed the outlook for patients with these tumours, which were previously often fatal.

The sex cord stromal tumours include granulosa cell or granulosa–theca cell tumours, which are of low grade. They produce oestrogens, and this may be associated with the development of a synchronous endometrial carcinoma. Sometimes, granulosa cell tumours are unexpected findings at hysterectomy for endometrial cancer. Surgery alone is usually adequate treatment for granulosa cell tumours, but late pelvic recurrence can occur, and oestrogen levels can be used as a tumour marker. Sertoli–leydig cell tumours, also called androblastoma or arrhenoblastoma are similar to granulosa cell tumours but tend to produce androgens and therefore often present with virilisation. They tend to occur most commonly in young adults, and are usually cured with surgery.

Other tumour types which can occur in the ovary are sarcomas, often mixed mesodermal tumours such as those which occur in the uterus, and high-grade non-Hodgkin's lymphomas, the management of which is described in Chapter 41.

CHAPTER 33

Other gynaecological malignancy

Carcinoma of the uterine cervix has been covered in Chapter 31 and ovarian cancer in Chapter 32. This chapter deals with endometrial cancer, uterine sarcomas, cancers of the fallopian tubes, vulva and vagina and gestational trophoblastic tumours.

ENDOMETRIAL CARCINOMA

Endometrial carcinoma is second to ovarian cancer in terms of incidence among gynaecological malignancies, with about 4,000 cases per year in the UK. It is most common among older women, the median age at diagnosis is 61 years. As many as 80% of patients are post-menopausal, and so it, usually, presents as post-menopausal bleeding. This is, usually, defined as vaginal bleeding occurring more than 6 months after the last period. About 10% of women with post-menopausal bleeding are found on investigation to have endometrial carcinoma. National criteria for urgent referral under the "2-week rule" (Chapter 5) to the gynaecological assessment service at the cancer unit for investigation are more than one episode, or a single heavy episode, of post-menopausal bleeding in a woman over the age of 55 years, who is not on hormone-replacement therapy (HRT).

However, many general practitioners (GPs) are more cautious than these guidelines suggest, and will refer any woman with even a single episode of post-menopausal bleeding, whatever her age. Women of a certain age who develop "menopausal" symptoms, such as hot flushes and are started on HRT may never experience a true menopause. Irregular bleeding in this group of women also has to be regarded with a degree of suspicion and merits early investigation.

Investigation will usually take the form of transvaginal ultrasound imaging, which will show the thickness of the endometrium and can be used to estimate the depth of myometrial penetration. Ultrasound alone can reliably exclude the presence of endometrial cancer in three-quarters of patients investigated for post-menopausal bleeding.

If the scan shows that the endometrium is more than 5 mm thick, outpatient aspiration biopsy should be performed. These two tests will not only confirm or refute the suspicion of cancer, but are used to stratify patients for risk and guide referral of more advanced cases to the cancer centre for surgery. Ultrasound and biopsy will not only confirm the presence of cancer (which is usually an adenocarcinoma), but will indicate the grade. Diagnostic dilatation and curettage (D&C) should be used only when outpatient aspiration biopsy is unsuccessful, and is particularly inappropriate for women under the age of 40 in whom the diagnosis of endometrial cancer is unlikely – fewer than 5% of cases occur in this age group.

SIMPLIFIED FIGO STAGING OF ENDOMETRIAL CANCER

I   Tumour confined to the corpus uteri
     IA: Tumour limited to the endometrium
     IB: Tumour invades up to less than one-half of the myometrium
     IC: Tumour invades to more than half of the myometrium
II   Tumour invades cervix, but does not extend beyond uterus
III   Local and/or regional spread
     IIIA: Tumour involves serosa and/or adnexa and/or cancer cells in ascites or peritoneal washings
     IIIB: Vaginal involvement
     IIIC: Metastasis to pelvic and/or para-aortic lymph nodes
IVA   Tumour invades bladder mucosal and/or bowel mucosal
IVB   Distant metastasis

About 40% of cases have disease, which is only Grade 1 or 2, and penetrates less than half the thickness of

---

TRANSVAGINAL ULTRASOUND IMAGING TO INVESTIGATE POST-MENOPAUSAL BLEEDING

- The negative predictive value of transvaginal ultrasound imaging – the accuracy for excluding a diagnosis of endometrial cancer in a woman with post-menopausal bleeding – is close to 100%

the myometrium. These cases are low risk, and total abdominal hysterectomy (TAH) and bilateral salpingo-oophorectomy (BSO) at the cancer unit is appropriate. No further treatment is likely to be necessary.

The grade of the tumour and the extent to which a tumour invades the muscle of the uterus are indicative of the likelihood of lymph node metastasis. If the scan shows a tumour reaching the outer half of the myometrium, or if the cancer is reported as Grade 3 by the pathologist, then the patient should be referred on to a specialist gynaecological cancer centre. Most of these patients will proceed to surgery with TAH and BSO (possibly with pelvic lymph node dissection), but radiotherapy is an alternative, if surgery is not appropriate for any reason, such as intercurrent illness.

In the light of the final pathology report, many higher-risk patients will be advised to have postoperative radiotherapy. This may involve a course of external beam radiotherapy to the pelvis, or one or more intracavitary caesium insertions to the vaginal vault or both.

Chemotherapy has no role in the initial radical treatment of women with endometrial cancer. It may have a very limited palliative role in those who present with metastatic disease, or in whom the disease recurs after initial treatment.

Progestogens were once offered as adjuvant therapy, but a number of randomised trials have shown no evidence of any benefit, and so this practice is no longer undertaken.

For patients who develop recurrent disease in the pelvis after initial treatment with surgery alone, radiotherapy may be beneficial.

Overall, 70–75% of women treated for endometrial carcinoma are cured. The likelihood of cure is related to grade and stage and treatment. Optimally treated patients with well-differentiated Stage I disease have a survival probability at 5 years of the order of 90%. Patients with more advanced disease fare worse: 5-year survival rates are 60–70% for patients with Stage II disease, 30–40% for patients with Stage III disease and about 10% for patients with Stage IV disease.

UTERINE SARCOMAS

Sarcomas account for less than 5% of cancers of the body of the uterus, and so are rare with an incidence in the UK of fewer than 200 cases per year. Presentation is usually with vaginal bleeding, or with pain or as a pelvic mass. An accurate preoperative diagnosis is made in only one-third of cases, and sometimes a sarcoma is diagnosed following hysterectomy in a woman thought to have fibroids. Initial treatment is with TAH and BSO, wherever possible. Staging is broadly according to the FIGO classification for endometrial cancers. Postoperative radiotherapy and chemotherapy are often given, but they may have no influence on survival.

Pathologically, there are several types, leiomyosarcoma being the commonest. The average age at presentation is about 50 years. Prognosis is related to histological grade. Overall, about a quarter of patients with leiomyosarcoma survive for 5 years.

Endometrial stromal sarcomas occur in a similar age group. Again, grade is the most powerful predictor of survival. About three-quarters of patients with low-grade tumours, but only about 20% with high-grade disease, will be cured.

Mixed Müllerian tumours (sometimes termed carcinosarcomas) occur in a slightly older age group, the median age at diagnosis is about 60 years. Overall, only about 20% of patients survive long term.

FALLOPIAN TUBE CARCINOMA

Primary carcinoma of the fallopian tube is rare, accounting for less than 1% of female genital tract cancer. The tubes are more commonly involved by spread from other gynaecological tumours, such as endometrial or ovarian cancer. The median age is around 60 years, but fallopian tube carcinoma can occur in much younger women. The disease may present with vaginal discharge or bleeding, or with pelvic pain or a mass, or with symptoms related to intraperitoneal spread, or metastases to pelvic and para-aortic lymph nodes.

Initial treatment is usually with TAH and BSO. The disease is staged in a similar way to ovarian cancer. Postoperatively, treatment with pelvic radiotherapy is often given, and chemotherapy schedules similar to those used for ovarian cancer may be recommended, although because of the rarity of the disease, there is relatively little evidence about efficacy. Stage and the completeness of surgical resection are the most powerful predictors of outcome. Overall, the 5-year survival probability is about one-third.

CARCINOMA OF THE VULVA

Vulval cancer is rare with only about 800 cases per year in England and Wales. The average GP may, therefore, only expect to see one case during a professional lifetime. It tends to affect older women – three-quarters of cases occur in women over 65. As with cervical cancer, the diagnosis of invasive vulval cancer may be preceded by the diagnosis of pre-invasive cancer – vulval intra-epithelial neoplasia or VIN. In two-thirds of cases, the cancer of the vulva affects the labia majora; in the remainder the clitoris, the labia minora, the fourchette or the perineum may be involved. Inguinal lymph nodes are involved in 30–40% of cases.

GPs should refer any woman with symptoms, which could be caused by vulval cancer, persistent itching, irritation or pain that fails to respond to local treatments, or ulceration or visible lesions with or without palpable enlarged groin nodes, to their local gynaecological oncology assessment unit for biopsy. When diagnosed, vulval cancer requires highly specialised treatment and all patients should be referred on for treatment in a specialist cancer centre. Malignant disease of the vulva is usually squamous cancer, but other tumours, such as malignant melanoma, basal cell carcinoma and adenocarcinoma, may occur.

Surgery is the mainstay of treatment for vulval cancer, irrespective of the age of the patient. This is most often a radical vulvectomy including lymph node dissection. Postoperative radiotherapy may be indicated for those with positive lymph nodes. Radical vulvectomy is mutilating and may remove all capacity for sexual enjoyment. In very carefully selected patients with less advanced disease, a lesser procedure preserving sexual function may be appropriate, but this clearly requires skilled decision-making based on specialist knowledge and experience, if cure is not to be compromised. For some patients with more advanced disease, radical radiotherapy or chemo-radiotherapy may be preferred to primary surgery.

Survival clearly correlates with stage. More than 80% of those without lymph node involvement will be expected to survive this disease, the likelihood of survival drops to only half that, if there is lymph node involvement. Overall, perhaps three-quarters of patients will be cured.

CARCINOMA OF THE VAGINA

Primary cancers of the vagina are rare, there are only about 200 cases per year in England and Wales. As with fallopian tube carcinoma, secondary involvement by other female genital tract cancers is more common. As with cervical and vulval cancer, invasive disease may be preceded by vaginal intra-epithelial neoplasia or VAIN. The disease is essentially one of elderly, often socially disadvantaged, women. Historically, there was an association with uterine prolapse and the use of ring pessaries. Vaginal adenocarcinomas used to be seen occasionally in teenagers and young women, who had been exposed *in utero* to diethylstilboestrol.

Presentation may be with vaginal bleeding or discharge or with fistula formation or ureteric obstruction in the case of advanced disease. Women with symptoms or signs suspicious of vaginal carcinoma, or other female genital tract malignancy, should be referred to their local gynaecological cancer assessment unit. The disease is staged according to an FIGO classification. One-third have Stage I disease, the majority have more advanced disease. If the diagnosis of vaginal cancer is confirmed, patients will be referred on to a specialist gynaecological centre for treatment. Most patients will be treated with radical radiotherapy, but some younger, fitter patients with less advanced disease will be suitable for radical surgery. Outcome is related to stage. Reported survival for Stage I disease varies widely from about 50% to 80%, but unfortunately the majority of patients with more advanced disease fare much worse.

GESTATIONAL TROPHOBLASTIC TUMOURS

Gestational trophoblastic tumours arise from the placenta, most usually early in pregnancy or after a first-trimester abortion. Much less commonly, they can arise some time after a normal-term delivery, usually within a year. There are a variety of different types, including hydatidiform mole, partial mole, invasive mole and choriocarcinoma.

Choriocarcinoma may develop after a normal pregnancy, a non-molar abortion, ectopic pregnancy or hydatidiform mole. Histologically, it is characterised by rapidly dividing and invasive villous trophoblast. It often metastasises widely to the lungs, brain and pelvic organs.

Management of these tumours is highly specialised, and patients with confirmed or suspected invasive mole or choriocarcinoma are referred for management to one of two centres in the UK in London or Sheffield. Patients are assessed and stratified into risk groups. Chemotherapy is the mainstay of treatment, and response is assessed by serial measurements of the tumour marker, human chorionic gonadotrophin (hCG). All patients in the low-risk group can expect to be cured, and over 90% of patients in the intermediate and high-risk groups will be cured, if they are managed properly in experienced centres. Most of the mortality comes when patients are not immediately referred to specialist centres, but are mis-managed until the disease is very advanced.

Skin cancer and melanoma

Skin cancer is the most common type of malignant disease. There are about 30,000 cases of skin cancer registered each year in the UK. This is, however, a gross underestimate of the real incidence of the disease. The true incidence is not known, as many small skin lesions are ablated *in situ* with physical treatments such as cautery, curettage or cryotherapy without any attempt being made to obtain a histological diagnosis. It has been estimated that about a million people in the US are diagnosed with skin cancer each year. Fortunately, the commonest types of skin cancer are usually totally curable, so the mortality from skin cancer is very low.

HISTOLOGICAL TYPES OF SKIN CANCER

> **RELATIVE INCIDENCE OF COMMON SKIN CANCERS**
>
> ◆ Basal cell carcinoma   30
> ◆ Squamous cell carcinoma   4
> ◆ Malignant melanoma   1

The skin is a complex organ with a variety of cell types, therefore there are several distinct types of skin cancer, with differing incidence rates and natural histories. The commonest skin cancers are basal cell carcinoma (BCC), squamous cell carcinoma (SCC) and malignant melanoma (MM). Rare skin cancers include Merkel cell carcinoma, cutaneous lymphoma and Kaposi's sarcoma. It is important to distinguish malignant skin tumours from benign tumours and pre-malignant change. Of course, the skin is not infrequently the site for metastases from various other cancers, but these are not considered here.

AETIOLOGY OF SKIN CANCER

Sun exposure and other sources of ultraviolet (UV) light are the principal cause of both malignant melanoma and non-melanoma skin cancer. Basal and squamous cancers seem to be related to cumulative exposure to UVB light. These cancers are most common on exposed parts of the body, such as the face and the back of the hands. They are more common in outdoor workers, and they are more common in countries, such as Australia, which are blessed with a more sunny climate than Britain. Natural skin pigmentation and tanning offer some protection, and fair-skinned races are much more vulnerable. The incidence of melanoma seems to correlate better with episodes of sunburn, especially in early life, than with cumulative sun exposure. General practitioners (GPs) should encourage their patients to avoid excessive sun exposure, especially around midday when the sun is at its highest, by wearing protective clothing, such as a wide-brimmed hat and large sunglasses, and using sunscreens. A good time for opportunist intervention is when patients attend for immunisation prior to foreign holidays. If the GP sees a young child in the surgery on a sunny day, he can use the opportunity to advise the parents of the dangers of the sun. In Australia, it is compulsory for schoolchildren to "slip, slop, slap".

> **SLIP, SLOP, SLAP TO PREVENT SUNBURN AND REDUCE SKIN CANCER INCIDENCE**
>
> ◆ Slip on a top
> ◆ Slop on sunscreen
> ◆ Slap on a hat

Less commonly, skin cancer may be related to physical or chemical carcinogens, but many of these now are only of historical interest. They include soot, mineral oils, arsenic, ionising radiation, scarring due to trauma (such as burns), and chronic inflammation (such as chronic granulomatous diseases, namely, syphilis, leprosy and cutaneous tuberculosis) and chronic ulcers or sinuses. Some cases of skin cancer may be related to human papilloma virus (HPV) infection, especially if there is chronic immunosuppression, such as in renal transplant recipients. There are a number of rare genetic conditions, such as xeroderma pigmentosum (a disorder of DNA repair) and Gorlin's syndrome where multiple skin cancers may occur.

DIAGNOSIS

Skin cancers can take a variety of forms. Although "rodent ulcer" is a commonly used synonym for BCC, the majority of early basal cell cancers are not ulcerated. They appear as nodules, most often on the face of older men and women whose skin may (but does not always) show general signs of excessive sun exposure.

LOCATION OF BCCs

- 90% occur on the head and neck
- 75% occur on the face

The nodules are often described as pearly in appearance, and they may be traversed by telangiectasia. Sometimes the nodule may be cystic, and sometimes it is pigmented. As it grows, it may ulcerate and a scab may form, with bleeding if it is displaced. Superficial BCCs, described as "morphoeic", may spread laterally without much by way of nodularity. The indistinct margins may become more apparent when the underlying skin is stretched. Very rarely one comes across a large, neglected "rodent ulcer" which may have been concealed for years, during which time it has destroyed a large part of the underlying skin, cartilage and bone. BCCs grow only very slowly, and for all practical purposes never metastasise, and so there is usually no need for urgent referral of a typical lesion.

SCC *in situ*, or Bowen's disease, typically appears as a flat red plaque with clearly defined edges. Usually, invasive squamous cancers appear on the sun-exposed skin of older people, for example the face or the dorsum of the hand, the extensor aspect of the forearm or the back of the neck. Other signs of sun exposure are dryness, photo-ageing and actinic keratoses. They may be nodular or ulcerated and are sometimes capped with keratin. Macroscopically it can, sometimes, be difficult to distinguish invasive squamous cancers from keratin horns, keratoacanthomas and actinic keratoses. Biopsy of part of a squamous lesion may be misleading, and it is often better, if possible, to excise the entire lesion for histology if it is small.

Patients in whom an SCC has been diagnosed from a biopsy in general practice should be referred for treatment to an oncologist or a dermatology clinic. As squamous cancers which develop in immunosuppressed patients can be unusually aggressive, it is recommended that transplant patients who develop new or growing cutaneous lesions should be referred for urgent assessment under the 2-week rule. Rarely, the patient may present with lymphadenopathy due to secondary spread from a cutaneous squamous carcinoma which, in itself, has seemed too trivial to merit medical attention, or was treated some time previously. These patients should, of course, be referred urgently for assessment.

Other patients with slowly growing, non-healing lesions with significant induration on palpation, and with documented expansion over 1 or 2 months, should also be referred urgently.

Malignant melanoma may present as a pigmented macule or nodule developing in an area of previously normal skin, or as a change in a pre-existing pigmented mole. Some melanomas are not pigmented. Melanoma may also arise within the eye, or on mucosal surfaces, such as that of the oral cavity or paranasal sinuses, the vagina or the anus. Sometimes, malignant melanoma may present with local lymph node enlargement, or with symptoms of distant metastases, before the primary tumour has been diagnosed.

Patients suspected to have a malignant melanoma should not undergo biopsy in the general practice setting, but should be referred urgently to a dermatologist for assessment under the "2-week rule" (Chapter 5). This would include any patient with a pigmented lesion on any part of the body which is either growing in size, changing in shape or has an irregular outline, changing in colour or has a mixed colour, or becomes ulcerated or inflamed. Early referral is the key to reducing mortality from malignant melanoma, and two useful tools have been devised which may aid appropriate referral. These are the "ABCD rule" and the "seven-point checklist" (see the boxes below).

THE ABCD RULE FOR REFERRING PATIENTS WITH SUSPECTED MELANOMA

- **A**symmetry
- **B**order irregularity
- **C**olour variation or dark black colour
- **D**iameter greater than 6 mm

SEVEN-POINT CHECKLIST: CLINICAL FEATURES OF EARLY MALIGNANT MELANOMA

- Major features
  1. Change in size of previous lesion or obvious growth of new lesion
  2. Irregular shape – asymmetry and an irregular outline of a newly developed pigmented lesion or appearance of this feature in an old lesion
  3. Irregular colour – a variety of shades of brown or black in a new or old lesion
- Minor features
  4. Largest diameter 7 mm or greater. Most benign acquired naevi are smaller than this.
  5. Inflammation – rare in benign lesions unless they are regularly traumatised
  6. Oozing, crusting or bleeding (not seen in naevi)
  7. Change in sensation – usually described as mild itch

There are four major subtypes of cutaneous malignant melanoma.

The majority, over half in most series, are superficial spreading melanomas. They usually manifest as an expanding, irregularly-shaped brown lesion or black lesion at the site of a pre-existing naevus. They are usually flat.

Nodular melanomas are the next most common type, accounting for about a quarter of cases. These present as rapidly growing nodules arising most often in previously normal skin. They are usually red, grey or black although sometimes they are not pigmented. They often bleed or crust at an early stage.

Acral lentiginous melanoma is comparatively less common than other melanoma subtypes in the white population. However, in black and Asian people in whom melanoma generally is less common, the acral lentiginous melanoma subtype accounts for a greater proportion of all melanomas. It may develop on the palms of the hands or the soles of the feet or in the nailbed. They are often large, and tend to occur in older people.

Lentigo maligna melanoma is uncommon. It tends to present on the face of elderly ladies, as a change in a lesion which may have been present for years.

TREATMENT OF BASAL CELL CARCINOMA

The treatment of many BCCs is based upon a clinical diagnosis. However, where clinical doubt exists because the appearances are atypical, or when patients are to be referred for specialised forms of treatment such as radiotherapy, initial biopsy is mandatory. Sometimes, of course, it may be reasonable not to offer treatment at all. If the patient is very frail or elderly and has a serious intercurrent illness, for example, the tumour may not be likely to cause significant morbidity in the patient's remaining lifespan. Individual tumours can be divided into low-risk and high-risk categories. The histological subtype has a direct bearing on prognosis, and other prognostic features are listed in the box below.

It is recommended that patients with high-risk tumours should be assessed in a joint consultation clinic staffed by a dermatologist, a plastic surgeon and a clinical oncologist to facilitate the selection of the most appropriate treatment. At some anatomical sites, for example at the medial canthus of the eye and adjacent to the nasal alae, BCCs may be more deeply penetrating than is clinically apparent. Appropriate imaging to exclude deep invasion

may, therefore, be required before a treatment plan can be decided on.

Low-risk tumours can be managed successfully by curettage, cautery, laser or cryotherapy in the majority of cases. Cure rates of more than 90% can be anticipated in carefully selected patients. Results with these techniques are much less good for high-risk tumours, and alternative methods should be employed.

Formal surgical excision an alternative for low-risk tumours, as well as being recommended for many patients with high-risk BCCs. Surgery has the advantage of permitting histological examination, not just to confirm the diagnosis, but also to monitor the adequacy of the excision margins. For small well-defined tumours, margins of 5 mm will be adequate in 95% of cases. In high-risk tumours a wider margin is needed to minimise the likelihood of recurrence. The cosmetic appearances will usually be good, even in difficult areas, such as around the nose and eyes, if the operation has been undertaken by an experienced surgeon who has made appropriate use of plastic reconstructive techniques with local skin flaps.

Moh's micrographic surgery is a special technique for use with high-risk tumours especially in challenging anatomical areas where it may be difficult to ensure adequate margins. It offers highly accurate yet conservative removal of BCCs, therefore allowing low rates of recurrence with maximal preservation of normal tissues. It involves close excision with frozen section histology being performed at the time of the operation. If the margins are involved, a further close excision is performed, and the process is repeated until the histopathologist is confident that complete removal with clear margins has been achieved. Needless to say, Moh's micrographic surgery is expensive compared with other treatments as it is so time consuming for both the surgeon and the pathologist.

Radiotherapy is a valuable treatment for high-risk BCCs. There is with radiotherapy the same difficulty as with surgery in defining accurately the margin of the tumour. It is, however, often possible to treat morphoeic tumours, for example, with a more generous margin of apparently normal tissue using radiotherapy than it is with surgery.

Radical radiotherapy for skin cancers often requires a shorter course of treatment than is needed for tumours at other sites, because the area to be treated is so small and superficial. Five fractions over a week, or 10 fractions over 2 weeks, depending on size are usually prescribed. Sometimes, in the old and infirm who are unwilling to travel repeatedly it is possible to consider a single treatment, but results in terms of cosmesis and recurrence are less good.

Radiotherapy is better avoided in some circumstances, such as for tumours of the limbs especially if overlying the tibia, tumours of the upper eyelid, in patients younger than 40 years, and in patients with an underlying predisposition syndrome who are likely to develop multiple tumours over the ensuing years.

Radiotherapy is a very effective treatment, curing over 90% of high-risk cases. Results are even better for low-risk tumours, but nowadays it is usual to recommend alternative treatments in this group of patients to avoid the late sequelae of radiotherapy which include atrophy of the skin with hypopigmentation and telangiectasia.

Various other treatments are, sometimes, used for BCCs instead of those already mentioned. These include topical chemotherapy with fluorouracil cream, especially useful for patients with multiple low-risk tumours affecting sites other than the face.

Follow-up of patients treated for BCCs is important. If the primary treatment has been carefully selected, cure rates should be well in excess of 90% for most lesions, nonetheless recurrence can occur, usually within the first 5 years of follow-up. Perhaps of greater importance is the fact that more than one-third of patients treated for one BCC will develop another, and one-fifth of patients will develop multiple lesions. It can often be difficult for a patient to pick up new lesions early on when the chances of successful treatment with the best possible cosmetic outcome are greatest, and so a follow-up visit at least annually may well be beneficial.

TREATMENT OF SQUAMOUS CELL CARCINOMA OF THE SKIN

As with BCCs, SCCs of the skin can be allocated to either low-risk or high-risk groups. The recognition of the risk category influences both treatment and outcome.

SCCs are often treated similarly to BCCs. Curettage and cautery even of low-risk SCCs is, however, associated with a higher rate of recurrence than surgical excision or radiotherapy, so the latter treatments are preferable. Surgical removal of low-risk SCCs with a 4 mm margin will usually be effective. Radiotherapy is also a safe and effective treatment for low-risk SCCs.

For high-risk tumours a wider surgical margin is indicated, and Moh's micrographic surgery has been shown to be associated with a significantly lower risk of

recurrence. Radiotherapy is not usually the sole treatment for high-risk tumours, but is sometimes recommended as an adjuvant if margins are dubious or if there is nodal involvement.

HIGH-RISK SCC OF THE SKIN

- Tumours arising in areas of chronic inflammation, prior radiation or thermal injury, Bowen's disease and non-sun-exposed sites, ear, lip, scalp and eyelids
- More than 2 cm diameter, 4 mm in depth or extending into subcutaneous fat
- Tumours with poor histological differentiation and/or perineural invasion
- Tumours arising in immunosuppressed individuals
- Recurrent tumours

Follow-up is even more important for patients with SCCs than for those with BCCs, as there is a risk of metastasis to the draining lymph nodes. Follow-up for 5 years is usually recommended, as local recurrence or metastasis, if going to happen, will almost always occur within this time frame. Patients at high risk of developing multiple tumours, for example those with severe actinic skin damage, may do better if followed indefinitely.

TREATMENT OF MALIGNANT MELANOMA

Excision biopsy is required for patients with suspected cutaneous malignant melanoma. This is necessary to confirm the clinical diagnosis and to stage the tumour. In turn, the stage will inform the decision about the extent of local treatment required, and is also the most powerful prognostic indicator.

CLARK'S CLASSIFICATION OF MALIGNANT MELANOMA

- Level I — Lesions involving only the epidermis (*in situ* melanoma), not an invasive lesion
- Level II — Invasion of the papillary dermis, but does not reach the papillary–reticular dermal interface
- Level III — Invasion fills and expands the papillary dermis, but does not penetrate the reticular dermis
- Level IV — Invasion into the reticular dermis but not into the subcutaneous tissue
- Level V — Invasion through the reticular dermis into the subcutaneous tissue

---

Originally, the stage of malignant melanoma was described by Clark's classification which determined by the extent of local invasion into the anatomical layers of the skin. Nowadays, it is more common to use in addition Breslow's classification which depends on the vertical thickness of the tumour in millimetres, as this more accurately predicts subsequent behaviour of the cancer.

> **BRESLOW'S CLASSIFICATION OF MALIGNANT MELANOMA THICKNESS**
>
> ◆ 0.75 mm or less
> ◆ 0.76–1.50 mm
> ◆ 1.51–4.0 mm
> ◆ 4.0 mm or greater

The pT-component of the TNM-staging classification for cutaneous malignant melanoma is based on a combination of both Clark's level of invasion and the Breslow thickness measurement, whichever is the greater.

> **pT-STAGING FOR CUTANEOUS MALIGNANT MELANOMA**
>
> ◆ pT1 ≤0.75 mm Breslow depth, not more than Clark level II
> ◆ pT2 >0.75–1.5 mm Breslow depth, not more than Clark level III
> ◆ pT3 >1.5–4.0 mm Breslow depth, not more than Clark level IV
> ◆ pT4 >4.0 mm Breslow depth or satellite nodules, or reaching Clark level V

Following initial excision biopsy, the primary tumour bed can be re-excised depending on the T-stage. Early tumours (pT1, pT2) need margins of 1 cm. More advanced tumours (pT3, pT4) need margins up to 3 cm. Often a skin graft or flap is required to close the defect caused by such a wide excision.

As lymph node involvement is common, sentinel lymph node biopsy (Chapter 7) is often undertaken when the primary tumour is greater than 1 mm thick. If the sentinel lymph node is free of disease, the patient is merely observed. If it is involved, therapeutic regional lymph node clearance is indicated. As lymph node involvement can be predictive of more disseminated disease, full staging investigations are often performed before lymph node clearance is performed.

There has been much interest in the systemic treatment of melanoma, both adjuvant therapy following surgery for localised poor prognosis (pT3, pT4 or with lymph node involvement), and also as palliation for metastatic disease present at presentation or diagnosed subsequently.

Unfortunately results have been disappointing. Melanoma is not a chemosensitive disease, and response rates are poor. Various chemotherapy regimens have been used. In general, the response rates of single agents are only between 10% and 20%, and the average response duration is only of the order of a few months. Single agent dacarbazine has become regarded as the standard treatment. Combinations may achieve higher response rates, but at the expense of greater toxicity and without any survival advantage. Most patients with visceral metastases from malignant melanoma will be dead within 2 years, regardless of whether their disease responds to chemotherapy.

Similarly, biological treatments such as interferon, interleukin-2 and modulators of the immune response such as BCG and levamisole and vaccines have been extensively investigated. Response rates similar to those achieved with chemotherapy may be seen. None of these biological treatments yet has an established place, alone or with chemotherapy, in either the adjuvant or the palliative setting. The use of all these agents should be confined to clinical trials.

> **FIVE-YEAR SURVIVAL OF PATIENTS WITH CUTANEOUS MALIGNANT MELANOMA**
>
> ◆ pT1 N0 M0   95%
> ◆ pT2 N0 M0   85%
> ◆ pT3 N0 M0   65%
> ◆ pT4 N0 M0   45%
> ◆ Nodes involved   35%
> ◆ Distant metastases   <5%

The prognosis of malignant melanoma is very dependent on the stage at presentation. The best hope is for early diagnosis at a stage when surgery is likely to be curative. Patients with advanced disease may well be candidates for clinical trials, but their prognosis is poor, and patients with metastatic disease will need good quality palliative care.

Malignant melanoma can occur at sites other than the skin. These include the conjunctiva and the choroid of the eye, and mucosal surfaces such as the oral cavity, nose and sinuses, vagina and anus. At most of these sites tumours are advanced at the time of diagnosis, with a correspondingly poor prognosis. Treatment is surgical excision where possible, or radical radiotherapy if it is not. Metastatic malignant melanoma is treated in the same way whether the primary was in the skin or not. Results are similarly disappointing.

MERKEL CELL CARCINOMA

Merkel cell carcinoma is a rare skin cancer of neuro-endocrine origin. It tends to present as a rapidly growing solitary cutaneous nodule in the older patient. Local treatment is with complete excision and postoperative radiotherapy. Regional lymph nodes may be involved at the time of diagnosis. When nodes are involved, lymph node clearance and radiotherapy are usually recommended. The prognosis is poor and distant metastases in liver, lung bone and other organs often appear. Intensive combination chemotherapy of the sort used to treat small cell lung cancer may be beneficial, but most patients will die of their disease.

CUTANEOUS LYMPHOMA

Several clinical syndromes exist in which the principal abnormality is involvement of the skin by a malignant lymphoid infiltrate. In almost all cases the abnormal cells are T-cells, and so this spectrum of disease is collectively known as cutaneous T-cell lymphoma (CTCL). The CTCL spectrum embraces mycosis fungoides, Sézary syndrome and other, less common entities. Patients are usually, although not exclusively, elderly.

The skin lesions of mycosis fungoides can be divided into three stages. Generally, there is a progression through these stages over a number of years, although all three stages may be present at the same time. In the pre-mycotic stage the disease is totally restricted to the skin, and the manifestations appear very non-specific resembling a chronic eczematous or psoriatic condition. Individual areas may heal spontaneously without scarring. In the plaque stage, well-demarcated erythematous plaques appear, most commonly on the buttocks, face and skin creases. They may be intensely itchy. Again there may be spontaneous healing starting at the centre of the lesions. The development of the tumour stage is heralded by the appearance of nodules within the plaques or in previously healthy skin. Some nodules may reach quite a size and the skin may well ulcerate.

The Sézary syndrome, which tends to affect elderly men, is characterised by generalised erythroderma. There may be a widespread thickening of the skin which leads to an alteration in the facial appearance. These changes are associated with lymphadenopathy and the appearance of atypical mononuclear cells in the blood.

CTCL is generally a slowly progressive and indolent disease with a natural history which may extend over many years. Patients, who are often elderly, may well die of intercurrent illness not their CTCL. Unlike most lymphomas, CTCL is not usually very chemosensitive. Radical treatment approaches are unlikely to be successful, and most available treatments are palliative in intent.

Various approaches are used, including phototherapy with PUVA as for psoriasis, topical chemotherapy, local radiotherapy and whole skin electron beam therapy. Many innovative treatments are also being evaluated.

KAPOSI'S SARCOMA

Kaposi's sarcoma has, in recent years, been associated with the AIDS epidemic (Chapter 42). However, it also exists in other forms, unassociated with HIV infection.

FORMS OF KAPOSI'S SARCOMA

- Classical Kaposi's sarcoma
- African Kaposi's sarcoma
- AIDS-related Kaposi's sarcoma

Classical Kaposi's sarcoma was the first recognised over 100 years ago. It is a rare, indolent disease, tending to affect elderly Jewish men from Eastern Europe and in the Mediterranean area with a particular HLA group. It usually occurs as pigmented nodules, particularly on the lower limbs.

African Kaposi's sarcoma was first recognised in equatorial Africa 50 or so years ago, where it is fairly common. It can appear in a nodular form affecting the legs of old men rather like the classical variety, but the natural history appears to be more aggressive. It may also present as a highly malignant form with lymph node involvement in younger patients, even children. Treatment is usually with radiotherapy, but sometimes chemotherapy is also used.

CHAPTER 35

Prostate cancer

Prostate cancer, which after lung cancer, is the second most common cause of death from malignant disease in men, is frequently only diagnosed once it has spread and become incurable. Its management is one of the greatest challenges in oncology. Early diagnosis would, therefore, seem to be of the utmost importance in diminishing the high levels of mortality and morbidity caused by this condition. Paradoxically, we do not know how best to treat – or even whether to treat – those cases which are diagnosed early.

Most general practitioners (GPs) can expect to see a newly diagnosed patient every year or so. As men become more interested in their own health and are more aware of the possible benefits of screening, GPs can enquire of older patients during a surgery visit about a totally unrelated matter if prostatic symptoms are present or if he wishes to be screened.

AETIOLOGY

The causes of prostate cancer are unknown. There is a big racial and geographical variation in incidence. It is more common in Europe and America than in the Far East, and black men have a higher incidence than white men. Epidemiological studies suggest that environmental influences are more important than genetic ones, for example, vegetarians are less likely to get prostate cancer than meat eaters. Nonetheless, it has become common practice in some places to offer screening to males over 40 years who are first-degree relatives of patients with prostate cancer. Although there has been much speculation about sexual activity in the pathogenesis of prostate cancer, there is very little evidence to implicate sexual lifestyle.

DIAGNOSIS

Despite the controversies surrounding the treatment of early prostate cancer, it still makes good sense to diagnose it early wherever possible. "Early" diagnosis of advanced disease can be beneficial as palliative treatment may prevent the development of unpleasant complications. Any man, whatever age, with new or changing urinary symptoms merits investigation. The most common symptoms of urinary outflow obstruction or "prostatism" – urinary frequency, nocturia, difficulty in initiating micturition,

poor stream, dribbling, pain on micturition, acute urinary retention – and other relevant symptoms, such as haematuria, are very non-specific. The differential diagnosis includes not only benign prostatic hyperplasia, of course, but also prostatitis, urinary tract infection, urothelial cancer, cardiac failure and diabetes mellitus.

Digital rectal examination by an experienced practitioner is important. With locally advanced prostate cancer, the gland may feel enlarged, hard, asymmetrical and nodular. The median sulcus is often lost, whereas it is typically preserved in benign hyperplasia. In many cases of early prostate cancer, however, the gland feels entirely normal. Only if, by chance, an early curable tumour lies in a subcapsular position in the posterior part of the gland will it be palpable. Many patients with prostate cancer diagnosed on rectal examination will have locally advanced or metastatic, and therefore incurable, disease.

The blood test for prostate-specific antigen (PSA) has now replaced measurement of acid phosphatase and can be a valuable aid in the diagnosis of prostate cancer. It too, however, (despite its name) is not specific for cancer. Although greatly elevated levels are virtually diagnostic, more than 10% of men over the age of 50 will have values above the normal range, and about a quarter of men with proven benign prostatic hyperplasia have at least marginally elevated levels. Prostatitis, prostatic surgery and biopsy can all cause transient elevation of PSA levels, but measurement of PSA after digital rectal examination is not thought to cause major problems.

SIGNIFICANCE OF PSA LEVELS

<4 ng ml^{-1}	normal range
4–10 ng ml^{-1}	25% chance of cancer
>10 ng ml^{-1}	60% chance of cancer

PSA measurement should be performed in men over 40 or 45 with urinary symptoms or an abnormal feeling prostate. Population screening with PSA is being investigated in the clinical trial setting in the UK, but cannot yet be recommended as routine practice in men without symptoms. Its use outside a clinical study as a screening investigation should be confined to those who wish its use, who have a family history of prostate cancer, and who have a good life expectancy, that is, are younger than, say, 70 and are free from other serious diseases which may shorten life. Patients should only receive a screening PSA estimation after they have been appropriately counselled.

Early prostate cancer may also be diagnosed incidentally, for example, on the histology of the transurethral resection chippings in a patient who has undergone surgery for benign prostatic hyperplasia, or in patients undergoing investigation of some other illness.

> Patient information prior to PSA screening should include:
>
> ♦ Transrectal ultrasound and biopsy may be needed to investigate an abnormal result which may then prove to be a false positive
> ♦ Early prostate cancer may be detected in about 5% of men aged 50–65 years
> ♦ We may not know how best to treat the cancer if one is found
> ♦ Some early tumours will not be detected
> ♦ Treatment of screen-detected early cancers carries risk and may not necessarily improve life expectancy

About half of all cases of prostate cancer are metastatic at presentation. Metastatic prostate cancer can, like early disease, also be a great mimic of other conditions. It most commonly presents with back pain due to bone metastases, but pain at other sites is also common. Lassitude or dyspnoea due to anaemia, anorexia, weight loss, the tiredness and sickness of chronic renal failure due to bilateral ureteric or bladder outflow obstruction and a lump in the neck due to nodal metastasis are other presentations. Occasionally inability to walk, sensory disturbances in the legs, or loss of normal bladder and bowel function may be due to spinal cord compression caused by vertebral metastatic disease.

INVESTIGATION

The patient suspected of having early prostate cancer should have the diagnosis confirmed histologically, usually by transrectal ultrasound guided needle biopsy. Examination of transurethral resection chippings is an alternative, and quite legitimate if the presenting symptom is bladder outflow obstruction which requires surgical relief in its own right. Necessary blood tests include, of course, PSA and urea, creatinine and electrolytes to evaluate renal function, full blood count and erythrocyte sedimentation rate (ESR) to exclude anaemia and "liver function tests" including alkaline phosphatase and calcium to evaluate the skeleton.

> ### STAGING INVESTIGATIONS IN EARLY PROSTATE CANCER
>
> ♦ Transrectal or transurethral biopsy
>   - To confirm diagnosis
>   - To grade tumour
> ♦ Blood tests
>   - PSA
>   - Full blood count ESR
>   - Urea, creatinine and electrolytes
>   - Alkaline phosphatase and calcium
> ♦ For assessing local extent
>   - Transrectal ultrasound
>   - CT of pelvis
>   - Abdominal ultrasound or IVU
> ♦ To evaluate the skeleton
>   - Bone scan
>   - Plain X-rays

Local staging will usually be by transrectal ultrasound to assess extracapsular spread and seminal vesicle involvement and/or computed tomography which will also evaluate the pelvic lymph node status. Excretion urography or alternatively ultrasound can be used to examine the upper tracts and to check for completeness of bladder emptying.

A bone scan will usually be performed as the skeleton is the commonest site for metastatic disease, but bone metastases are unlikely if there is no bone pain and the alkaline phosphatase and acid phosphatase levels are normal and the PSA is low. Bone scan may be omitted with a well-differentiated cancer and a PSA of less than $20 \, \text{ng ml}^{-1}$.

Plain X-rays should be carried out to evaluate abnormal areas shown on bone scan, as false-positive scans are not uncommon. Bone metastases from prostate cancer are usually sclerotic, and therefore, have quite characteristic X-ray appearances.

STAGING OF PROSTATE CANCER

> ### T-STAGING OF PROSTATE CANCER
>
> ♦ T1 Incidental
>   T1a Three foci or fewer
>   T1b More than three foci
> ♦ T2 Clinically or grossly limited to the gland
>   T2a = 1.5 cm
>   T2b > 1.5 cm/>one lobe
> ♦ T3 Invades prostatic apex/beyond capsule/ bladder neck/seminal vesicle/not fixed
> ♦ T4 Fixed or invades other adjacent structures

Prostate cancer is staged by the TNM system. T1 disease is an incidental finding. About 10% of men undergoing prostate surgery for bladder outflow obstruction thought to be due to benign prostatic hypertrophy will be found to have an incidental cancer. T2 disease is a clinically evident cancer confined to the prostate gland. In T3 disease there is extension to the bladder neck or seminal vesicles. T4 disease is fixed to or invades other local structures such as the rectum. The various N categories denote progressively greater lymph node involvement. M0 indicates the absence, and M1 the presence, of haematogenous metastases, most commonly in bone.

HISTOLOGY AND GRADING OF PROSTATE CANCER

Prostate cancer is nearly always adenocarcinoma. Rarely other types such as transitional cell carcinoma are observed. The degree of differentiation of prostatic adenocarcinoma is of prognostic significance. There are several systems for the histopathological grading of prostate cancer. The most widely used is that described by Gleason, with Grade 1 representing a well-differentiated tumour with a good prognosis, and Grade 5 indicating a very poorly differentiated carcinoma with a correspondingly poor outlook.

TREATMENT POLICIES

The treatment of prostate cancer remains controversial. For any particular clinical scenario there are a number of options.

> **KEY DETERMINANTS OF TREATMENT POLICY IN PROSTATE CANCER**
>
> - Tumour-related factors
>   - Stage
>   - Grade
> - Patient-related factors
>   - Age
>   - Co-morbidity
>   - Personal preferences
> - Medical opinions

In early disease with a good prognosis, the choice lies between observation only or immediate treatment with radical prostatectomy or radical radiotherapy, with or without adjuvant hormonal manipulation. In advanced disease the choice lies between immediate or deferred hormone therapy. If hormone therapy is to be given, the choice lies between orchidectomy or medical therapy.

The main factors determining treatment are the stage and grade of the tumour, the age and general health of the patient, together with the opinion of various specialists and the wishes of the patient. Individual patient management options should be discussed in a multidisciplinary setting with urologists, oncologists, radiologists and pathologists. The final decision should be made in consultation with the openly counselled patient, who should be offered the opportunity to participate in clinical trials where appropriate.

TREATMENT OF EARLY DISEASE

> **TREATMENT OPTIONS IN LOCALISED DISEASE**
>
> - Observation until progression
> - Radical radiotherapy
> - Radical prostatectomy
> - Hormone manipulation

The key to decision-making in early prostate cancer is the life expectancy of the patient, which is related both to his age and to any other illnesses. For T1a disease, the likelihood of tumour progression without treatment is usually less than 10%, and the time to progression is often 5–10 years or more. A policy of observation in these patients is thus justifiable, especially as we do not know whether treatment influences life expectancy. An exception may be in fit men under the age of 70 years, whose life expectancy of 15 or more years means that they have a higher risk of disease progression during their lifetime. A decision to treat will also be supported if the tumour is less than well differentiated.

With more advanced T1 tumours and with T2 tumours there is a greater likelihood of local progression, and so while observation probably remains the policy of choice in the elderly, radical local treatment is more likely to be preferred in younger and slightly older patients. Both radiotherapy and surgery can be offered. Each offers the prospect of improved local control, although the likelihood of an improvement in survival is less clear cut. There is no evidence to say that one modality is better than the other, but the side-effect profile differs. As well as the acute surgical complications common to many major operations, especially in the elderly, radical prostatectomy can lead to incontinence, impotence and urethral stricture. Radiotherapy may cause acute side-effects of dysuria, tenesmus and skin erythema and desquamation. In the long term a small proportion may suffer from urethral or rectal stricture, haematuria and rectal bleeding and urinary frequency. Modern radiotherapy techniques, such as brachytherapy and conformal external beam treatment, may have a lower risk of late complications.

There is no evidence to suggest that routine postoperative radiotherapy improves survival after initial surgery. Certainly the complications of combined modality therapy are likely to be greater. Similarly, there is no evidence for a survival benefit when radiotherapy is used as salvage for localised relapse after surgery, or if surgery is used for salvage of local recurrence after primary radiotherapy.

Whether or not adjuvant hormone therapy should be given to patients with localised disease is controversial. Its use is more likely to be justified in more advanced disease which is still localised (T2b), or if the tumour is less well differentiated, as the likelihood of systemic relapse is greater. Adjuvant hormonal therapy may prolong the time to progression, but whether it results in longer survival compared with its introduction at the time of progression is less clear. Hormone therapy can be used as first line treatment in patients with localised disease, where it is wished to avoid radical treatment but observation is not considered to be appropriate.

TREATMENT OF LOCALLY ADVANCED DISEASE

By locally advanced disease, we mean T3 or T4 tumours, without evidence of nodal or distant metastases. Radical surgery is not an option, but transurethral resection may be indicated for relief of bladder outlet obstruction. Radical radiotherapy is the principal treatment. As the side-effects of radiotherapy are related to the volume of tissue irradiated, some advantage may be gained by initial hormone therapy which causes the tumour to shrink before radiotherapy is given, allowing a smaller volume to be treated. In addition, hormone therapy may be of value because of the greater incidence of occult nodal disease, and the greater likelihood of systemic relapse than is the case with early localised tumours.

TREATMENT OF PATIENTS WITH METASTATIC DISEASE

Hormone manipulation is the first line treatment for patients presenting with metastatic disease, and for metastatic relapse in patients who have not previously been exposed to hormonal treatment. Some people prefer to defer treatment in asymptomatic patients until symptoms appear, but the consensus favours immediate treatment in the majority of patients. Surgical orchidectomy has traditionally been the initial procedure to deprive the body of testicular androgens. Subcapsular orchidectomy is as effective as total orchidectomy, and is usually preferred by patients as it does not leave an empty scrotum.

Medical treatment with luteinising hormone releasing hormone (LHRH) depot analogues is an equally effective

alternative to surgery. Goserelin is the most widely used compound, and is available as monthly or 3-monthly depot injections. Initial use of LHRH agonists may be associated with tumour flare. To prevent this an anti-androgen such as cyproterone acetate 100 mg three times a day should be given for at least 3 days prior to, and 3 weeks after, the first use of the LHRH antagonist.

PRINCIPAL HORMONAL OPTIONS IN PROSTATE CANCER

◆ Surgical orchidectomy
◆ LHRH agonists
◆ Anti-androgens
◆ Combined androgen blockade

The testes are not the only source of endogenous androgens: some are produced by the adrenal glands. Because of this, total androgen blockade – where an LHRH agonist is combined with an anti-androgen such as flutamide or bicalutamide – is being compared with LHRH agonist monotherapy in clinical trials. At the moment there is insufficient evidence to justify the use of combined androgen blockade outside the clinical trial setting.

Oestrogens were formerly widely used in the management of prostate cancer, but the associated thrombo-embolic risk, accentuated by the presence of malignancy and possibly immobility, has lead to their replacement with the safer drugs described above.

TREATMENT OF HORMONE REFRACTORY PROSTATE CANCER

Although hormone treatment will produce a response in about 80% of patients, disease progression occurs after a median interval of about 18 months. Response rates to second line hormone therapy are poor, of the order of 10%. Chemotherapy has similarly disappointing results in prostate cancer, but it is occasionally used especially in younger patients.

COMPLICATIONS OF BONE METASTASES

◆ Pain
◆ Pathological fracture
◆ Hypercalcaemia
◆ Spinal cord compression

The patient with relapsed hormone refractory prostate cancer requires essentially palliative treatment and good symptom control. Painful bone metastases are the most common problem, and appropriate analgesics and anti-inflammatory drugs are indicated. Localised bone pain can be treated with radiotherapy. Sometimes, patients with diffuse bone pain benefit from hemi-body treatment. The characteristically osteoblastic bone metastases take up bone-seeking isotopes and enable effective radionuclide treatment strontium-89. Biphosphonate infusions also help to reduce bone pain. Sometimes, an actual or threatened pathological fracture may require orthopaedic intervention. Two particular complications related to bone metastases are often seen in prostate cancer: spinal cord compression and hypercalcaemia. Both merit urgent treatment as described in Chapter 49.

Symptoms related to the primary tumour such as urinary outflow obstruction or haematuria may benefit from palliative radiotherapy, if the primary site has not already been treated, or transurethral resection. Incontinence greater than can easily be dealt with by pads merits urethral or suprapubic catheterisation. Pelvic lymphadenopathy can lead to leg oedema and ureteric obstruction. Again palliative radiotherapy may be beneficial. Obstructed ureters can be stented. This may be appropriate in a newly diagnosed patient with advanced disease, but should only be undertaken after careful thought in patients with relapsed disease.

OUTCOME

It is very difficult to give a figure for overall survival in prostate cancer, as so much depends on the grade and stage of the tumour, and different reported series vary in the case mix. At one end of the spectrum, most patients with incidentally diagnosed well-differentiated tumours are more likely to die from other causes than they are from prostate cancer, at the other extreme, many patients with advanced disease have a life expectancy of less than a year at the time of diagnosis.

Bladder cancer

Carcinoma of the urinary bladder is typically a transitional cell carcinoma arising from the urothelium which extends from the renal pelvis to the urethra. It is a disease which varies at the time of diagnosis from a superficial well-differentiated cancer (sometimes, erroneously called a "benign papilloma") to aggressive muscle-invasive disease with a high chance of metastatic disease and the potential for a rapidly fatal outcome. The variations in reported incidence are to some extent explained by whether or not early cancers are diagnosed and recorded. About 10,000 cases are diagnosed each year in the UK, representing approximately 5% of the total cancer incidence. Worldwide, the incidence of bladder cancer is increasing, although there have been small declines in the UK and other developed countries.

Bladder cancer is two to three times more common in men than women. It is also more common in white than black populations. It tends to be a disease of the elderly, and it is rarely seen in people under the age of 50 years.

The most important cause of bladder cancer nowadays is cigarette smoking. Smokers have an up to five fold increased risk of developing bladder cancer compared with non-smokers, depending on the type and quantity of tobacco smoked. A number of important occupational carcinogens have been identified, including aromatic amines in the dye and rubber, and allied industries. In the developed world, health and safety legislation means that these should no longer be a cause of bladder cancer, but the same is almost certainly not true in many other countries. In Egypt, and other countries where infection with schistosomiasis is endemic, there is a greatly increased incidence of squamous cell carcinoma (SCC) of the bladder. Other recognised but uncommon causes include the obsolete analgesic phenacatin, alkylating chemotherapeutic agents such as cyclophosphamide, and ionising radiation, as in prior treatment for carcinoma of the cervix.

> **CAUSES OF BLADDER CANCER**
>
> - Cigarette smoking
> - Industrial carcinogens, aromatic amines, aniline dyes
> - Schistosomiasis (SCC)
> - Cyclophosphamide
> - Radiation

PRESENTING FEATURES

The most common presenting symptom of bladder cancer is haematuria. Sometimes, the diagnosis of bladder cancer may be delayed by the concurrent diagnosis of a urinary tract infection which may be associated with infection. The haematuria associated with bladder cancer is classically described as being "painless, periodic and profuse." However, pain can be a feature, for example if there is infection present, if blood clots cause urinary retention or if there is bladder spasm.

Adult patients presenting to their general practitioner (GP) with definite painless macroscopic haematuria should be referred to a urologist or haematuria clinic for investigation under the 2-week rule (Chapter 5). If asymptomatic haematuria is detected on a routine medical examination in an adult, an MSU should be checked, twice if necessary, and any infection which is detected should be treated. After treatment of a urinary tract infection, urinalysis should be repeated, and if it remains positive for the presence of blood, the patient should again be referred urgently for investigation.

Tumours deeply invading or blocking of a ureter may also cause pain, as can nodal or distant metastases. Rarely, patients will present with symptoms of renal failure caused by an obstructive uropathy.

INVESTIGATION

Many hospitals will have rapid access clinics for the investigation of haematuria. Macroscopic haematuria at any age, or microscopic haematuria in people over 50 are indications for the urgent referral of patients with suspected cancer under the 2-week rule (Chapter 5). Bladder cancer at presentation is not usually associated with any physical signs.

The minimum investigation to exclude the presence of a cancer will be an intravenous urogram (IVU) or abdominal and pelvic ultrasound to examine the upper tracts and bladder, followed by an outpatient flexible cystoscopy if the bladder appears normal on imaging. Urine cytology may be helpful, but a normal result does not exclude the presence of urothelial malignancy. If there is an abnormality in the bladder seen on imaging or detected on flexible cystoscopy, formal cystoscopy and examination under anaesthesia (EUA) will be required to obtain tissue for histology, and to allow for diathermy or transurethral resection of disease.

If cancer of the bladder is confirmed, a computed tomography (CT) scan of the abdomen and pelvis and a chest X-ray will be required as the minimum staging investigations in addition to routine bloods. Other investigations, such as a bone scan, may be appropriate, if there are additional symptoms which need to be investigated.

PATHOLOGY AND STAGING

Macroscopically, bladder tumours may be single or multiple, and they may be papillary or solid in appearance. Papillary tumours are the most common type, accounting for about 75–80% of cases. They are often multiple and usually superficial. Only a small proportion of these will go on to become aggressive, invasive cancers. Solid tumours are more likely to be less well differentiated and invasive. This type accounts for about one-fifth to one-quarter of cases. In most cases, patients with solid, invasive cancers do not have a past history of superficial bladder cancer. Both types may, however, co-exist.

PATHOLOGY OF BLADDER CANCER

- Macroscopic appearances
  - Papillary or solid
  - Solitary or multiple
- Histological types
  - Transitional cell carcinoma
  - SCC
  - Adenocarcinoma

Histologically, most bladder cancers are transitional cell carcinomas which arise from the urothelium lining the urinary tract. Cancers of similar histology arise in the renal pelvis, the ureters and the urethra, but the majority arise in the bladder. In the UK, perhaps 1 in 10 will be a squamous carcinoma, but this is the predominant pathological type in areas where schistosomiasis is found. Rarely, an adenocarcinoma will be identified. Adenocarcinoma is often found in an urachal remnant connecting the bladder to the umbilicus and is more common in those who have had a congenital urinary tract abnormality, such as exstrophy of the bladder.

The pathologist will identify and comment on two particular characteristics of transitional cell carcinomas. These are the grade (well, moderately and poorly differentiated – G1, G2, G3 – or undifferentiated) and the depth of invasion. Has the cancer breached the lamina propria? Is it invading the muscle? These are the most important prognostic features. Sometimes flat areas of carcinoma *in situ* are diagnosed on biopsy. These may be multiple and part of a field change, and often co-exist with more

advanced disease. These features determine the T-stage of the cancer (see box below), which cannot accurately be decided without histological assessment of the depth of invasion.

T-STAGING OF BLADDER CANCER

- Ta   Non-invasive papillary carcinoma
- Tis Carcinoma *in situ*: "flat tumour"
- T1   Tumour invades subepithelial connective tissue
- T2   Tumour invades muscle
       T2a Tumour invades superficial muscle (inner half)
       T2b Tumour invades deep muscle (outer half)
- T3   Tumour invades perivesical tissue
       T3a Tumour invades microscopically
       T3b Tumour invades macroscopically (extravesical mass)
- T4   Tumour invades any of the following: prostate, uterus, vagina, pelvic wall, abdominal wall
       T4a Tumour invades prostate or uterus or vagina
       T4b Tumour invades pelvic wall or abdominal wall

The lymph node status will be assessed on CT, if invasive bladder cancer has been diagnosed. Pathological confirmation of the N-stage (see box below) will be performed after surgery, if a cystectomy is performed. The regional lymph nodes are those of the true pelvis. Metastases in para-aortic lymph nodes count as distant metastatic spread.

N-STAGING OF BLADDER CANCER

- N0   No regional lymph node metastasis
- N1   Metastasis in a single lymph node 2 cm or less in greatest dimension
- N2   Metastasis in a single lymph node more than 2 cm but not more than 5 cm in greatest dimension, or multiple lymph nodes, none more than 5 cm in greatest dimension
- N3   Metastasis in a lymph node more than 5 cm in greatest dimension

---

TREATMENT OF SUPERFICIAL BLADDER CANCER

Patients with superficial bladder cancer can be allocated to one of three risk groups.

Low-risk superficial bladder cancers are those where there is a single, low histological grade, Ta tumour. This will have been ablated at the first cystoscopy following biopsy. The first check cystoscopy is likely to be negative, following which only occasional surveillance cystoscopies will be called for, and the prognosis is likely to be extremely good.

Intermediate-risk tumours can require repeated interventions but are not commonly life threatening. Patients falling into this group have multiple low-grade Ta tumours. Intravesical treatment with chemotherapy or BCG immunotherapy is needed after initial surgery in this group.

High-risk superficial bladder cancer constitutes a threat to the bladder, and by the possibility of progression to muscle-invasive disease, to life also. Patients in this category often have multiple, high-grade tumours which may be associated with areas of atypia, dysplasia or carcinoma *in situ*. Following endoscopic surgical treatment, intravesical therapy, usually with BCG, is used. If an initial course is not successful, this may be repeated before resorting to more drastic measures, such as surgery.

Intravesical chemotherapy has been used for treatment of superficial bladder cancer for many decades now. It is effective at reducing the likelihood of recurrence of low-grade, low-stage tumours after an initial endoscopic procedure. It is less likely to be successful if used to eradicate existing disease. Intravesical therapy with BCG is used as first line therapy for high-risk superficial bladder cancer, or where disease recurs after initial treatment with intravesical chemotherapy. A commonly used schedule is weekly treatment for 3 consecutive weeks repeated 6 monthly for 3 years. Treatment may be complicated by systemic symptoms, such as fever, or rarely by local problems, such as granulomatous prostatitis or ureteric obstruction.

Follow-up after treatment is generally with regular cystoscopies. In low-risk patients, annual cystoscopy for 10 years may suffice if the first check was clear. In high-risk patients, checks should be 3 monthly to begin with, gradually increasing to annual cystoscopies, if all remains well. Surveillance is often for life. Urine cytology is, sometimes, used in addition in patients with high-risk tumours.

TREATMENT OF MUSCLE-INVASIVE BLADDER CANCER

Staging is used to stratify patients with muscle-invasive bladder into two groups. Fit patients with T2 or T3 disease confined to the bladder (N0, M0) are suitable for treatment with curative intent. Some patients with T4 disease by virtue of prostatic involvement whose disease is still localised may also be amenable to radical treatment. Patients with intercurrent illness who are medically unfit for radical treatment, and those with involved lymph nodes or distant metastases are probably only suitable for a palliative approach.

Radical treatment options in muscle-invasive bladder cancer are surgery and radiotherapy either alone or in combination. There is no clear difference in survival between these approaches. The integration of chemotherapy into radical treatment is under investigation but is not yet established practice.

In Britain, primary radical radiotherapy is the most commonly used treatment. A course of 4–6-weeks treatment is usually given. Acute side-effects of radiotherapy include frequency, dysuria and tenesmus. Late side-effects can include a shrunken bladder resulting in frequency, nocturia and urgency. Haematuria may be due to telangiectasia within the bladder, but vigilance needs to be maintained as this may herald recurrence or a second primary tumour in the upper tracts. Radiation proctitis may cause rectal bleeding.

With modern CT-planning techniques, radical radiotherapy will achieve local control in about half those treated. About one-third of patients will be cured and retain an intact bladder. Salvage cystectomy can be considered in those with an incomplete response to radiotherapy and in those whose disease subsequently recurs. Metastatic relapse is common. Survival is related to T-stage at presentation, with about half of those with T2 tumours being cured compared with only about one-quarter of those with T3 disease.

Primary surgery more commonly used in younger and fitter patients. Often it is advisable to perform a urethrectomy as well as cystectomy. In the past, all patients undergoing cystectomy were left with an ileal conduit and collected urine in a bag. Nowadays, it is possible in some patients to fashion a new bladder from gut and probably retain continence. Although micturition with a reconstructed bladder is not normal, quality of life is better than with a urinary stoma. Sexual function is affected in both men and women. The vagina will be narrowed, possibly resulting in dysparunia, and most men will become impotent. As with primary radiotherapy, even when surgery controls local disease, metastatic relapse is common.

TREATMENT OF ADVANCED DISEASE

The most common site for metastases in patients with bladder cancer are the lungs and lymph nodes. Metastases in other sites, such as bone, brain and liver, are less frequently seen. The general palliative care of patients with distant metastases is covered in Chapter 49, and treatment of specific symptoms, such as pain, is covered in Chapter 50. The specific treatment of patients with metastatic bladder cancer is difficult. Many patients are elderly, and co-morbidity is frequently present. Renal function is often reduced as a result of previous treatment. Nonetheless, bladder cancer can be surprisingly chemosensitive, and combinations of drugs, such as methotrexate, vinblastine, doxorubicin and cisplatin, can provide good palliation and prolongation of survival in carefully selected, fit patients. The prognosis for patients with metastatic disease is poor, and only a few will survive longer than a year.

Palliative treatment may also be needed for patients with local symptoms, such as haematuria due to uncontrolled disease in the bladder. Options include transurethral resection and diathermy, a short course of palliative radiotherapy to the pelvis, systemic chemotherapy, irrigation of the bladder with alum or formalin, and palliative cystectomy. The choice of treatment depends on the fitness of the patient, their wishes, and, of course, prior treatment.

Some patients may develop obstructive uropathy due to extensive pelvic tumour. In most cases, intervention to relieve this would not be justifiable. Occasionally, however, as in an young, otherwise fit patient in whom there are still untried treatment options, a more aggressive approach may be indicated. Decision-making in this sort of situation is difficult, and it may be helpful for the hospital specialist to discuss the case with the GP as well as with the patient and family members before reaching a definite decision.

Kidney cancer

Cancers of the kidney are not common, comprising only about 2% or 3% of the cancer incidence in the UK. They occur more commonly in men.

CLASSIFICATION OF CANCERS OF THE KIDNEY

Adult types
- Renal cell adenocarcinoma   90%
- Transitional cell carcinoma of
  the renal pelvis   8%
- Squamous cell carcinoma (SCC)   2%

Childhood types – see Chapter 46

Adenocarcinoma, also called renal cell or clear cell carcinoma or hypernephroma accounts for about 90% of cases. Transitional cell carcinoma and much more rarely SCC of the renal pelvis account for most of the rest. Wilms' tumour and other renal tumours of childhood are discussed in Chapter 46.

CLINICAL PRESENTATION

Haematuria is a common feature, and may cause clot colic. Loin pain may also be due to haemorrhage into the tumour or local extension of the cancer. Extension along the renal vein and into the vena cava may cause a hydrocoele or features of inferior vena cava obstruction. Systemic features, such as pyrexia, malaise, hypercalcaemia and polycythaemia or anaemia, may be present. The disease may present with symptoms of bone or lung metastases. On examination, there may be a palpable mass and hypertension may be detected.

INVESTIGATION

Various imaging tests may be used to show the presence of a renal tumour and to define its nature and extent, including ultrasound, intravenous urography, computed tomography and sometimes angiography. These tests will identify whether or not there is any vascular invasion or para-aortic lymphadenopathy. Other investigations will be required to show the presence or absence of distant metastases, which are most common in the lungs and bone.

STAGING SYSTEM

Renal cell cancer is staged by the TNM classification. The T-stage relates to the size of the primary tumour and local extension into surrounding tissues. The N-stage relates to whether there is more than one regional lymph node involved, only one, or none at all. The M-stage relates to the presence or absence of haematogenous spread (Chapter 8). There is also a stage grouping system whereby localised tumours with no lymph node involvement or distant spread are Stage I or II, more extensive local disease or lymph node involvement are categorised as Stage III and those with very extensive local or nodal involvement and all patients with haematogenous spread are put into Stage IV.

Transitional cell carcinoma of the renal pelvis and ureter has a different but similar staging classification.

TREATMENT OF RENAL CELL CARCINOMA

Surgery remains the standard treatment for patients with localised (Stages I and II) renal cell carcinoma. The operation of radical nephrectomy removes the tumour along with the kidney and ipsilateral adrenal gland and the surrounding fat and fascia. Usually adjacent lymph nodes are removed as well, although the true benefit of lymphadenectomy remains uncertain. When the tumour is very small, or when disease is bilateral, a partial nephrectomy may be performed to spare functioning renal parenchyma and avoid the need for dialysis or transplantation.

With more advanced Stage III disease, radical nephrectomy is again the treatment of choice. Sometimes, external beam radiotherapy may be used in conjunction with surgery in selected patients, but there is little evidence to say that this adds to the benefit of surgery.

Patients with Stages I to III renal cell carcinoma, who are medically unfit for radical surgery, can have symptoms of local disease palliated by external beam radiotherapy or embolisation of the tumour.

Patients with Stage IV disease are for all practical purposes incurable. However, the rare observation of spontaneous remission of metastatic disease has lead to an interest in biological therapy using drugs, such as interferon alpha and interleukin-2. The role of nephrectomy in patients with metastatic disease at presentation is controversial. It may be performed on the grounds that it lessens the likelihood of local symptoms progressing or that it leaves less tumour burden in the body for other modalities of treatment to deal with. Whether or not it materially influences the prognosis is a different matter.

Renal cell carcinoma is not usually responsive to cytotoxic chemotherapy. Reported response rates are only of the order of 10%. Progestogens have often been administered to patients with metastatic renal cell cancer because of their low toxicity and some early reports which indicated a benefit, but the frequency of response is disappointingly low. Interferon alpha has about a 15% response rate in selected fit individuals although remissions are rarely complete or sustained for a long time. Interleukin-2 has a similar response rate to interferon alpha, but about 5% of the appropriately selected patients have durable complete remissions. Higher doses of interleukin-2 are associated with higher response rates, but much greater toxicity. Combinations of interleukin-2 and interferon are no better than interleukin-2 alone.

Patients with renal cell carcinoma of any stage at presentation, whose disease relapses or progresses after initial treatment, have a poor prognosis. Treatment needs to be carefully selected depending on age, fitness and prior treatment. In many, symptom control measures alone will be the best policy, but some may benefit from a trial of interleukin-2.

TREATMENT OF TRANSITIONAL CELL CARCINOMA OF THE RENAL PELVIS AND URETER

The whole of the urinary tract from the renal pelvis, down the ureters, through the bladder to the urethra is lined by transitional cell epithelium or urothelium. Tumours arising in the urothelium at any site are usually transitional cell carcinomas, occasionally squamous carcinomas. The factors predisposing to the development of urothelial cancers have been set out in Chapter 36; the most important of these is smoking.

A particular characteristic of urothelial cancers is that they are often multifocal. This is why patients presenting with bladder cancer must have the upper tracts and urethra examined for synchronous primary tumours, the presence of which may alter management. Similarly, when a patient presents with an upper tract transitional carcinoma, a cystoscopy is indicated to evaluate the urethra and bladder, and the contralateral upper tract must also be assessed.

The majority of upper tract cancers arise in the renal pelvis. Ureteric cancers are rare. The key factors in upper tract cancers are the degree of differentiation and the depth of invasion. These two characteristics often go hand in hand, so deeply invasive tumours are more likely to be poorly differentiated, while superficial tumours are most often well differentiated.

The principal treatment for localised upper tract cancer is surgery. The operation is nephro-ureterectomy which involves total excision of the ureter with a bladder cuff, renal pelvis and the kidney. More conservative surgery is being explored, but the precise place of lesser procedures than nephro-ureterectomy is still not well defined. It is particularly important to consider the feasibility of a more conservative approach, if the patient has already lost the opposite kidney.

Radiotherapy and chemotherapy (as described in Chapter 36) may be used for the palliation of transitional cell carcinomas which are too advanced for radical surgery, or which recur after surgery.

PROGNOSIS OF RENAL CELL CARCINOMA

Patients presenting with Stage I disease have a 50% chance of survival at 5 years following radical nephrectomy. More advanced stages do less well. No adjuvant therapies have an established place, although clinical trials continue. Most patients with metastatic disease will die from their cancer, but indolent behaviour leading to long survival durations in some patients is well recognised.

PROGNOSIS OF TRANSITIONAL CELL CARCINOMA OF THE RENAL PELVIS AND URETER

Outcome is related to stage and tumour grade. Upper tract tumours are curable in more than 90% of patients, if they are superficial and confined to the renal pelvis or ureter. Patients with deeply invasive tumours that are still confined to the renal pelvis or ureter have a 10–15% likelihood of cure. Patients with cancers which have penetrated through the urothelial wall or have metastases are usually beyond cure.

It is important to be vigilant about metachronous primary transitional cell carcinomas. Only about 2% of patients will develop a contralateral upper tract primary tumour after successful treatment of transitional cell carcinoma of the kidney or ureter. But as up to 50% may develop a bladder cancer subsequently, regular surveillance cystoscopy is indicated.

Testicular tumours

The treatment of testis cancer is one of the great success stories of modern oncology. Thanks to the development of platinum-based chemotherapy, coupled with the careful use of imaging technology and tumour marker assays to stage the disease and monitor response to treatment, cure rates in excess of 90%, even with metastatic disease, can be expected. The quality of life of survivors is attested to by the fact that treated patients have gone on to win such sporting classics as the Grand National and the Tour de France.

The disease principally affects younger men aged between 20 and 40 years, although any age may be affected. It comprises about 1% of cancers in adult men. The tumours are usually germ cell tumours, seminoma or non-seminomatous germ cell tumours, commonly called teratoma. Rarely, and usually in old men, lymphoma of the testis may occur (see Chapter 41).

PRESENTATION

The most common presenting symptom, accounting for up to 90% of cases, is the discovery of an enlarged, hard testicle, which is characteristically painless. Sometimes, a hydrocoele develops, which may obscure an underlying mass. Occasionally, the first symptom is back pain, due to metastases in para-aortic lymph nodes. Other less common presentations include the development of gynaecomastia due to the production of the hormone beta human chorionic gonadotrophin (bhCG).

Patients presenting with a swelling in the scrotum should be examined carefully and an attempt made to distinguish between lumps arising from the body of the testis and other intrascrotal swellings. Those patients suspected of having a lump in the testis, and those with doubtful epididymo-orchitis or orchitis not resolving within 3 weeks of treatment should be referred urgently for assessment by a urologist.

Men, especially those aged from 20 to 40 years who are in the highest-risk group, should be encouraged by their general practitioner (GP) regularly to check their testicles for lumps. This type of opportunistic intervention can conveniently take place at a new patient medical examination, when a young man registers for the first time with a practice.

INVESTIGATION

Following history and examination, the specialist will arrange for an ultrasound examination of both testicles and the abdomen, chest X-ray and measurement of blood tumour markers alpha fetoprotein (AFP), beta human chorionic gonadotrophin (βhCG) and lactate dehydrogenase (LDH).

Tumour marker assays have revolutionised the management of germ cell tumours. They are, however, not entirely sensitive (in other words, false-negative results can occur) and they are not completely specific (that is levels can be raised for other reasons). Either hCG or AFP or both are elevated in three-quarters of patients with teratoma. In about one-third of seminomas the hCG may be mildly elevated. The initial values are of prognostic significance, as is the rate of decline in levels after surgery, and whether or not levels normalise with surgery alone. If levels are initially elevated, they can be used to monitor response to treatment. When remission is achieved, tumour markers can be used for surveillance to detect relapse. LDH is another non-specific marker of tumour bulk, useful also in lymphoma. High levels are of adverse prognostic significance in metastatic seminoma, particularly.

Definitive diagnosis is made by the pathologist after the operation of inguinal orchidectomy. A prosthetic testicle may be placed in the scrotum.

PATHOLOGY

The main distinction is between seminoma, and non-seminomatous germ cell tumours (teratomas). Mixed tumours are regarded as teratomas, and this group includes any apparently pure seminomas with a raised AFP. The peak incidence of teratomas is in the mid-20s, seminoma tends to occur in an older age group with the peak incidence in the mid-30s.

The pathologist will not only classify the tumour type but also comment on pathological features predictive of prognosis, such as the invasion of surrounding structures, involvement of the spermatic cord and vascular or lymphatic invasion.

CLASSIFICATION OF TESTICULAR GERM CELL TUMOURS

- Seminoma
- Non-seminomatous germ cell tumour (teratoma)
  - Teratoma differentiated (mature teratoma)
  - Malignant teratoma intermediate (teratocarcinoma)
  - Malignant teratoma undifferentiated (embryonal carcinoma)
  - Yolk sac tumour
  - Malignant teratoma trophoblastic (choriocarcinoma)

STAGING

The stage of the cancer is dependent on the preoperative levels of the tumour markers and the rate of decline after surgery, pathological features of the resected tissue, and computed tomography (CT) scanning of the abdomen, pelvis and thorax.

There is a TNM-staging classification, but in the UK the traditional staging system has been the Royal Marsden Hospital classification. This is now supplemented by the International Germ Cell Consensus Classification (IGCCC) prognostic grouping to allocate treatment strategies.

ROYAL MARSDEN HOSPITAL STAGING CLASSIFICATION

- Stage I   No evidence of disease outside the testis
  IM As above, but tumour markers fail to normalise after surgery
- Stage II   Lymph node involvement below the diaphragm
  A <2 cm diameter
  B 2–5 cm diameter
  C 5–10 cm diameter
  D >10 cm diameter
- Stage III Lymph node involvement above the level of the diaphragm
- Stage IV Haematogenous spread, for example to lung or brain

For seminoma, the IGCCC prognostic grouping allocates patients to the intermediate group if there are any non-pulmonary visceral metastases. The primary site and marker levels are not relevant. All other patients are in the good prognostic group. There is no poor prognostic group for seminoma.

IGCCC PROGNOSTIC GROUPING FOR TERATOMA (BOTH TESTICULAR AND NON-TESTICULAR)

- *Good prognosis*
  Testicular or retroperitoneal primary and no non-pulmonary visceral metastases and all of
  AFP < 1,000 ng ml^{-1}
  hCG < 5,000 IU l^{-1}
  LDH < 1.5 × upper limit of normal

- *Intermediate prognosis*
  Testicular or retroperitoneal primary and no non-pulmonary visceral metastases and any of
  AFP > 1,000 and < 10,000 ng ml^{-1}
  hCG > 5,000 and < 50,000 IU l^{-1}
  LDH > 1.5 and < 10 × upper limit of normal

- *Poor prognosis*
  Mediastinal primary or non-pulmonary visceral metastases and any of
  AFP > 10,000 ng l^{-1}
  hCG > 50,000 IU l^{-1}
  LDH > 10 × upper limit of normal

TREATMENT OF SEMINOMA

In Stage I seminoma, the initial treatment will be inguinal orchidectomy. Without further treatment there is about a one in five chance of recurrence. Postoperative radiotherapy to the para-aortic lymph node area is usually recommended to prevent recurrence. Only a relatively low dose is needed, and toxicity is very limited. Anti-emetics, such as granisetron, may be required to prevent acute vomiting.

Surveillance with regular CT scanning instead of radiotherapy is not advisable except in exceptional circumstances as recurrences beyond 5 years may occur, so surveillance would need to be for a prolonged period. If radiotherapy is contraindicated, adjuvant chemotherapy offers an alternative to surveillance, but should be considered experimental.

In metastatic seminoma (Stages II, III and IV), chemotherapy is usually the treatment of choice. A combination of cisplatin and etoposide is normally used. Radiotherapy may be an alternative for small volume disease (Stage IIA).

TREATMENT OF TERATOMA

In Stage I teratoma, the initial treatment will be inguinal orchidectomy. Without further treatment, there is about a one in three chance of recurrence. Most relapses occur early, within the first year. Surveillance involves a combination of monthly chest radiography and tumour markers and 3-monthly CT scans. These allow for early treatment of those who do relapse while sparing others the toxicity of chemotherapy. Adjuvant chemotherapy can be offered to the subset of patients with pathological features predictive of a high risk of recurrence. Two courses of bleomycin, etoposide and cisplatin (BEP) are effective in this situation.

Good prognosis metastatic disease (including patients with Stage IM disease) should be treated with three courses of BEP chemotherapy.

For patients with intermediate or poor prognosis metastatic disease, the standard initial treatment remains BEP. Many other schedules have been tested, but more intensive regimens seem to produce similar results with greater toxicity. Alternative drug schedules and high-dose chemotherapy are being evaluated for the treatment of resistant or relapsed disease. Any residual tumour masses after chemotherapy for advanced disease should be resected. If orchidectomy was not done earlier, it should be performed after completion of chemotherapy. Patients with brain metastases should be treated with radical intent. Surgery should be considered for operable lesions, and radiotherapy may also play a role.

PROGNOSIS

The likelihood of disease-free survival for Stage I seminoma with surgery and postoperative radiotherapy is in excess of 95%. The small number who relapses can usually be salvaged with chemotherapy. The 5-year survival for the 90% of patients with good prognosis seminomas is over 85%, and for those in the intermediate prognostic group it is about 75%.

With metastatic teratoma, only 10% of those achieving a complete remission will relapse. More than half of those with teratomas have good prognosis disease. For these, the 5-year survival is over 90%. Over a quarter of patients with teratomas have intermediate prognosis disease, with a likelihood of survival at 5 years of 80%. About 15% have poor prognosis teratomas, and around half of these may be cured.

Brain tumours

The most common brain tumours in adults are cerebral metastases. Primary brain tumours are rare and account for the minority of intracranial tumours. They form only about 3% or 4% of cancers. Brain tumours are relatively common in children and are considered in Chapter 46. In adults, the peak incidence is in people in their 60s and 70s. There is a slightly higher incidence in men. The majority are sporadic, but a small proportion are associated with underlying genetic abnormalities, such as neurofibromatosis.

PRESENTATION

The history is usually short, measured in weeks, and presentation is usually with raised intracranial pressure, focal neurological deficit or seizures, or a combination of these.

> **PRESENTING FEATURES OF BRAIN TUMOURS**
>
> ◆ Raised intracranial pressure
> ◆ Focal neurological deficit
> ◆ Seizures

Raised intracranial pressure is characterised by headaches, principally present in the early morning or causing early waking but which settle through the day, and vomiting which is often said to be effortless or not associated with nausea. There may be blurred vision due to papilloedema or a squint due to a sixth cranial nerve palsy. Finally, consciousness may be impaired.

> **PREVALENCE OF SYMPTOMS AMONG PATIENTS PRESENTING WITH BRAIN TUMOURS**
>
> ◆ Focal neurological deficit   >50%
> ◆ Seizures   25–30%
> ◆ Headache   25–35%
> ◆ Papilloedema   25–50%
> ◆ Mental changes   15–20%

A variety of focal neurological deficits may be produced. Tumours affecting the motor cortex may result in weakness of an upper motor neurone type affecting the face and limbs, typically on one side only. If the brain stem is affected there may be cranial nerve palsies as well as long tract signs, and the facial weakness may be on the opposite side to the limb weakness. A cerebellar tumour may result in ataxia.

> **ARE NEW SEIZURES DUE TO A TUMOUR?**
>
> ◆ New seizures in adults – 5% risk of underlying brain tumour
> ◆ New status epilephicus – 10% risk of underlying brain tumour

Siezures may be focal or Jacksonian, grand mal convulsions or status epilepticus. They tend to be associated with more slowly growing low-grade tumours, and a history of siezures may be longer than a history of raised intracranial pressure. The likelihood of a new onset seizure disorder of any type in an adult being due to a brain tumour is only about 5%. The development of new onset status epilepticus is due to a brain tumour in only about 10% of cases.

> **GUIDELINES FOR URGENT REFERRAL OF PATIENTS WITH SUSPECTED BRAIN TUMOURS**
>
> ◆ Subacute progressive neurological deficit developing over days to weeks (e.g. weakness, sensory loss, dysphasia, ataxia)
> ◆ New onset seizures characterised by one or more of the following:
>   – Focal seizures
>   – Prolonged post-ictal focal deficit (longer than 1 hour)
>   – Status epilepticus
>   – Associated inter-ictal focal deficit
> ◆ Patients with headaches, vomiting and papilloedema
> ◆ Cranial nerve palsy (e.g. diplopia, visual failure including optician-defined visual field loss, unilateral sensorineural deafness)
>
> *Consider* urgent referral for
> ◆ Patients with non-migrainous headaches of recent onset, present for at least 1 month, when accompanied by features suggestive of raised intracranial pressure (e.g. woken by headache, vomiting, drowsiness)

Magnetic resonance imaging (MRI) is the best investigation to confirm the presence of a suspected brain tumour. A computed tomography (CT) scan is an alternative screening investigation when MRI is not immediately possible. If the CT is abnormal, an MRI scan will usually be performed prior to any surgical intervention; but will not be required if the patient is too old or too neurologically disabled for a neurosurgical procedure to be considered. If the CT scan is normal, this may provide reassurance if the index of suspicion is low, but if, clinically, a brain tumour seems to be the likely diagnosis, then an MRI will be required.

If a patient has symptoms and signs of raised intracranial pressure then initial treatment with steroids, say dexamethasone 16 mg daily in divided doses may be appropriate while investigations are being arranged. In an acute emergency, the patient should be hospitalised and treatment with intravenous mannitol given.

As there are many different types of brain tumour, histology is necessary to characterise any imageable abnormality fully. The exception to this is in the case of typical brain stem tumours where the procedure would be associated with a significant hazard. The neurosurgeon will make a judgement as to whether the first procedure should be biopsy only, or whether an attempt at removal of the abnormality is indicated.

CLASSIFICATION

The most common type of primary brain tumour is the glioma (of all grades), accounting for about half of all adult brain tumours. About 20% are meningiomas. Pituitary adenomas and acoustic schwannomas come next. Other types, such as primitive neuroectodermal tumours (PNETs, e.g. medulloblastoma), craniopharyngioma, intracranial germ cell tumours are all rare in adults, although relatively more common in children (Chapter 46). Primary central nervous system (CNS) lymphoma is rare, and is more commonly associated with human immunodeficiency virus (HIV) infection (Chapter 42).

Gliomas

Gliomas are a group of tumours comprising astrocytomas, oligodendrogliomas and ependymomas. Astrocytomas form about two-thirds of all gliomas and can be divided into a number of subtypes depending on histological grade. Astrocytomas Grades I and II have a better prognosis, and are more common in childhood than adults. Anaplastic astrocytoma (Grade III) is more malignant. Glioblastoma multiforme (Grade IV) is the most common type in adult life and is almost universally fatal.

Low-grade astrocytomas, the commonest form of childhood brain tumour, are much less common in adults. They are more likely to occur in the cerebral hemispheres than in the posterior fossa. In adults, treatment consists of surgery, either debulking or total resection if feasible, or biopsy alone if the tumour is at a site where an attempt at resection would pose too great a hazard. Radiotherapy may be given immediately postoperatively, or held in

reserve until there is evidence of tumour progression. It is not clear which approach is better. Chemotherapy is not usually used as first-line treatment. Some patients, perhaps about half, will be cured, but in others there will be recurrence. Further surgery may be indicated, or radiotherapy if it has not already been used. Chemotherapy may be used if there are no other options. Sometimes, low-grade gliomas may become more transform into frankly malignant tumours with time.

GLIOMAS

- Astrocytoma
  - Grade I
  - Grade II
  - Grade III   Anaplastic astrocytoma
  - Grade IV   Glioblastoma multiforme
- Oligodendroglioma
  - Low-grade oligodendroglioma
  - Anaplastic oligodendroglioma
- Ependymoma
  - Low-grade ependymoma
  - Anaplastic ependymoma

Anaplastic astrocytomas are treated with a resection as good as possible, followed by radiotherapy. Again the place of chemotherapy as first-line treatment is not clear. About 20% of patients with Grade III astrocytomas will be cured with local therapy, but the majority will relapse. Further surgery can be considered, followed by chemotherapy, but the real aim of treatment is palliation only, and the main benefit is to prolong life. The most commonly used chemotherapy is the combination procarbazine, vincristine and lomustine (PCV), but recently the National Institute for Clinical Excellence (NICE) has recommended temozolamide as second-line chemotherapy for use in the treatment of high-grade gliomas which have progressed on PCV.

AIMS OF SURGERY IN THE MANAGEMENT OF BRAIN TUMOURS

- To obtain tissue for a histological diagnosis
- To relieve direct pressure effects from the tumour
- To relieve obstructive hydrocephalus
- To remove the tumour where possible
- To reduce the tumour bulk to make radiotherapy and chemotherapy more effective

---

Glioblastoma multiforme is usually very extensive at presentation, and though a debulking operation is useful to relieve pressure symptoms, complete excision is only rarely possible. Radical radiotherapy will prolong survival, but the majority of patients are dead within 2 years. Palliative chemotherapy with PCV or temozolamide may be offered as an adjuvant or on progression, but the results are disappointingly short lived.

Oligodendrogliomas are generally well-circumscribed, low-grade tumours with a long natural history. Anaplastic oligodendrogliomas behave more like high-grade astrocytomas. Surgery and radiotherapy are the principal treatments. Again, palliative chemotherapy may be used to treat tumour progression.

Ependymomas arise from the ependyma lining the ventricles. They may occur in the cerebral hemispheres or in the posterior fossa. Radical surgery is essential for cure, and is usually followed by radiotherapy to the tumour bed. Ependymoma is usually a low-grade tumour. Anaplastic ependymoma carries a worse prognosis, but is treated in the same way.

Meningiomas

Meningiomas arise from the meninges surrounding the brain and spinal cord and are generally slow growing. There are other variants that constitute a group called malignant meningioma, which are more likely than ordinary meningiomas to metastasise within the craniospinal axis.

Meningioma is a benign tumour, usually curable with surgery, if the initial resection is complete. Radiotherapy is used in selected cases, such as for patients with known or suspected residual disease or with recurrence after previous surgery. Radiotherapy alone is sometimes used, if the disease is not amenable to surgery.

Patients with malignant meningioma are treated in the same way as ordinary meningiomas, although the prognosis is worse because complete resections are less common and the mitotic activity is greater.

Pituitary adenomas

Pituitary adenomas are reasonably common benign brain tumours. They may present with endocrine effects, such as acromegaly, Cushing's syndrome and hyperprolactinaemia. Non-functional adenomas may not present until they have reached a size where they cause pressure effects, such as visual field loss due to compression of the optic chiasm. Medical management is possible for some smaller secreting tumours, but those with mass effects need surgical removal. This is often done via the trans-sphenoidal route, but some larger tumours may need a transfrontal approach. Although these are benign tumours, radiotherapy may be needed if there continues to be an abnormal level of hormone production.

Acoustic schwannomas

Like meningiomas and pituitary adenomas these are benign tumours. They may be associated with neurofibromatosis type 2, and if so they can be bilateral. They present with sensorineural deafness or the cerebellopontine angle syndrome, hopefully these days before pressure effects have produced a seventh nerve palsy as

well. Treatment is usually surgical, but fractionated stereotactic radiotherapy or radiosurgery are sometimes used.

Primitive neuroectodermal tumours

Intracranial PNETs occur most commonly in childhood, but also occur in young adults. PNETs can occur at different sites within the brain, and have been known by various names. The most common type, found in the cerebellum, is medulloblastoma. It is associated with a more favourable outcome than supratentorial PNETs, such as the pineoblastoma and the ependymoblastoma and central neuroblastoma. These tumours have a propensity for spread through the cerebrospinal fluid (CSF) pathways and so a staging MRI scan is needed to look for intracranial or spinal metastases. The principals of treatment are radical surgical removal, if possible, followed by craniospinal radiotherapy with a boost to the tumour bed, and adjuvant chemotherapy. Survival rates are approximately 50% for all PNETs, being best for completely resected cerebellar tumours with no metastatic spread, and worse in those with supratentorial tumours, if there is residual disease after surgery and if there are metastases present.

Craniopharyngioma

Craniopharyngioma is a tumour which occurs most often in children, but may also present in adult life. It occurs in the suprasellar and pituitary region. It may present with endocrine dysfunction, visual field defects as a result of chiasmatic compression or with raised intracranial pressure. The tumours are usually partly solid and partly cystic. Although histologically benign, complete resection is difficult. Attempts at resection can result in very significant morbidity, especially if the hypothalamus is involved. It is often better to decompress the cysts and treat with radical radiotherapy. If the tumour is resectable, postoperative radiotherapy is still advised as without it the risk of recurrence is high.

Intracranial germ cell tumours

These too are more common in adolescence, but also occur in young adults. They usually occur in the pineal or suprasellar regions, and have a tendency to metastasise through the CSF pathways. There are two main types, pure germinoma and secreting tumours. Germinoma is usually curable with craniospinal radiotherapy alone. Secreting tumours produce high levels of either alpha fetoprotein (AFP) or beta human chorionic gonadotrophin (bhCG) or both. If these tumour markers are elevated, surgery is not necessary to make the diagnosis. They are more malignant than germinomas and require combined modality therapy with chemotherapy and radiotherapy and sometimes surgery if there is a residual mass left after initial non-surgical treatment. About two-thirds will be cured.

Leukaemia is the generic name given to a wide variety of cancers of the haemopoietic stem cells in the bone marrow and blood. It is not a common malignancy, accounting for only about 3% of the total cancer incidence or about 5,000 cases per year in the UK. This chapter relates principally to leukaemia occurring in adults, childhood leukaemia is covered in Chapter 46.

Although there are many different types of leukaemia, for most practical purposes it is sufficient to classify the disease by whether it is acute or chronic, and by whether the cell type is myeloid or lymphoid.

> ## CLASSIFICATION OF LEUKAEMIA
>
> ◆ Acute myeloid leukaemia (AML)
> ◆ Acute lymphoblastic leukaemia (ALL)
> ◆ Chronic myeloid leukaemia (CML)
> ◆ Chronic lymphatic leukaemia (CLL)

Patients with acute leukaemia are often very unwell at the time of diagnosis and give only a short history. Untreated, most would die within a couple of months. Chronic leukaemia tends to be a disease of older people. It may present as an incidental finding in an asymptomatic patient. Alternatively, symptoms may have been present for months at the time of diagnosis of chronic leukaemia. Without treatment, the life expectancy of a patient with chronic leukaemia may be measured in years.

In acute leukaemia, there is an uncontrolled proliferation of haemopoietic stem cells (or blasts) in the bone marrow and usually spilling over into the peripheral blood. In AML, these cells are myeloblasts, and in ALL they are lymphoblasts. Due to confusing medical fashion for naming diseases by what they are not, rather than by what they are, AML is sometimes referred to as acute non-lymphocytic leukaemia (ANLL).

In chronic leukaemia, the excess cells seen in the blood and bone marrow are more mature, being neutrophils or granulocytes in CML (hence, the alternative term chronic granulocytic leukaemia, CGL), and lymphocytes in CLL.

PRESENTING FEATURES OF ACUTE LEUKAEMIA

The clinical presentation of acute leukaemia is similar, regardless of whether the cell type is myeloid or lymphoblastic. The features are essentially those of bone marrow failure with one or more of anaemia, thrombocytopenia or infection. Anaemia may result in tiredness and breathlessness or in extreme cases angina or heart failure. Thrombocytopaenia will manifest as bruising or petechial haemorrhages. Swollen, bleeding gums are characteristic, although not always present. There may also be a sore mouth or throat, fever, or other signs of infection at presentation.

ACUTE MYELOID LEUKAEMIA

When a patient presents with symptoms which might be due to acute leukaemia, a full blood count is the first investigation. This is likely to show anaemia and thrombocytopenia, and an elevated white blood count with an excess of blasts. Following urgent referral to a haematologist for investigation, a full bone marrow examination will be performed to confirm the diagnosis and characterise the disease. If it is acute leukaemia, deciding whether it is AML or ALL has important therapeutic and prognostic implications. Four out of five adults with acute leukaemia have AML. Various subtypes of AML are recognised depending on the degree of differentiation along different cell lines and the extent of cellular maturation. These are numbered M0 to M7 according to the French, American, British (FAB) classification.

> ## PRINCIPAL SUBTYPES OF AML – THE FAB CLASSIFICATION
>
> ◆ AML with minimal differentiation (M0)
> ◆ Myeloblastic leukaemia without maturation (M1)
> ◆ Myeloblastic leukaemia with maturation (M2)
> ◆ Promyelocytic leukaemia (M3)
> ◆ Myelomonocytic leukaemia (M4)
> ◆ Monocytic leukaemia (M5)
> ◆ Erythroleukaemia (M6)
> ◆ Megakaryoblastic leukaemia (M7)

These AML subtypes can have different clinical features. For example, patients with promyelocytic leukaemia (M3) are often very ill at presentation as it is usually associated with disseminated intravascular coagulation. Patients with monocytic leukaemia (M5) characteristically have gum infiltration, and patients with erythroleukaemia (M6) often have a degree of fibrosis in the marrow and are less likely to achieve remission with standard therapy, but the distinction between the subtypes is of lesser practical importance than between AML and ALL.

Rarely, a patient may present with an isolated tumour of myeloblasts called a granulocytic sarcoma or chloroma. This may be visceral, in soft tissue or skin, head or neck, bone, or in the central nervous system (CNS). Patients with these tumours are not cured by local therapy, and they should be treated with aggressive chemotherapy as if they had AML.

Treatment of AML falls into a number of phases. First comes remission induction, where a two or three drug regimen is used to clear detectable malignant cells from the blood and bone marrow. Once the disease is in remission, additional chemotherapy is given to reduce the likelihood of relapse. This consolidation treatment is either conventional dose chemotherapy alone, or it may be followed by high-dose chemotherapy and an autograft or bone marrow transplantation from a relative or matched unrelated donor (MUD). Transplants are usually restricted to patients under the age of 60 years. Transplants from sibling donors are associated with fewer complications than MUD transplants. If there is CNS involvement, intrathecal chemotherapy is used in addition. As the incidence of CNS disease is much lower in AML than in ALL, CNS directed therapy is only given to patients with detectable CNS disease and not used in all patients as a matter of routine. If the disease relapses, then treatment can begin again, and a bone marrow transplant (if a suitable donor can be identified) is often recommended in second remission if it has not been used before.

KEY ELEMENTS IN AML TREATMENT

- Remission induction
- Consolidation
- Bone marrow transplantation
- Treatment of CNS disease
- Supportive care

As was said earlier, patients with acute leukaemia are often very sick at presentation with features of bone marrow failure, infection and coagulopathies. The treatment of AML is very intensive, and adds to the problems with prolonged periods of profound myelosuppression requiring blood product support and treatment of opportunistic infections. There is a significant possibility of death from the disease during the early stages of remission induction,

and there is an appreciable treatment-related mortality, highest when MUD transplants are used. Morbidity and mortality rates are greater in older patients. Patients should only be managed in specialist malignant haematology centres, as adequately resourced and experienced personnel are essential for high-quality supportive care (Chapter 17).

AML is nowadays a curable disease in many cases, but a number of features are recognised which predict for a poor outcome.

ADVERSE PROGNOSTIC FACTORS IN AML

- Older age at presentation
- Presenting white cell count greater than $100 \times 10^9 l^{-1}$
- Systemic infection at presentation
- Cytogenetic abnormalities
- History of myelodysplastic syndrome
- AML related to previous chemotherapy
- CNS involvement

Overall, about two-thirds of patients with AML enter first remission. The chances of entering remission are greater in the absence of the adverse prognostic factors listed above. Of those who do remit, between a quarter and a third are likely to be cured. The chance of cure is greater in those who have had a successful transplant.

ACUTE LYMPHOBLASTIC LEUKAEMIA

The presenting features of acute leukaemia usually give no clue as to whether the disease is AML or ALL. Only 20% of adults with acute leukaemia have ALL. The diagnosis is confirmed by examination of the blood and bone marrow including immunological and cytogenetic studies. Treatment and prognosis are guided by the immunological cell type and cytogenetic features.

CLASSIFICATION OF ALL

By cell lineage
- Pre-B-cell or common ALL   80%
- B-cell   5%
- T-cell   15%

By cytogenetic analysis
- Philadelphia chromosome positive (Ph+)   25%

As in childhood ALL, treatment of pre-B-cell or common ALL in adults is divided up into four principal phases, remission induction, consolidation, CNS directed therapy and maintenance. As with AML, careful supportive care (Chapter 17) is necessary to minimise the morbidity and mortality of treatment. Key features include the prevention of tumour lysis syndrome, treatment of infection and blood product support.

> **TREATMENT OF ALL**
>
> - Remission induction
> - Consolidation
> - CNS directed therapy
> - Maintenance
> - Supportive care

Successful treatment of ALL implies eradication of malignant cells in the blood and bone marrow, and also in "sanctuary" sites, such as the meninges which conventional chemotherapy fails to penetrate adequately. Chemotherapy, usually comprising a combination of three or four drugs including an anthracycline, vincristine and corticosteroids, will achieve remission (the absence of detectable leukaemia cells in the blood and bone marrow) in up to 80% of patients. Further blocks of chemotherapy called intensification or consolidation follow at intervals to treat undetectable residual disease. Intrathecal chemotherapy and cranial radiotherapy are used to treat established CNS disease, or are employed prohylactically to reduce the likelihood of CNS relapse in patients whose CNS was clear at diagnosis. Maintenance or continuing chemotherapy is low-intensity oral chemotherapy, with the dose adjusted according to the blood count, carried on until 2 or 3 years from diagnosis. This prolonged phase of maintenance chemotherapy is very important in eradicating undetectable leukaemia cells and thereby improving the prospects for cure.

Patients with B-cell or T-cell variants of ALL do not fare well with this pattern of treatment and will be treated on alternative, intensive shorter duration protocols. Patients with Ph+ ALL similarly do not do well with conventional ALL treatment and are often offered transplantation in first remission if a suitable donor can be found. Patients who relapse, especially while on treatment, have a poor prognosis, and are often offered transplantation as well.

The outcome for adults with ALL is nowhere near as good as it is for children with the same disease (Chapter 46). Nonetheless, about 40% may be cured. Outcome is clearly worse in patients who have one or more of the adverse prognostic factors listed below.

> **ADVERSE PROGNOSTIC FACTORS IN ALL**
>
> - Older age at presentation
> - Presenting white cell count greater than $50 \times 10^9 \, l^{-1}$
> - Cytogenetic abnormalities especially Ph+
> - CNS involvement

CHRONIC LYMPHOCYTIC LEUKAEMIA

CLL is essentially a disease of older people, occurring with increasing frequency in successive decades of life. Only 5% are under the age of 50 years at diagnosis. It is characterised by a malignant proliferation of mature B-cell lymphocytes and there is a spectrum of disease activity ranging from an incidental finding on a blood count performed for another reason in a patient without symptoms, to a life-threatening disease with generalised lymphadenopathy, splenomegaly and pancytopaenia caused by marrow infiltration. Coombs-positive haemolytic anaemia, immune thrombocytopenia, and depressed immuno-globulin levels may complicate CLL and enhance the problems of anaemia, haemorrhage and infection.

There is no real distinction to be drawn between CLL (a blood and bone marrow disease where there may be lymphadenopathy) and lymphocytic lymphoma (Chapter 41) (where the presentation may be with lymphadenopathy and the marrow may also be involved). These are essentially two aspects of the same disease, which is treated in the same way.

Staging of some sort is useful for stratifying patients for treatment and to gauge prognosis. There is no universally recognised system, but several classifications are used, taking into account anaemia, thrombocytopenia and hepatosplenomegaly as the most important factors. Auto-immune haemolytic anaemia and thrombocytopenia are less important prognostically than anaemia and thrombocytopenia due to marrow infiltration.

The pace of the disease is often slow, with a natural history measured in years. Patients with asymptomatic lymphocytosis only, have a median survival of the order of 10 years. As most patients are elderly (Chapter 48) and cure is not possible, treatment strategies are very conservative. Disease discovered at an early stage does not necessarily require treatment.

> **INDICATIONS FOR INITIATING TREATMENT FOR CLL**
>
> - Constitutional symptoms: fever, night sweats, weight loss
> - Symptomatic lymphadenopathy or splenomegaly
> - Marrow infiltration causing anaemia or thrombocytopaenia
> - Auto-immune haemolysis or thrombocytopaenia

Constitutional symptoms, such as fever, night sweats or weight loss ("B" symptoms); progressive or painful lymphadenopathy or splenomegaly; anaemia or thrombocytopaenia due to marrow infiltration; or auto-immune haemolysis or thrombocytopaenia may indicate the need for treatment. When treatment is required, simple oral chemotherapy regimens such as chlorambucil with or without steroids (especially if there are auto-immune features) are often sufficient as first-line therapy. There is no evidence that starting treatment early, or using more aggressive combinations of chemotherapy drugs improves outcome. Careful attention to early treatment of infective complications, such as shingles and thrush is necessary.

TREATMENT STRATEGIES FOR CLL

- Observation or "watchful waiting"
- Single agent chemotherapy with oral chlorambucil or cyclophosphamide
- Steroids especially if there are features of auto-immune anaemia or thrombocytopaenia
- Combination chemotherapy, for example, cyclophosphamide, vincristine and prednisolone (CVP) or doxorubicin, cyclophosphamide, vincristine and prednisolone (CHOP)
- Purine analogues, such as fludarabine
- Low-dose radiotherapy to lymph node masses or the spleen
- Monoclonal antibody therapy, such as rituximab
- Bone marrow transplantation approaches are experimental in the very rare young fit patient

---

If first-line treatment with intermittent courses of oral chlorambucil with or without prednisolone is not satisfactory, then more intensive combinations including a vinca alkaloid such as vincristine and perhaps an anthracycline such as doxorubicin may be helpful.

Care should be exercised when treatment is initiated in patients with a significant tumour burden, as rapid breakdown of cells may lead to the tumour lysis syndrome (Chapter 17). Patients at risk may need intravenous fluids, allopurinol and close monitoring of blood biochemistry.

Fludarabine is an antimetabolite recommended for use in patients with CLL after failure of alkylating agent therapy. It is given orally daily for 5 days each month. Myelosuppression and other side-effects, such as peripheral neuropathy and pulmonary toxicity, are more marked than with chlorambucil.

Rituximab, a humanised monoclonal antibody directed against antigens on B-cells, has found a place in the treatment of follicular lymphoma and high-grade B-cell NHL. It is also being investigated in refractory CLL.

Radiotherapy is a good palliative treatment for patients distressed by lymph node masses or splenomegaly. Splenectomy is an alternative treatment for troublesome splenomegaly in a patient who is fit for surgery.

Most patients with CLL are elderly and may well have co-morbidity. As the patient may co-exist peacefully with the disease for many years, aggressive treatments aimed at cure are not usually indicated. In the few very young patients with this disease, much more aggressive strategies have been tried. These include high-dose chemotherapy with autologous or allogeneic bone marrow transplantation, accepting that the potential long-term benefits of achieving a cure may offset the risk of early treatment-related mortality. However, the real place of such treatments is not yet known.

CHRONIC MYELOID LEUKAEMIA

CML, like CLL, accounts for about one-quarter of adult leukaemia cases. The peak incidence in the fifth decade of life, is somewhat younger than that of CLL. CML is one of a group of diseases called myeloproliferative disorders, all of which may terminate in the development of acute leukaemia after a chronic phase of variable duration.

MYELOPROLIFERATIVE DISORDERS

- CML
- Myelofibrosis
- Polycythaemia rubra vera
- Essential thrombocythaemia

CML was the first disease to be shown to be associated with a characteristic chromosomal abnormality. The so-called Philadelphia chromosome was identified in 1960, and is present in 95% of cases of CML as well as in a proportion of some other disorders such as ALL (above). It is caused by a reciprocal translocation between parts of the long arms of chromosomes 9 and 22. This cytogenetic abnormality is important, not just for diagnosis and prognosis, but also for treatment. As a consequence of the translocation, a fusion gene named *bcr-abl* is produced. The abnormal protein encoded by this fusion gene is a constitutively active tyrosine kinase, C-KIT, which influences cellular proliferation, differentiation and survival. Cells containing the abnormal gene and protein replicate quickly and may be protected from programmed cell death. They, therefore, become predominant, initially in the bone marrow and subsequently in the blood stream, impairing the production of normal white cells. Patients with CML may be considered Ph+ either by virtue of a visible Philadelphia chromosome on conventional cytogenetic studies, or if the *bcr-abl* fusion gene can be demonstrated by molecular biology techniques in the absence of a conventionally detectable abnormality.

CML is a disease which progresses through three identifiable phases, chronic phase, accelerated phase and blast crisis. The chronic phase is the initial phase of CML, lasting for a variable duration with an average of 3–5 years. About 5–10% of patients progress from chronic phase to accelerated phase in each of the first 2 years after diagnosis, subsequently, the rate of progression is about 20% each year. The accelerated phase is often heralded by increasing splenomegaly, the development of drug resistance, a greater number of immature white blood cells, or the development of anaemia and thrombocytopenia with a normal white count. This phase generally lasts for a number of months or a year before progression to the inevitably fatal blast crisis occurs.

PHASES OF CML

- Chronic phase
- Accelerated phase
- Blast crisis

Many patients with chronic phase CML are asymptomatic at presentation. A full blood count performed for another reason may be abnormal, leading to the diagnosis of CML, or perhaps an enlarged spleen, present in the majority of patients, is an incidental finding on a medical examination. Sometimes, patients present with symptomatic splenomegaly, anaemia, infections or other signs of bone marrow failure. Less commonly the patient may present with neurological symptoms due to leucostasis.

Allogeneic bone marrow transplantation from related or MUDs is the only known curative therapy for CML. The aims of allogeneic bone marrow transplantation are: eradication of the clone of leukaemic cells with myeloablative doses of chemotherapy and radiotherapy, which also provide the immunosuppression necessary for engraftment; restoration of normal haemopoiesis by the donor marrow and exploitation of the graft versus leukaemia effect of the donor marrow to suppress or destroy any remaining leukaemic cells. The use of allogeneic bone marrow transplantation is associated with a significant procedure-related mortality. Usually only otherwise healthy patients under the age of 55 or 60 years will be considered for bone marrow transplantation, for whom a suitable donor will be found in only about three-quarters of cases. Results are best when the transplant is performed within a year of diagnosis. Bone marrow transplantation is substantially less effective when it is used in the accelerated phase or in blast crisis.

Various treatments are available for CML when transplantation is not an option, and these may also be used in potential transplant patients while the search for a suitable donor takes place.

TREATMENT STRATEGIES IN CML

- Allogeneic bone marrow transplantation in selected patients with a donor
- Interferon alfa
- Chemotherapy with hydroxyurea (or less commonly busulfan)
- Imatinib
- Supportive care with blood products

Conventional oral single agent chemotherapy, historically with busulfan, more recently with hydroxyurea, has been the mainstay of treatment for decades. Chemotherapy is effective at lowering the abnormal white cell count in chronic phase, but is not curative. The main aim is to prevent symptoms from a raised white blood cell count.

Interferon alfa is a more effective treatment in reducing the abnormal white cell count in chronic phase, and can result in complete haematological and cytogenetic remission, with normal peripheral blood and bone marrow, no splenomegaly and no detectable Ph+ cells. This treatment may prolong survival, and the risk of mortality is about one-third lower each year for patients treated with interferon compared with hydroxyurea or busulphan. However, the disease eventually relapses and progression to blast crisis ensues. Interferon alfa has significant toxic effects, and the incidence of complications is greater in elderly patients. Toxicity may require dose modification or discontinuation of therapy in many cases. Common side-effects include an influenza-like syndrome, nausea, anorexia, weight loss, and neuropsychiatric symptoms, all of which are completely reversible with cessation of therapy. Immune-mediated complications, such as hyperthyroidism, haemolysis, and connective tissue diseases may occur rarely after long-term treatment.

Imatinib is a specific inhibitor of the tyrosine kinase protein produced from *bcr-abl* fusion protein on the Philadelphia chromosome. It is a new and effective treatment for patients with Ph+ CML. Imatinib has recently been recommended for use by the National Institute for Clinical Excellence as a treatment option for the management of Ph+ CML in chronic phase in adults who have failed, or who cannot tolerate the use of, interferon alfa therapy. Imatinib is also recommended as a treatment option in patients with accelerated phase or blast crisis provided that they have not received it at an earlier stage.

The lymphomas

Lymphoma is a malignant proliferation of lymphoid cells, which usually presents as enlargement of lymph nodes. Other non-nodal lymphoid structures, such as the pharyngeal lymphoid tissue known as Waldeyer's ring and the spleen, can be primarily involved. Occasionally, non-lymphoid structures, such as the skin and the brain, may be the site of the presenting disease.

> **THE LYMPHOMAS**
>
> - Hodgkin's disease
> - Non-Hodgkin's lymphoma (NHL)

Lymphoma is not a single disease, but a variety of different clinico-pathological entities with widely varying natural histories. The London physician, pathologist and Quaker philanthropist, Thomas Hodgkin, described six patients with lymphadenopathy in 1832. Four of these cases have, more recently, been proven to be due to lymphoma. Nowadays, lymphomas are divided into Hodgkin's disease, a reasonably clearly defined entity, and NHL, which is a collection of many distinct diseases. As one of Hodgkin's six original patients had what we now call NHL, it might have been better if the term Hodgkin's disease was applied to all types of lymphoma; however, common practice leaves us with Hodgkin's disease and NHL.

HODGKIN'S DISEASE

Hodgkin's disease can occur at any age, although it is rare in children under 5 years of age. There is a rising incidence in older adolescents and younger adults, with a peak between the ages of 20 and 30 years. After that it becomes less common, although the incidence rates rise again in old age. Males are more commonly affected than females. The cause is not known, but several epidemiological features suggest a complex interaction between genetic and environmental factors.

Presentation

The majority of patients present with painless enlarged lymph nodes, most commonly in the neck. The size of the nodes may wax and wane over a period of months before the diagnosis is made. Mediastinal lymph nodes are commonly involved, and the presentation may be with superior vena cava obstruction. Infradiaphragmatic lymph node involvement is less common. While involvement of the para-aortic nodes is not infrequently found by staging investigations, an inguinal presentation is rare.

> **APPROXIMATE FREQUENCY OF LYMPH NODE INVOLVEMENT IN HODGKIN'S DISEASE**
>
> - Cervical nodes: 70%
> - Mediastinal nodes: 50%
> - Axillary nodes: 30%
> - Para-aortic nodes: 30%
> - Inguinal nodes: 10%

Involvement of extra-nodal lymphatic tissue is well recognised. The spleen is most commonly affected. Involvement of Waldeyer's ring is, however, unusual. It is much less common in Hodgkin's disease than in NHL. Involvement of non-lymphoid tissue, such as liver, bone or bone marrow, is recognised as being of importance, but is unusual at presentation.

> **APPROXIMATE FREQUENCY OF NON-LYMPH NODE INVOLVEMENT IN HODGKIN'S DISEASE**
>
> - Spleen: 30%
> - Liver: 5%
> - Bone marrow: 5%
> - Waldeyer's ring: 1–2%

Systemic symptoms are reported in up to one-third of patients. These include the so-called B-symptoms of weight loss, fever and night sweats, which affect the staging classification.

> **B-SYMPTOMS IN HODGKIN'S DISEASE**
>
> - Fever
> - Weight loss
> - Night sweats

Other symptoms, such as pruritis and the rarely encountered but classical phenomenon of pain after drinking alcohol, are not regarded as B-symptoms. Breathlessness may occur for various reasons including pleural or peri-cardial effusion, and anaemia may be due to bone marrow infiltration or a Coombs positive auto-immune process.

Pathology

While the history and examination findings may be highly suggestive of Hodgkin's disease, a lymph node biopsy is necessary to confirm the diagnosis. The typical lymph node architecture is destroyed by a mixture of cells comprising predominantly normal reactive cells and a lesser proportion of abnormal lymphoid cells. The malignant population comprises the classical multinucleate cells first recognised by Sternberg and Reed, and, therefore, called Reed–Sternberg cells, and their mononuclear variant, called the Hodgkin cell. Hodgkin's disease has been subdivided according to the predominant cell types, and the presence or absence of fibrosis. These varieties are of prognostic significance.

> **CLASSIFICATION OF HODGKIN'S DISEASE**
>
> ◆ Lymphocyte predominant (rare)
> ◆ Nodular sclerosing (most common): Type 1 and Type 2
> ◆ Mixed cellularity (less common)
> ◆ Lymphocyte depleted (rare)

Staging

It is important in Hodgkin's disease to define its anatomical extent or stage (Chapter 8). Formerly, when diagnostic imaging was less accurate and the principal treatment was radiotherapy, laparotomy with splenectomy and multiple biopsies were performed for pathological assessment to identify abdominal disease in patients with clinically more localised disease. Although the staging laparotomy for Hodgkin's disease is now redundant, there are still survivors in the community who underwent this procedure years ago. Splenectomy leads to long-term immunodeficiency, particularly with regard to fulminant septicaemia caused by encapsulated bacteria, such as pneumococcus and meningococcus, which can be rapidly fatal. Patients who have undergone splenectomy, therefore, require life-long penicillin prophylaxis, and regular immunisation against pneumococcal infection.

Nowadays, clinical staging is usually all that is required. Computed tomography (CT) scans of the neck, thorax, abdomen and pelvis will show the extent of the nodal disease. Other investigations, such as a bone scan may be called for by symptoms such as pain. Bone marrow aspirate and trephine is no longer routinely performed in early stage disease, but may be indicated, for example, if there are B-symptoms, anaemia or a markedly raised ESR.

A stage number from I to IV is then allocated according to the Ann Arbor system. The stage number is given a suffix A or B depending whether (B) or not (A) constitutional symptoms of fever, night sweats or weight loss are present.

> **ANN ARBOR STAGING CLASSIFICATION FOR HODGKIN'S DISEASE**
>
> ◆ I: Involvement of a single extra-nodal site (I_E) or a single lymph node region (e.g. cervical, axillary, inguinal, mediastinal, hilar) or lymphoid structure such as spleen, thymus or Waldeyer's ring
> ◆ II: Involvement of two or more lymph node regions or lymph node structures on the same side of the diaphragm, or localised involvement of an extra-nodal organ or site and of one or more lymph node regions on the same side of the diaphragm (II_E)
> ◆ III: Involvement of lymph node regions or lymph node structures on both sides of the diaphragm
> ◆ IV: Diffuse or disseminated involvement of one or more extra-nodal organs or tissues with or without associated lymph node involvement
> ◆ A or B: The suffix A is used in the absence of, and the suffix B is used in the presence of, any of the following three constitutional symptoms:
> - Otherwise unexplained weight loss of more than 10% over the previous 6 months
> - The presence of an otherwise unexplained persistent or recurrent, fluctuating fever (>38°C) during the previous month
> - Recurrent drenching night sweats during the previous month

Treatment and prognosis

The likelihood of cure in clinically staged patients is the same as for comparable populations, who have been pathologically staged. This is because it is now possible to select out those clinically staged patients, who have a significant likelihood of having more extensive disease and require more intensive treatment. The adverse prognostic factors include B-symptoms, large mediastinal masses, involvement of many lymph node groups, unfavourable histology and old age. In these patients, chemotherapy should be the principal treatment, and the precise anatomical extent of disease is irrelevant. Radiotherapy can be reserved as the principal treatment for patients with localised, biologically favourable disease. If they relapse because of undetected intra-abdominal disease, salvage chemotherapy offers a high likelihood of cure.

The initial treatment choices in Hodgkin's disease lie between radiotherapy and chemotherapy or combined modality treatment. There are few hard and fast rules, and various alternative strategies are acceptable and produce good results.

For adult patients with localised (clinical Stage I or II) disease without adverse features, radiotherapy alone is often used. This may be wide-field treatment, encompassing not only known sites of disease, but also adjacent nodal groups, which are not clinically involved, but could harbour occult foci of disease. Most commonly, for supra-diaphragmatic disease this would involve radiotherapy to the "mantle" field. This encompasses glands in the neck, mediastinum and axillae. For those few patients with infra-diaphragmatic presentations, an "inverted Y" field is used, covering the para-aortic, iliac and inguinal node regions. For patients with favourable prognosis, Stage I disease, involved field radiotherapy, covering only the node group known to be affected is good treatment associated with less morbidity.

Patients with Stage III or IV disease, and patients with earlier stage disease and unfavourable features will receive initial combination chemotherapy. Advanced Hodgkin's disease was first recognised as chemocurable over 30 years ago. Since then, many chemotherapy schedules have been evaluated. Usually, when chemotherapy is used, six to eight courses are sufficient.

Combined modality therapy refers to the elective use of chemotherapy and radiotherapy, usually in that order. It can be used to intensify treatment in patients with poor prognosis disease, or with the aim of diminishing treatment-related morbidity. For example, combined modality therapy may allow a reduction in the dose of radiotherapy and the volume irradiated and/or a reduction in the number, of courses, of chemotherapy compared with, if either modality was used alone.

One of the biggest advances in recent years has been the introduction of high-dose chemotherapy with allogeneic bone marrow or peripheral blood stem cell support. This has been shown to improve outcome in patients with relapsed or poor prognosis disease.

With modern treatment, the majority of patients with early stage, good prognosis disease will be cured. The prospects for cure in patients with more advanced disease or with adverse prognostic factors is clearly less good, nonetheless a significant proportion should still be cured.

NON-HODGKIN'S LYMPHOMA

NHL is not one disease, but many, and so a lot of individual subtypes are actually quite rare. It embraces a spectrum from low grade, indolent disease with an untreated natural history, which may be measured in decades through to aggressive types, which, if untreated, may prove fatal within days of presentation. NHL as a whole is three or four times as common as Hodgkin's disease, but many of the subtypes are relatively rare. NHL seems to be becoming significantly more common, but the reasons for this are not clear.

Usually, NHL is a disease of lymph nodes, but extra-nodal NHL is significantly more common than extra-nodal Hodgkin's disease. Children (Chapter 46) are more likely than adults to present with extra-nodal disease. NHL can present at virtually any age, but different types are more common at different ages. For example, in children, high-grade lymphoblastic lymphoma predominates. Low-grade NHL is exceptionally rare in childhood, and very uncommon in young adults, but is frequently encountered in the elderly. For most categories of NHL, there is a small but distinct male predominance.

There is a geographical variation in the type of NHL encountered. For example, T-cell disease is more common in Japan (about 50% of NHL cases) than in Europe (about 15%); Burkitt's lymphoma is more common in parts of Africa; and human T-cell lymphotrophic virus type 1 (HTLV-1)-related T-cell lymphoma is more common in the Carribean. For the most part, the aetiology of NHL is unknown, but some types are clearly related to viral infections such as HIV (Chapter 42), EBV and HTLV-1.

Presentation

Nodal NHL typically presents with painless enlargement of superficial lymph nodes in the neck, less commonly in the axillae or groins. The enlargement may be slow or rapid. The enlarged nodes tend to be rubbery rather than hard. They may mat together rather than remain discrete, and sometimes the masses may become very large. Sometimes, mediastinal lymphadenopathy may lead to symptoms of superior vena cava compression (Chapter 22), and para-aortic or iliac lymphadenopathy may present with an abdominal or pelvic mass or obstructive uropathy. Classical B-symptoms, or other vague and non-specific symptoms, such as tiredness and lethargy, may draw attention to ill health before any lymph node enlargement is apparent.

Extra-nodal NHL may manifest in many ways, depending on the site affected. In almost every case, there is a broad differential diagnosis including other types of malignancy and sometimes benign disease. Often, the diagnosis of lymphoma comes as a surprise after the biopsy.

Extra-nodal NHL of the head and neck may present in a similar way to squamous head and neck cancer of the nose and sinuses or pharynx (Chapters 26, 27 and 30). For example, there may be nasal obstruction and discharge, deafness as a result of Eustachian tube blockage, dysarthria, pain in the face, ear or jaw, proptosis or facial swelling.

Cutaneous lymphoma may present as a localised or generalised skin abnormality with areas of erythema or rash, indurated plaques of cutaneous infiltration, superficial swellings and ulceration.

Primary lymphoma of bone, solitary plasmacytoma and multiple myeloma may present with localised or diffuse bone pain or pathological fracture. In myeloma, anaemia, hypercalcaemia and renal failure may also feature.

Primary central nervous system (CNS) lymphoma will usually present as a brain tumour with headache and vomiting and other signs of raised intracranial pressure (Chapter 39). Sometimes, there may be a focal neurological deficit.

Thyroid lymphoma will usually present as a rapidly enlarging goitre, often in association with dyspnoea and stridor. Testicular NHL will present with testicular enlargement, as other testicular cancers do (Chapter 38).

Gastro-intestinal tract NHL often presents as an acute emergency with gastro-intestinal haemorrhage, perforation, intussusception or obstruction. Sometimes, the onset is more insidious with dyspepsia, abdominal pain or a mass.

Classification and staging

> **PRINCIPAL TYPES OF NHL – APPROXIMATE INCIDENCE**
>
> *Low-grade NHL*
> - Follicular lymphoma: 20%
> - Small lymphocytic lymphoma: 5%
> - Mantle cell lymphoma: 5%
> - Marginal zone or mucosa-associated lymphoid tissue (MALT) lymphomas: 5%
> - Cutaneous T-cell lymphoma: 5%
> - Plasmacytoma and multiple myeloma: 5%
>
> *High-grade NHL*
> - Diffuse large B-cell lymphoma: 40%
> - Burkitt's lymphoma: 5%
> - Lymphoblastic lymphoma: 5%

Over the years, many different classifications of NHL have been used. For pathologists, the classification of NHL appears to be a source of perpetual joy. For clinicians, the regular arrival of new classifications often leads to confusion rather than enlightenment. Despite the profusion of classification systems with counter-intuitive nomenclature, NHL can, for practical clinical purposes, largely be divided into just two groups: high-grade NHL and low-grade NHL.

The various classifications have come about partly as a result of increasing understanding about the biology of NHL and newer diagnostic techniques, such as immunocytochemistry and cytogenetics, and partly because of a sensible desire to harmonise the nomenclature used by different groups in various countries. Problems have arisen because the same terminology is used in different classifications to describe separate clinico-pathological entities, and what is regarded as one entity in one system is split into several subtypes in another. Currently, one of the most widely used classifications is the REAL (Revised European American Lymphoma) classification. Whichever system is used, the simplistic division of NHL into high-grade and low-grade subsets remains for the most part entirely valid. A detailed description of the classification of NHL is not appropriate for this book. Instead, clinical features of the principal types will be discussed.

Once NHL has been diagnosed, it is important to ascertain the stage of the disease. Nodal and extra-nodal NHL in adults are staged in the same way as Hodgkin's disease, using the Ann Arbor classification. B-symptoms are less common in advanced NHL than in Hodgkin's disease. In addition to CT scanning, other investigations, such as bone marrow aspirate and trephine biopsy are often called for, as marrow involvement (Stage IV disease) is common. In patients with certain high-grade NHL, CNS spread is common and a lumbar puncture is part of the staging process.

If a plasma cell tumour is diagnosed, it is important to find out whether it is a solitary plasmacytoma or whether there is any evidence of multiple myeloma. Blood should be sent for plasma protein electrophoresis and immunoglobulin measurements, and urine sent for Bence Jones protein estimations. Bone marrow aspirates and trephines should be performed, and a radiological skeletal survey is better able to show bone involvement than a bone scan, as the lesions encountered in myeloma are not usually osteoblastic and do not provoke a periosteal reaction.

Once a patient with NHL has had the tumour characterised, classified and staged, it is possible to think about what treatment may be appropriate. As with any other cancer, it is necessary also to take into account the patient's age, performance status, co-morbidity, lifestyle factors, social support and personal wishes, before deciding on treatment.

Some of these factors, like staging and histology, relate to prognosis. A number of prognostic indices have been developed, which take into account details of age, stage, pathology, performance status, biochemical parameters and others to assign patients to a particular prognostic group.

FOLLICULAR LYMPHOMA

Follicular lymphoma is a low-grade B-cell lymphoma, accounting for one in four or five patients with NHL. It is characterised histologically by nodules of follicle centre cells, a mixture of centrocytes, which are smaller, and centroblasts, which are larger. Usually, it presents as lymph node enlargement in the elderly. Splenomegaly may be a feature. Only about 20% of patients with follicular NHL have localised (Stage I) disease. These patients may be treated by involved field radical radiotherapy, and about half will not relapse.

More commonly, however, follicular NHL is advanced at presentation, with bone marrow involvement (Stage IV). This disease is, generally, indolent, and as it must be considered incurable, it may not actually require specific treatment following diagnosis, unless or until symptoms require palliation. Simple chemotherapy with oral chlorambucil and prednisolone may be all that is required to make the patient symptom-free and achieve a long remission. The use of interferon alfa may prolong remission. At relapse, if symptoms dictate, then the same treatment can be repeated. Alternatively, more intensive, but still relatively gentle chemotherapy with intravenous regimens, such as cyclophosphamide and vincristine with oral prednisolone may be chosen. Low-dose palliative radiotherapy is often effective at shrinking tumour masses and relieving symptoms. Eventually, the remission duration may shorten, the disease may become refractory to treatment, and in about half, it may transform into a high-grade NHL. At this stage, treatment with alternative drugs, such as fludarabine-, rituximab- or anthracycline-containing regimens with their greater toxicity may be called for. The median survival of follicular NHL is of the order of 10 years. As many patients are elderly, a substantial proportion will die of other causes before their lymphoma catches up with them.

More aggressive initial treatment policies involving high-dose chemotherapy with autologous bone marrow or peripheral blood stem cell support have been investigated in younger fitter patients with low-grade NHL. Although some long-term remissions have been seen, this approach is associated with substantial treatment-related morbidity and even mortality, and it is not clearly superior to a more conservative treatment policy.

SMALL LYMPHOCYTIC LYMPHOMA

Small lymphocytic lymphoma is another form of low-grade NHL, accounting for about 5% of NHL. It is essentially a disease of older people. It is really the same disease as chronic lymphatic leukaemia (Chapter 40) and is treated

in the same way. The only difference is that it presents as a lymphoma in that the predominant symptoms are lymphadenopathy, although the marrow is usually involved and the blood picture is often abnormal. On the other hand, chronic lymphatic leukaemia presents with the finding of an abnormal blood count, although lymphadenopathy and splenomegaly often feature.

MANTLE CELL LYMPHOMA

Mantle cell lymphoma is another B-cell NHL. It is essentially a low-grade lymphoma in that its course is slow, although often relentless. It is like follicular lymphoma and small lymphocytic lymphoma, a disease of the elderly. Men are affected more often than women. It is often Stage IV at presentation, and extra-nodal deposits are common. It responds poorly to treatment, and remissions are often incomplete and rarely last longer than a year or two. The best approach seems to be with anthracycline-based regimens, and rituximab may have a role. The median survival is only 3 years, and only a few patients will survive more than 8 years.

MARGINAL ZONE OR MALT LYMPHOMAS

Marginal zone lymphomas are low-grade NHL, which have a propensity for extra-nodal sites, and often arise in areas of mucosa associated lymphoid tissue (MALT). MALT lymphomas are often found in the gastro-intestinal tract, and infection with *Helicobacter pylori* has been causally implicated. Sometimes, eradication of *H. pylori* with triple therapy is enough to make gastric MALT lymphomas regress completely. Localised MALT lymphomas may sometimes be cured with local therapy, such as surgery or radiotherapy. More advanced disease may call for chemotherapy with single agent chlorambucil or an anthracycline-based combination depending to some extent on the fitness of the patient. About three-quarters of patients with MALT lymphomas will become long-term survivors. Patients with non-MALT marginal zone lymphoma continue to be at risk of relapse or transformation to a high-grade NHL and so the survival curve never flattens out. The median survival is of the order of 10 years, and few patients will live longer than 20 years from diagnosis.

CUTANEOUS T-CELL LYMPHOMA

Cutaneous T-cell lymphoma comprises Mycosis Fungoides (MF) and Sézary Syndrome. Patients with MF are generally elderly, and present with localised plaques, nodules or tumours of the skin, and sometimes with generalised erythroderma. Nodal involvement is not a usual feature, but many patients will have inflammatory rather than malignant, dermatopathic lymphadenopathy. Visceral involvement is a late feature and may mark transformation to high-grade disease. Sézary syndrome is essentially T-cell leukaemia.

MF is a chronic condition, and treatment is palliative. First-line treatment is psoralens phototherapy (PUVA) as used by dermatologists for other skin diseases, such as psoriasis. Topical or systemic chemotherapy may be called for, and radiotherapy either to localised tumours or with electrons to the whole skin may be beneficial.

MULTIPLE MYELOMA AND SOLITARY PLASMACYTOMA

As plasma cells are of lymphoid origin, plasma cell neoplasms are, strictly speaking, types of lymphoma, although they are often thought of as distinct diseases. Isolated extra-medullary plasmacytomas most often present in the head and neck region. If there is no evidence of dissemination, radiotherapy will result in a good chance of local control, and sometimes cure; although more often after a number of years, the disease relapses as multiple myeloma.

Patients more commonly present with multiple myeloma than with solitary plasmacytoma. Most patients are elderly, and they present with bone pain and signs of marrow infiltration, such as anaemia and thrombocytopenia. Sometimes, pathological fracture or spinal cord compression may be the initial symptom. Because plasma cells produce immunoglobulins, the diagnosis is supported by the demonstration of a monoclonal band on plasma protein electrophoresis. Sometimes, immunoglobulin fragments, called Bence Jones Proteins, can be demonstrated in the urine. A bone marrow examination showing an excess of primitive plasma cells confirms the diagnosis.

Treatment is essentially palliative, and as many of the patients are old and frail, gentle oral chemotherapy with melphalan and prednisolone is usually the treatment of choice, along with palliative radiotherapy and analgesia for bone pain. Sometimes, orthopaedic intervention may be necessary, if there is an established or imminent pathological fracture. Hypercalcaemia may be a feature, and bisphosphonate therapy (Chapter 14) may be beneficial in normalising calcium levels, alleviating bone pain and reducing the risk of fracture.

In the minority of younger fitter patients, more intensive intravenous chemotherapy regimens, or high-dose chemotherapy with peripheral blood stem cell support, may be used and give more durable remissions. Interferon is being explored as a way of prolonging remission.

DIFFUSE LARGE B-CELL LYMPHOMA

Diffuse large B-cell lymphoma is the commonest high-grade lymphoma, accounting for about 40% of cases.

It may arise *de novo* or be the final diagnosis after transformation of a previous low-grade lymphoma. In about two-thirds of cases, the presentation is nodal; in one-third, it is extra-nodal. Similarly, in about two-thirds of cases it is advanced, and in one-third it is localised.

Many different chemotherapy schedules of varying intensity have been compared, but nothing seems to be significantly better than a combination of cyclophosphamide, vincristine, doxorubicin and prednisolone (CHOP), which must, therefore, count as the gold standard against which any new treatments must be compared. In localised disease, or where there was initially bulky disease, chemotherapy may be followed by radiotherapy to the sites of disease at presentation. Hybrid regimens with alternating weekly combinations of myelosuppressive and non-myelosuppressive drugs may be better tolerated in older patients than CHOP. Recently, the addition of rituximab to standard chemotherapy had been suggested as better treatment. The place of high-dose chemotherapy with peripheral blood stem cell support has been investigated in younger, fitter patients with high-risk disease, but its exact place remains to be determined. CNS-directed therapy with regular intrathecal chemotherapy may be needed in patients at high risk of developing meningeal disease.

Overall, about half of those with diffuse large B-cell lymphoma will be cured. Most of those destined to die will succumb within 2 years. Prognosis is better in those with localised disease, of whom about 80% will be long-term survivors. Only about 30% of those with advanced disease will be cured. Cure is not expected in patients, who develop high-grade lymphoma following transformation of low-grade NHL.

BURKITT'S LYMPHOMA

This type of high-grade B-cell NHL was first described by Sir Dennis Burkitt, a missionary surgeon, in African children. Epstein–Barr virus infection is involved in its development (Chapter 1). It accounts for about 5% of NHL in adults, but is proportionately more common in children (Chapter 46). Its presentation is mostly extra-nodal, most commonly with abdominal swelling due to involvement of the caecum and mesentery. Less common is the form affecting the head and neck described by Burkitt.

Burkitt's lymphoma calls for very intensive chemotherapy. Even in otherwise fit patients, this is a risky approach and there is an appreciable treatment-related mortality. The tumour is often very bulky at presentation, and rapid cell breakdown with chemotherapy will cause the tumour lysis syndrome (Chapter 17). Patients will require hydration and allopurinol and careful monitoring of blood biochemistry. Admission to an intensive care unit and haemodialysis may be required. If the bowel wall is involved, there is a significant risk of effective chemotherapy leading to perforation as the tumour cells lyse.

With appropriate chemotherapy, however, about half those with Burkitt's are cured. The elderly tolerate such intensive chemotherapy poorly, and have a poor prognosis. Those with marrow or CNS disease at diagnosis, and those in whom Burkitt's appears after transformation from low-grade disease, also have a very poor prognosis.

LYMPHOBLASTIC LYMPHOMA

Lymphoblastic lymphomas are diseases of children and young adults. Most commonly, they develop from T-cells. B-cell lymphoblastic lymphoma does occur, but is much less common. Together they account for about 5% of lymphomas in adults, and a much greater proportion in children (Chapter 46). A bulky mediastinal tumour is usually present, and presentation may be with superior vena cava obstruction. There is a significant likelihood of bone marrow and CNS disease, both of which are associated with a worse prognosis. Patients are treated with acute lymphoblastic leukaemia protocols (Chapter 40), regardless of whether or not the marrow is involved. About 80% will achieve remission, but there is a significant relapse rate and only about half can expect to be cured. It is possible that high-dose chemotherapy and autologous or allogeneic transplantation improves the prospects for cure.

CHAPTER 42

AIDS-related cancer

The acquired immune deficiency syndrome (AIDS) was first recognised in 1981. It is caused by infection with the T-cell lymphotrophic retrovirus called human immuno-deficiency virus (HIV). AIDS is, however, not synonymous with HIV infection. It is only diagnosed when the CD4+ T-lymphocyte subset count falls below $0.2 \times 10^9 l^{-1}$ or an AIDS-defining illness develops. These include various opportunistic infections, for example pneumocystis carinii pneumonia (PCP) and cancers including Kaposi's sarcoma (KS) and non-Hodgkin's lymphoma (NHL).

KAPOSI'S SARCOMA

KS was first described in 1872 by the Austro-Hungarian dermatologist, Moritz Kaposi. From that time until the AIDS epidemic began, KS remained a rare tumour. While most of the cases seen occurred in elderly men of Mediterranean or Jewish origin, KS also occurred in several other distinct populations. These included black African adult males and kidney transplant patients and others receiving immunosuppressive therapy. The form of KS associated with HIV infection is referred to as epidemic KS to distinguish it from the classic, African and transplant-related varieties. Although the histopathology of the different types of KS is essentially identical in all of these groups, the clinical manifestations and course of the disease differ dramatically.

> **TYPES OF KAPOSI'S SARCOMA**
>
> ◆ Classic or endemic KS
> ◆ African KS
> ◆ Transplant-related KS
> ◆ Epidemic or AIDS-related KS

Classic Kaposi's sarcoma

Classic KS occurs more often in males, with a ratio of between 10 and 15 to 1. The usual age at onset is between 50 and 70 years. Patients often have an Ashkenaze Jewish or Italian background. Classic KS usually presents with asymptomatic red, purple or brown skin lesions, often localised to one or both legs, especially involving the

ankle and soles. Classic KS most commonly runs a relatively indolent course for 10–15 years or more with slow enlargement of the original tumours and the gradual development of additional lesions. Venous stasis and lymphoedema of the involved limbs are frequent complications. In chronic cases, systemic lesions can develop. Some patients will develop a second malignant neoplasm.

African Kaposi's sarcoma

Fifty years ago, KS became recognised as a relatively common cancer endemic in equatorial Africa. African KS is seen as either a slowly progressive neoplasm identical to the classic disease or as an aggressive disease with fungating and exophytic tumors that may invade the subcutaneous and surrounding tissue. In Africa, both the indolent and locally more aggressive forms of KS occur with a marked male preponderance, but at a much younger age than classic KS. A rapidly fatal childhood form of KS is also seen in Africa, again more commonly in males. Characteristically, there is generalised lymphadenopathy, often with visceral involvement.

Transplant-related Kaposi's sarcoma

KS in association with therapeutic immunosuppression was first recognised shortly after the introduction of renal transplantation. The incidence of KS in immunosuppressed organ transplant recipients has been estimated at up to 200 times than expected. The average time from transplantation to the development of KS is less than 2 years. Although KS in immunosuppressed organ transplant patients may remain localised to the skin, there may be widespread dissemination. Regression of tumours has been seen following reduction in immunosuppressive therapy.

Epidemic Kaposi's sarcoma

Epidemic KS, the form of KS associated with AIDS, often has a much more fulminant course than classic KS. It is usually characterised by multifocal, widespread lesions at the onset of illness. The sites of involvement are many and varied. They may involve the skin, oral mucosa, lymph nodes and viscera, including the gastro-intestinal tract, lung, liver and spleen. Most patients with AIDS who present with the mucocutaneous lesions of KS feel healthy and are usually free of systemic symptoms, compared with those who first develop an opportunistic infection. Patients who present with localised mucocutaneous disease will almost inevitably develop disseminated disease.

The epidemiology of HIV infection and AIDS is complex, and sheds light on to the role of factors apart from HIV itself in causing other manifestations of AIDS, such as KS. AIDS was first recognised among male homosexuals in cities, such as New York and San Francisco. Other groups recognised early on as being at risk included blood product recipients, especially haemophiliacs, whose factor VIII preparations were prepared from pooled blood donations, and intravenous drug abusers, who shared syringes and needles.

At the outset of the AIDS epidemic, KS was the AIDS-defining illness in almost half of those affected. By the late 80s, the cumulative proportion of AIDS patients with KS had diminished to less than 20%. The incidence of KS in intravenous drug abusers was only about one-tenth of that in homosexual men. In addition, there are a small number of homosexual men who have KS, but are persistently HIV negative. This suggests that another sexually transmitted infection may be a co-factor with HIV in the development of KS. A key piece to the puzzle of KS pathogenesis was the discovery, in 1994, of human herpes virus type 8 (HHV-8). HHV-8 has been identified in KS tissue biopsies from patients with all types of KS and so is also known as the KS herpes virus.

Over the last decade, the amount of KS seen in relation to AIDS in the UK has greatly diminished. This is as a result of the high mortality in the early years of the epidemic, a greater understanding of the mechanisms of transmission of HIV and effective public health programmes, and the development of highly active anti-retroviral therapy (HAART). On a worldwide scale, however, HIV/AIDS remains a problem of enormous significance. The prevalence of the disease in sub-Saharan Africa is greater now than was ever the case in Europe or North America, and public health measures to limit transmission of HIV, and the identification and treatment of infected individuals is pitifully inadequate. Migration from Africa means that AIDS, and KS, will continue to be diseases requiring treatment in this country.

Treatment of epidemic KS

Patients with AIDS-related KS should be managed by a multidisciplinary team including an HIV physician and an oncologist. The degree of social deprivation common to many African immigrants in this country means that community support is essential, and so the general practice team will usually be heavily involved.

Treatments for epidemic KS have evolved over two decades in parallel with advances in the management of the underlying HIV infection, and associated opportunistic infections. Historically, most patients with KS died not as a direct result of the infection, but from opportunistic infections. Nowadays, as the underlying immune dysfuntion and associated infections are better controlled, a patient may live with KS for a longer time, and require more treatment over the years.

There is no universally accepted staging system for KS, but clearly, it is important in each patient to ascertain how widespread the disease is, what symptoms it is causing, and the severity of immunodeficiency and other problems. Disseminated KS, low CD4+ count and the presence of systemic illness are all independent predictors of a poor prognosis.

Treatment of patients with epidemic KS clearly requires anti-retroviral therapy to control the underlying HIV infection and prophylaxis or treatment of opportunistic infections, as well as treatment directed against the KS itself. Treatment of KS in AIDS patients will not cure the disease, and must, therefore, be considered as only palliative.

Limited, localised areas of cutaneous KS are very effectively treated with superficial radiotherapy or electron treatment. Only a single treatment, or a short, low-dose course is required to control an individual lesion. Often any exophytic component regresses well, but the area may be permanently discoloured. Radiotherapy is also effective for the treatment of localised mucosal disease, but treatment can be complicated by a much more severe and prolonged mucositis than would be expected in a healthy individual given the same low-dose treatment. For limited disease, intralesional chemotherapy with vinblastine has been used with good effect, although it is associated with pain and ulceration.

For more generalised disease, especially if there is visceral involvement, chemotherapy can be used. Because of the established cellular immunodeficiency, it is important to try and avoid adding to the risk of infection by causing severe neutropenia as well. A variety of schedules have been shown to be safe effective involving drugs, such as doxorubicin, bleomycin, vinblastine, vincristine, paclitaxel and etoposide, either alone or in combinations. Liposomal anthracyclines have a more favourable side-effect profile and a better therapeutic ratio. Interferon has been shown to have some effect against KS, but its role is at present not clearly defined.

NON-HODGKIN'S LYMPHOMA

Primary central nervous system (CNS) NHL, which is otherwise a very rare entity, was recognised as a feature of AIDS early in the epidemic. Subsequently, it became clear that the incidence of non-CNS NHL was also significantly raised, and NHL became an AIDS-defining illness in HIV-positive patients. The histology of AIDS-related NHL is nearly always of the high-grade B-cell type including diffuse large

B-cell lymphoma and Burkitt's lymphoma (Chapter 41). There is a strong association with EBV infection, suggesting that this virus may be a co-factor with HIV in the development of NHL in this group of patients.

In about one-third of patients with AIDS and NHL, the development of lymphoma in a previously fit patient leads to the discovery of the underlying HIV/AIDS diagnosis. In two-thirds of patients, NHL develops in someone who was already known to have HIV infection or AIDS. Because of the introduction of HAART, NHL is now less frequently seen. NHL seems to affect all groups of people with AIDS equally, unlike the tendency of KS to occur with increased frequency on homosexual men.

The clinical picture of NHL in patients with AIDS is very different from that in the normal lymphoma patient (Chapter 41). AIDS-related NHL is almost always histologically aggressive, usually presents at an advanced stage, and is much more commonly extra-nodal. Unusual extra-nodal sites, such as the anus, heart, bile duct, gingiva and muscles are not uncommonly involved. AIDS-related NHL is less responsive to chemotherapy than common NHL, and patients with immunodeficiency are less well able to tolerate the intensive chemotherapy, which would normally be recommended.

NHL is staged with the Ann Arbor System in the same way as usual (Chapter 41), but most patients have advanced disease. The most commonly used chemotherapy regimen is CHOP, but lower doses are used than in immunocompetent patients. G-CSF support may be used to reduce the likelihood of complications due to neutropenia. Remissions are often seen, but they may be incomplete and are rarely durable. The role of rituximab in addition to chemotherapy in this setting is being investigated. As the likelihood of CNS involvement is high, CNS directed therapy with intrathecal chemotherapy is often recommended. Radiotherapy may be used for established CNS disease.

For all these reasons, the treatment of NHL in patients with AIDS is for the most part palliative. Patients with limited stage disease and a high CD4+ count and no complicating factors will do better than average, but they are in the minority. The median survival is less than 6 months after the diagnosis of NHL complicating AIDS.

AIDS-related primary CNS lymphoma

Until 20 years ago, primary CNS lymphoma was a rare disease. There has since been a dramatic increase in this disease in association with AIDS. Primary CNS lymphoma, however, accounts for less than 1% of initial AIDS diagnoses, but is the second most frequent CNS mass lesion in adults with AIDS. These patients usually have evidence of far advanced AIDS, are severely debilitated, and present with convulsions, focal neurological symptoms or raised intracranial pressure. Computed tomography and magnetic resonance imaging scans usually show large contrast-enhancing mass lesions. The major clinical and radiographic differential diagnosis is cerebral toxoplasmosis. Histologically, cerebral lymphomas in AIDS patients are high-grade B-cell tumours.

Patients with AIDS-related primary CNS lymphoma clearly require holistic care with attention to control of opportunistic infections and optimal anti-retroviral therapy. Radiotherapy alone has usually been used for treatment of the lymphoma itself, but the median survival is only of the order of 3 or 4 months. Survival is longer in younger patients with better performance status and absence of opportunistic infection.

OTHER CANCERS IN PATIENTS WITH AIDS

Cancer of the uterine cervix occurs more commonly in women with HIV than in the general population, and has been recognised as an AIDS-defining illness. Management of the disease has to take into account management of the underlying HIV infection and any associated opportunistic infections. In relatively fit patients with early cervical cancer, management is as outlined in Chapter 31. In patients with very advanced AIDS complicated by a low CD4+ count, opportunistic infections and poor performance status, palliative treatment only may be possible.

Other squamous cancers, such as of the skin and anus are also more common in patients with underlying immunodeficiency, including transplant recipients as well as AIDS patients. Again, the principles of management are to involve a multidisciplinary team including an HIV physician, an oncologist and an appropriate surgeon. When the management of the underlying disease has been optimised, attempts can be made to treat the cancer radically, if possible. These cancers are often more aggressive in their course than similar cancers occurring in immunocompetent patients.

Hodgkin's disease is also more common in patients with HIV infection than would be expected by chance, but the increased risk is much less than that of NHL. The disease is often more advanced and aggressive than in immunocompetent people. As with NHL, care has to be taken to ensure that treatment of the underlying infection and any associated infections is as good as possible, and then the Hodgkin's disease can be treated on its own merits as set out in Chapter 41.

Soft tissue sarcomas

Sarcoma is the name given to malignant tumours of mesenchymal, that is connective tissue, origin. Sarcomas can be divided into two broad groups: bone sarcomas, which are the subject of Chapter 44, and soft tissue sarcomas, which are considered here. Soft tissue sarcomas can occur at any age. The most common sarcoma in paediatric practice is the rhabdomyosarcoma, which is covered in Chapter 46. Only the non-rhabdomyosarcoma soft tissue sarcomas, which occur more commonly in adults, are described here, although they too can, very occasionally, occur in children.

The management of soft tissue sarcomas is complex for three main reasons: firstly, they are very rare, accounting for less than 1% of all cancers; secondly, within the group, there is a wide range of different histological types with a varying degree of malignancy; and finally, they can occur in almost any part of the body, so patients presenting with symptoms (which later prove to be due to a soft tissue sarcoma) may be referred to a variety of specialties for investigation.

DIFFICULTIES IN MANAGING SOFT TISSUE SARCOMAS

- Rare tumours: less than 1% of all cancers
- Various histological types with different natural histories
- Various anatomical presentations

For optimal outcomes, it is important for patients with proven soft tissue sarcomas, and even with suspected sarcomas, to be referred to a specialist sarcoma team for investigation and treatment.

PRESENTATION

The most common presenting symptom is a painless lump, which has been present for weeks or months, or rarely longer. Sometimes, there may be pain caused by pressure on adjacent structures or by erosion of bone. Internal tumours may present with symptoms of blood vessel compression, or obstruction of a viscus, such as the ureter or the gut, or with haemorrhage. Uterine sarcomas (see Chapter 33) usually present like fibroids.

The early referral guidelines (Chapter 5) suggest that patients with a soft tissue mass should be referred for investigation under the 2-week rule, if it is larger than 5 cm, painful, enlarging, situated deep to the fascia or has recurred after an earlier excision.

GUIDELINES FOR URGENT REFERRAL OF PATIENTS WITH SUSPECTED SOFT TISSUE SARCOMA

- Size greater than 5 cm
- Pain
- Increasing in size
- Deep to fascia
- Recurrence after previous excision

Although they can occur virtually anywhere in the body, the lower limb is the commonest site for soft tissue sarcomas. Generally, they grow by local infiltration, infiltrating local tissues and structures. Often, they remain confined within the tissue compartment of origin, extending along the muscle bundle without breaching the fascial planes. Nodal metastases may occur. Distant metastases are uncommon at presentation, fewer than 10% will be found to have lung or other distant deposits on staging investigations. Distant metastases are more likely, if the tumour is very large or of a high-grade histology.

ANATOMICAL LOCATION OF SOFT TISSUE SARCOMAS

- Lower limb: about 45%
- Torso: about 20%
- Upper limb: about 15%
- Head and neck: about 10%
- Retroperitoneum and other: about 10%

INVESTIGATION

Following a history and clinical examination, careful imaging of the suspected tumour is essential. These days, MRI is the favoured technique for assessment of the primary tumour. The lungs are the most common site for distant metastases. Computed tomography will be used to search for pulmonary metastases, as it is a much more sensitive technique than plain chest radiography.

It is worth emphasising again that sarcomas are best managed by experienced multidisciplinary sarcoma teams. It is preferable for the specialist sarcoma surgeon to see the patient before any interventional procedure is undertaken. Biopsy is usually performed prior to surgery as knowledge of the tumour type may help in planning the extent of surgery. Knowledge of the type of operation, which may be most appropriate, will influence the choice of biopsy technique. A core needle biopsy may be taken, or possibly the surgeon will elect to perform an open biopsy. The surgeon will wish to excise the biopsy scar or needle track when the definitive operation is performed. Only occasionally, if the lesion is small and accessible, will the surgeon choose to excise it completely for histological assessment without prior biopsy.

HISTOLOGICAL CLASSIFICATION

Soft tissue tumour histopathology is difficult and complex, requiring special techniques and great expertise in interpretation. The final diagnosis should always be reviewed by a pathologist experienced in this type of work. The first distinction is between benign soft tissue tumours (of which there are perhaps 100 different types) and malignant tumours, the soft tissue sarcomas. There are almost as many types of sarcoma as there are benign tumours of soft tissue. The principal category is those that are differentiating so as to resemble normal connective tissues, for example, liposarcoma (fat), leiomyosarcoma (smooth muscle), malignant peripheral nerve sheath tumour and so on. Other tumours may differentiate along lines which have no normal counterpart, and some may be completely undifferentiated.

The proportion of different tumour types varies widely between different reported series. Usually, malignant fibrous histiocytoma, fibrosarcoma and liposarcoma together account for more than half of all cases. The many other tumour types including leiomyosarcoma, synovial sarcoma, alveolar soft part sarcoma, soft tissue primitive neuroectodermal tumours, each account for fewer than 10% of cases.

The most important contribution of the pathologist, other than identifying the tumour as a sarcoma, is, however, not the precise type, but the grade. The grade is of much more value in guiding management and predicting outcome than the name of the tumour. In fact, the grade is rather unusually incorporated into the TNM staging classification. Three grades are recognised. Grade 1 is well differentiated, Grade 2 is moderately differentiated, and Grade 3 is poorly differentiated or undifferentiated. Grade 3 tumours are much more likely to have metastasised at the time of presentation and are associated with a much worse outcome than Grade 1 tumours.

STAGING

The reasons why accurate staging is necessary have been set out in Chapter 8. As local control rates are good, the most important factor in the staging of localized soft tissue sarcomas is the likelihood of distant failure. This can be predicted by size and grade.

APPROXIMATE LIKELIHOOD (%) OF DISTANT METASTASES DEVELOPING BY 5 YEARS		
	Grade 1	Grade 2 or 3
Size 5 cm or less	0	15
Size >5 cm	5	50

So the principal factors taken into account with soft tissue sarcomas are the size of the primary tumour, the histological grade and the presence of nodal and distant metastases.

SIMPLIFIED STAGING SYSTEM FOR SOFT TISSUE SARCOMAS

- ◆ Stage I: Grade 1, no nodal or distant metastases
- ◆ Stage II: Grade 2, no nodal or distant metastases
- ◆ Stage III: Grade 3, no nodal or distant metastases
- ◆ Stage IV: Any grade with nodal or distant metastases

TREATMENT

Decisions about treatment of adult soft tissue sarcomas are undertaken by the multidisciplinary team, based on the nature of the primary, including, of course, tumour size, grade, stage and location; and the age and fitness of the patient. For most localised tumours, radical surgery should be undertaken, if possible. The extent of operation necessary may range from conservative excision through compartmental excision to amputation. Postoperative radiotherapy will be advised if the tumour was high grade or if there was any doubt about adequacy of the resection margins. This means that the majority of patients will receive postoperative radiotherapy, the exceptions being completely excised Grade 1 tumours.

For patients with tumours of borderline operability, preoperative radiotherapy or neoadjuvant chemotherapy may be attempted in an attempt to shrink the tumour and make complete excision more likely. For patients with inoperable tumours, radical radiotherapy may lead to effective local control in up to one-third of patients.

Chemotherapy, often including a combination of anthracyclines and alkylating agents, such as doxorubicin and ifosfamide, has activity against soft tissue sarcoma;

about half respond. Chemotherapy can, therefore, provide valuable palliation for some patients with metastatic or recurrent sarcomas. This treatment can, however, be quite toxic, and so the risks and benefits, and the individual's wishes, should be carefully considered before recommending such treatment to elderly or frail patients with incurable disease.

The role of adjuvant chemotherapy following local treatment of sarcomas is still not fully established. Most centres would offer treatment to young, fit patients with Stage II or III sarcomas following local treatment with surgery and radiotherapy.

Bone sarcomas

Most tumours occurring in bones are metastases from the common epithelial malignancies, such as prostate, breast and lung cancer. Primary bone tumours are rare, and most are classified as sarcomas which may affect patients of almost any age. The different types of primary bone tumour often present in a similar way, with the classic triad of pain, swelling and loss of function (such as difficulty walking) depending on the anatomical site involved.

PRESENTATION OF BONE TUMOURS

- Pain
- Swelling
- Loss of function

As other clinical features and management are dependent on the histological classification, the rest of this chapter considers primary bone sarcomas according to histology. These distinct entities tend to occur in specific age groups.

CLASSIFICATION OF BONE SARCOMAS

Osteosarcoma	30%	10–25 years and elderly
Chondrosarcoma	20%	50–70 years
Ewing's sarcoma	15%	5–30 years
Osteoclastoma	10%	20–50 years
Malignant fibrous histiocytoma	10%	Any age, peak in middle age

RARER TYPES OF BONE SARCOMA

- Chordoma
- Peripheral primitive neuroectodermal tumour

Haematological malignancies, such as lymphoma and myeloma, can also occur as isolated bone lesions with no evidence of dissemination (e.g. primary lymphoma of bone and solitary plasmacytoma). These have been considered in Chapter 41.

OSTEOSARCOMA

Osteosarcoma accounts for about one-third of primary bone tumours, nonetheless it is rare, and an average general practitioner (GP) will probably see only one case in a lifetime's practice. It usually arises in the limbs, most commonly in the distal femur or the proximal tibia in relation to the knee joint. Only 10% occur in the axial skeleton. There is a peak incidence in adolescence, earlier in females than males because the female pubertal growth spurt occurs earlier. There is a second larger peak in the elderly in association with Paget's disease of bone. Males are more commonly affected than females. There is sometimes a genetic basis. It may occur as part of the Li Fraumeni syndrome when there is familial clustering of breast cancer, brain tumours, leukaemia and bone and soft tissue sarcomas, often occurring at younger ages in each succeeding generation.

Osteosarcoma is the most common type of second malignant neoplasm in patients who have been treated for the familial type of retinoblastoma, usually presenting about 10 years after the original tumour.

The other classic cause of osteosarcoma is irradiation, but hopefully this is now a rarity as the dangers of radiation exposure have been known for some time and are, to a large extent, avoidable.

Presentation is most often with pain and swelling around the knee, associated with difficulty in walking. The pain may precede swelling or any visible signs of disease, and characteristically may be worse at night. Sometimes, knee pain can be referred from the hip, and patients being investigated for pain in the knee should also have their hips examined clinically and radiologically. The diagnosis is often made late, as pain is ascribed to trauma, "growing pains" or psychological causes.

AN X-RAY IS ALWAYS WORTHWHILE

- All patients with demonstrable skeletal radiological abnormalities including bone destruction, new bone formation, soft tissue swelling and periosteal elevation should be referred urgently to an orthopaedic surgeon or paediatrician for further investigation.

An X-ray is always worthwhile, and may show cortical bone erosion, osteoblastic changes, periosteal reaction and exophytic new bone formation, sometimes with the classical "sun-ray" appearance. Although often characteristic, radiographic appearances can be misleading; abnormalities with a benign appearance may be due to a malignant tumour, and benign disease may be mistaken for malignancy.

Patients with imaging suggesting osteosarcoma or another primary bone tumour will usually be referred on by the local team before biopsy to one of the major bone tumour centres for confirmation of the diagnosis, staging and planning of treatment. There is clear evidence that for rare tumours requiring complex, specialised, multidisciplinary management, outcomes are better in dedicated units with special experience and expertise.

Histological confirmation of the radiological diagnosis will be required. Osteosarcoma is usually a high-grade malignant tumour, but there are various subtypes of low-grade osteosarcoma which carry a better prognosis.

Full staging of the disease is essential. Metastases occur most commonly in the lungs, less frequently in the skeleton, and these markedly worsen the prognosis.

Primary surgery is rarely appropriate. Nowadays, almost all patients are treated initially with chemotherapy. Surgery is performed after two or three courses of chemotherapy. Following surgery, more chemotherapy is given. Advances in conservation surgery with metal bone and joint replacements have made amputation less common. In children, who have not yet reached their final height, it is possible to insert "growing" endoprostheses which can be lengthened periodically to match growth of the opposite limb. The interval between diagnosis and definitive surgery, while chemotherapy is being administered, allows time for the preparation of an individualised endoprosthesis to be custom built for the patient. Another advantage of giving chemotherapy prior to surgery is that the histopathologist is able to study the effect the chemotherapy has had on the tumour. Extensive tumour necrosis is a good prognostic feature. The presence of residual viable tumour following chemotherapy identifies a sub-group of patients with a poor prognosis who might benefit from intensification of treatment or novel approaches after surgery. Innovative approaches include high-dose chemotherapy and immunological methods involving vaccines and derivatives of BCG which may stimulate the immune response.

Patients with pulmonary metastases which do not disappear with chemotherapy, or which develop following initially successful treatment, may often be controlled by resection. Repeated thoracotomy and resection, even of multiple or bilateral pulmonary metastases, is generally well tolerated and may result in prolonged remission and occasionally contribute to cure.

Prior to the introduction of chemotherapy, surgery alone, which usually entailed amputation of the affected limb, cured about 20% of patients. The introduction of intensive chemotherapy has improved the survival rate to about 60% now.

Unfortunately, despite much international endeavour over the last two decades, this cure rate has stubbornly remained at about 60%. A good proportion of patients, over one-third, are, therefore, at present destined to die from their disease. High-quality palliative care input is essential in this group of patients. Many are young and have had to cope with intensive treatment, perhaps including amputation, in an attempt to cure them, and their psycho-social needs will be as great as their purely physical ones. The disease is not often rapidly progressive, and the period during which they require palliative care may well be prolonged.

Osteosarcoma in the elderly presents special challenges. Over half of cases will be associated with Paget's disease, and a few may be second malignant tumours arising many years after radiotherapy successfully cured them of a previous tumour. Tumours are more likely to affect the axial skeleton, where surgical resection will be more difficult or impossible. Age and co-morbidity often mean that intensive chemotherapy is out of the question. Palliative care is often the mainstay of patient management following diagnosis. The prognosis is poor with a median survival of only 12–18 months; patients with Paget's disease fare worse.

CHONDROSARCOMA

Chondrosarcoma is the second most common primary bone tumour, comprising about one-fifth of cases. The peak incidence is in the middle aged and elderly, and again there is a male predominance. The pelvis, the femur and the humerus are the most commonly affected sites. The presenting symptoms will be similar to those of other bone tumours, pain, swelling and loss of function.

There is a spectrum of malignancy varying from well-differentiated tumours which have a tendency to recur locally but rarely metastasise, to highly malignant forms where metastasis is the rule. In the absence of demonstrable metastases, surgery is the principal treatment when the anatomical location and fitness of the patient permit. Chemotherapy is probably indicated in fit patients with high-grade tumours, and radiotherapy should be used for local control unless it has been possible to perform radical surgery.

Grade is the best predictor of the likelihood of distant metastasis, and correspondingly the best prognostic indicator. Metastases occur in only 5% of low-grade chondrosarcomas, and the cause specific survival at 10 years is of the order of 80%, as some patients will die from uncontrolled local disease in the absence of distant metastases. Intermediate-grade tumours have a metastatic risk of about 15%, and cause-specific survival figures of about 60%, can be anticipated. High-grade chondrosarcomas metastasise in three-quarters of cases and so only about one-quarter will be long-term survivors.

EWING'S SARCOMA

Ewing's sarcoma is less common than osteosarcoma and chondrosarcoma, comprising about 15% of all primary bone tumours, but it is the second most common bone tumour type in childhood and adolescence. It occurs between the ages of 5 and 30 years, with a peak incidence between 10 and 15 years, more frequently in males. In about half of all cases, the long bones of the limbs are affected (40% in the leg, 10% in the arms), the remainder affect the axial skeleton (about 20% each in the pelvis and the chest wall and shoulder girdle, and 10% in the spine and skull). Rarely, Ewing's sarcoma may arise in soft tissues with no demonstrable bone involvement.

Patients typically present with persistent pain and a tender swelling at the affected site, with loss of function. Nerve compression and pathological fracture are sometimes associated features. A proportion of patients may be non-specifically unwell at the time of diagnosis with fever and anaemia.

It is important to remember that children and young people are always getting knocks in the rough and tumble of life. Traumatic swellings are often associated with visible bruising. A history of trauma does not mean that there cannot be a tumour present. Often it is the knock which brings the swelling to the patient's attention, but is not its cause. Due to the rarity of cancer in children and young people compared with the relative frequency of bone and soft tissue injury consequent on trauma, the diagnosis of Ewing's sarcoma and other primary bone tumours is often delayed.

Remember that the 2-week rule guidelines (Chapter 5) for children include bone pain (especially, if it is diffuse or involves the back, persistently localised at any site, requiring analgesia or limiting activity) and a soft tissue mass (particularly, if it shows rapid or progressive growth, is greater than 3 cm in size, is fixed to or deep to fascia or is associated with regional lymph node enlargement).

If the GP has any suspicion of a bone tumour, or if there is a need to exclude a bone injury caused by trauma, an X-ray should be requested. Remember if the patient presents with knee pain but there are no physical signs to suggest a problem in the knee, the pain may well be referred from the hip and this too should be X-rayed. Radiographs of Ewing's sarcoma may show a patchy destructive abnormality in the bone, sometimes with a characteristic "onion-skin" appearance due to a layered periosteal reaction. An associated soft tissue extension may be apparent. The principal radiological differential diagnosis (apart from other types of bone tumour) is osteomyelitis.

Following referral to an orthopaedic surgeon or a paediatrician for investigation, further imaging with magnetic resonance imaging (MRI) or computed tomography (CT) scanning is likely to be undertaken which will define the site and extent of the problem more accurately, and will give additional clues about the diagnosis. Biopsy, however, is essential to confirm the suspected diagnosis (Chapter 7). Histologically, Ewing's sarcoma is one of the small round blue cell tumours, like rhabdomyosarcoma, neuroblastoma and lymphoma. Characteristic immunohistochemistry and an associated chromosomal abnormality are helpful in making the diagnosis.

Following diagnosis and staging, chemotherapy is almost always the first line of treatment. This treats both the local disease as well as obvious or undetected distant metastases. Subsequently, local control is obtained with surgery or radiotherapy. Where possible without undue functional or cosmetic loss, surgery is recommended for local control, with postoperative radiotherapy if there is any doubt about completeness of excision. Ewing's sarcoma is substantially more radiosensitive than osteosarcoma; and radical radiotherapy is a good local treatment, if surgery is not thought to be appropriate, as for example may be the case in most spinal and pelvic sites. Further chemotherapy then follows.

The advent of intensive, prolonged multi-agent chemotherapy has transformed the outlook for patients with Ewing's sarcoma, with survival rates rising from only about 10% in the era of local treatment alone to about 70% currently.

The principal adverse prognostic factors are the presence of distant metastases and a large primary tumour volume. Metastases are present in up to one-third of patients at the time of diagnosis. They are most commonly found in the lungs, other bones and the bone marrow. Tumour volume is often related to site and the ability to perform radical surgery. Tumours of the axial skeleton, such as the pelvis, are often enormous at the time of diagnosis, and are rarely resectable; so the prognosis of patients with tumours of this type is generally poor. On the other hand, tumours of the distal appendicular skeleton, such as the radius or the fibula, tend to present early, are often resectable, and are associated with a better than average prognosis.

OSTEOCLASTOMA

Osteoclastoma or giant cell tumour of bone accounts for 5–10% of primary bone tumours. It is most commonly seen in younger adults, between 20 and 50 years of age. Unlike most bone tumours, women are affected more commonly than men. Long bones, particularly those around the knee, are most commonly involved. The tumour may be multifocal.

Surgery is the principal treatment; radiotherapy is, sometimes, used, if complete surgery is not possible. It is a tumour of variable malignancy. Most commonly, it is a low-grade lesion with a tendency to recur locally, if the surgery has been inadequate. Rarely, high-grade tumours, which may metastasise to the lungs, are encountered.

MALIGNANT FIBROUS HISTIOCYTOMA OF BONE

Malignant fibrous histiocytoma is now recognised as one of the commonest soft tissue sarcomas (Chapter 45). It may also occur in bone, and it comprises about 10% of primary bone tumours. It may present at any age, but it is more common in the middle aged; men are affected more often than women. It presents, as do other bone tumours, with pain, swelling and functional impairment. The long bones are most commonly affected, and the region around the knee is the commonest site. Histologically, it tends to be a high-grade spindle cell neoplasm, with a potential to recur locally and metastasise rapidly to lymph nodes and the lungs. Following diagnosis and staging, it should be managed in a similar way to osteosarcoma, with intensive chemotherapy in fit patients and radical surgery wherever possible; the prognosis is poor, with only about one-third surviving long term.

CHORDOMA

Chordoma is so called because it is a tumour which is assumed to arise from notochord remnants along the spine. Half occur on the sacrum, one-third in the clivus or base of skull, and the remainder in the cervical, thoracic or lumbar spine. It is usually a low-grade malignant tumour. Surgery is the recommended treatment wherever possible, but there is a tendency to local recurrence even after apparently satisfactory resection. Radiotherapy is used after incomplete resection, in inoperable cases and for palliation of recurrent disease. However, high doses are required and cure is seldom achieved. There is some suggestion that heavy particle (proton beam) therapy may be advantageous, but this is not available in the UK. Distant metastases may occur. Although chemotherapy has been used, it has no clearly defined rôle.

PERIPHERAL PRIMITIVE NEUROECTODERMAL TUMOURS

Primitive neuroectodermal tumours (PNETs), arising in bone or soft tissue peripherally, are distinct from the intracranial PNETs, such as medulloblastoma, but the identical name often leads to confusion. Peripheral PNETs arising in bone present in a similar way to other bone tumours with pain and swelling. They are aggressive malignant tumours with a tendency to metastasise. Histologically, they are characterised by small round blue cells, and so resemble Ewing's sarcoma, but neural differentiation may be a more prominent feature, and there are characteristic features on immunohistochemistry and cytogenetic analysis. Tumours arising around the chest wall, often associated with an intrathoracic mass and pleural effusion, were once grouped together as Askin's tumour, but this is now recognised to be just one clinical presentation of peripheral PNETs. Tumours of this type, following biopsy and staging, are treated with intensive multimodality therapy with initial chemotherapy, radical surgery wherever possible, and often radiotherapy for local control in a very similar fashion to Ewing's sarcoma. There is a significant mortality from this tumour, but cure can be expected in over half.

A miscellany of rare tumours

All the common and many of the rarer cancers have been considered in some detail in the earlier chapters of Section IV of this book. There are some other tumour types – all rare – which did not naturally fall into these chapters, but did not quite seem to merit a chapter of their own. These are considered here – in alphabetical order, for want of a better way to organise them.

ANAL CARCINOMA

Carcinoma of the anus occurs in both men and women, usually in the middle aged and elderly, but younger adults may be affected. There is an association with human immunodeficiency virus (HIV) infection and receptive anal intercourse, and with anal condylomata and human papilloma virus (HPV) infection.

Anal carcinoma usually presents with anal pain and bleeding, and there may be an associated mass at the anal orifice. Pruritis and discharge may feature. Tumours within the anal canal may be associated with tenesmus. Advanced disease may present with faecal incontinence or a fistula into the vagina. There may be secondary involvement of the inguinal lymph nodes.

The principal differential diagnosis is piles, and all patients with symptoms should have a careful anal and rectal examination. Features which suggest malignancy include an indurated mass with ulceration and a raised, everted edge. If the cancer is within the anal canal, it may not be visible but should be palpable. Pain may prevent a thorough digital examination. Enlarged groin nodes may be palpable. If there are any suspicious signs, or if a complete examination has not been possible, urgent referral to a coloproctologist is indicated.

The referring surgeon will examine and biopsy the patient under anaesthesia. Imaging investigations may be undertaken to assess the extent of local infiltration. Histologically, these cancers are usually poorly differentiated squamous, cloacogenic or basaloid (together termed epidermoid) carcinomas. Adenocarcinomas may arise in the upper part of the anal canal, but this histology usually indicates distal extension of a primary tumour in the rectum. Occasionally, a malignant melanoma may be found. A distinction is, sometimes, made between cancers of the anal canal and cancers of the anal margin. Canal tumours are more likely to be less well differentiated

and, if so, may have a worse prognosis than well-differentiated squamous carcinomas of the anal margin or perianal skin.

Cancers will need staging by the TNM classification to define the extent of local spread and to determine if the inguinal nodes are involved. Distant metastases are unusual at presentation, but are more common in those dying from uncontrolled local disease.

The traditional treatment for anal canal cancers was surgical, with abdomino-perineal excision of the lower rectum and anal canal and the formation of a permanent end colostomy. Nowadays, surgery is used for the small proportion of well-differentiated localised (T1 N0) cancers amenable to local excision with preservation of anal function, and for salvage of those who fail initial non-surgical treatment.

The standard of care for most patients with epidermoid anal cancer is now accepted as primary chemoradiotherapy. A large randomised trial was run in the UK between 1987 and 1994 which convincingly showed the benefit of chemoradiotherapy over radiotherapy alone. This trial was remarkable for the fact that an exceptionally high proportion, over one-third, of all patients in the country were accrued. In total, 856 patients were registered of whom 585 were randomised patients, giving greater power to the trial than might have been anticipated for such a rare disease. The risk of local failure was 59% in the radiotherapy group compared with only 36% among those treated with chemoradiotherapy. There was no difference in overall survival, reflecting the power of surgery to salvage local failures. Approximately, half of all patients were alive at 5 years, regardless of the initial treatment.

CARCINOID TUMOURS

Carcinoid tumours are neuroendocrine tumours which may occur at a number of sites in the body. The gastrointestinal tract is the most common primary site, accounting for 85% of cases. Within the gut, the appendix is the most common primary site, followed by the rectum and the ileum. Bronchial carcinoids account for 10% of cases and the remainder occur in the skin, kidney, ovary or at miscellaneous other sites. Metastases to local lymph nodes may occur, followed by haematogenous spread to the liver and lungs.

Carcinoid tumours are characterised by the production of hormones, particularly serotonin (5-hydroxytryptamine, 5-HT), other vaso-active amines and peptides. A metabolite of 5-HT, 5-hydroxy indole acetic acid (5-HIAA) is excreted in the urine and 24-hour urinary 5-HIAA measurements are useful tumour markers.

Carcinoid syndrome is a condition characterised by sudden red flushes which can be very dramatic, diarrhoea and bronchospasm. In long-standing cases, abnormalities of the cardiac valves can develop. Carcinoid syndrome is caused by surges of 5-HT and other hormones produced by carcinoid tumours. Carcinoid tumours do not always cause carcinoid syndrome. Small, non-metastatic, tumours are usually "silent" from the endocrine point of view. Carcinoid syndrome is most likely to be seen when there is extensive metastatic disease in the liver.

Carcinoid tumours are, sometimes, incidental findings in appendices removed for appendicitis. Sometimes, they may present with abdominal symptoms. If the tumour is localised and completely excised, the prognosis is very good.

If there is established metastatic disease, cure is not likely, and treatment aims are essentially palliative. The pace of disease, however, is often very slow and patients may live for a number of years. In a proportion of patients, the tumours take up radiolabelled mIBG or octreotide, and this can be used for scanning and is an option for therapy. Interstitial ablation of liver metastases can provide good palliation. Conventional cytotoxic chemotherapy produces responses in about a quarter of patients. Drug treatments aimed at reducing the symptoms of carcinoid syndrome, but which have no effect on the progress of the tumour, include the somatostatin analogues, namely octreotide and lanreotide.

CHOLANGIOCARCINOMA

Cholangiocarcinoma is an adenocarcinoma arising within the bile ducts. It affects men and women more or less equally, and the average age at presentation is about 60 years. It accounts for about one in five primary liver tumours in the UK, the proportion is lower in countries where hepatocellular carcinoma is much more common.

Very rarely, a small, asymptomatic tumour may be discovered by accident when potentially curative surgery is possible. However, it usually presents with right upper quadrant pain and jaundice, often in association with malaise, anorexia and weight loss. Unfortunately, by the time these symptoms are present, the disease is usually too extensive for any attempt at radical treatment. There is often metastatic disease present in lymph nodes around the porta hepatis, and lung and intraperitoneal metastases may also be present.

Imaging investigations will show the extent of the disease, and a biopsy will confirm the diagnosis. The

tumour markers CEA and CA 19-9 may be elevated, but alpha fetoprotein (AFP), characteristic of hepatocellular cancer is usually normal.

Palliative procedures include biliary drainage and stenting to relieve obstructive jaundice. Intraluminal brachytherapy has been used with some success. Conventional chemotherapy may produce a few responses, but these are usually short lived. The median survival is reported to be between 6 and 12 months. Only one in four of the small proportion of patients undergoing potentially curative resection is likely to be alive at 5 years.

GALL BLADDER CANCER

Cancer of the gall bladder tends to be a disease of elderly women. Gallstones are the most commonly implicated cause. Presenting symptoms are likely to include pain, jaundice, malaise and weight loss. The disease is usually very advanced locally at the time of diagnosis, with direct local infiltration of the liver and involvement of the lymph nodes at the porta hepatis. Very rarely, an early cancer may be identified in a gall bladder removed because of gallstone disease.

For the most part the only treatment options available are palliative, with measures to relieve obstructive jaundice and pain. Palliative chemotherapy may be attempted in fitter patients, but the benefits are not clear-cut. In patients with early disease surgically removed, there is no known advantage from adjuvant therapies, and it is sensible just to observe and await events.

The prognosis is very poor, with a median survival of only a few months. Only about 10% of patients will still be alive at 1 year.

HEPATOCELLULAR CARCINOMA

The majority of "liver cancers" are not primary hepatic tumours but metastases from a variety of primary sites, such as the bowel, stomach, lung and breast. In the UK, primary hepatocellular carcinoma is rare. Worldwide, it is much more common, with various countries in Asia and Africa having a particularly high incidence.

In the majority of cases it arises in cirrhotic livers, with alcohol and hepatitis B being the most common causes. Hepatitis B may be the most important factor in countries where there is a particularly high incidence. Haemochromatosis and hepatitis C can also predispose to cirrhosis and hepatocellular carcinoma. It tends to be a disease of the middle aged and elderly, and men are more commonly affected than women.

It often presents with abdominal pain and hepatomegaly or a palpable mass, perhaps in association with lethargy and weight loss. In patients known to have cirrhosis of the liver, deterioration of previously stable hepatic function may herald the development of a hepato-cellular carcinoma.

Most hepatocellular carcinomas are very extensive at presentation, and they are often multifocal within the liver. Diagnosis is by biopsy after imaging investigations and AFP measurement. The AFP level is often raised in a variety of liver diseases including cirrhosis and chronic hepatitis, and so a mildly abnormal AFP reading is not of itself diagnostic. However, a very greatly raised value makes a diagnosis of hepatocellular carcinoma likely.

Most patients with hepatocellular carcinoma will have disease which is too extensive for curative therapy, or their intercurrent illness and poor hepatic function will make radical therapy inappropriate. Surgery will be indicated in very carefully selected patients, and transplantation may, occasionally, be undertaken. Palliative chemotherapy may prolong survival in some patients with unresectable tumours. As with surgery, poor performance status and hepatic dysfunction may preclude aggressive chemotherapy.

For most patients, the survival duration will be measured in months, and in these circumstances good quality community palliative care is essential.

MESOTHELIOMA

Mesothelioma is a malignant tumour arising from the serosal lining of body cavities. It most commonly affects the pleura, but it can also originate in the peritoneum, the pericardium and rarely in the tunica vaginalis around the testis.

The principal cause has been identified as asbestos exposure, although about one-third of patients have no identifiable asbestos exposure. The relationship with asbestos was first recognised in 1960. Since then, there has been an epidemic of mesothelioma occurring as an industrial disease in those people occupationally exposed in the shipbuilding and demolition industries, as well as in the asbestos industry itself. There are several varieties of asbestos and the dangerous form is crocidolite or blue asbestos. White asbestos or chrysotile has a different structure and is not implicated in the development of mesothelioma. The latent period between exposure to asbestos and the development of mesothelioma is very long, at least 20 years. The epidemic will, therefore, continue for decades, even though effective occupational hygiene measures are in place in developed countries to eliminate exposure to dangerous varieties of asbestos.

Presentation depends on the part of the body involved. The onset of symptoms related to pleural mesothelioma may be insidious. There may be increasing dyspnoea, possibly in a patient with pre-existing pulmonary disease, cough and poorly localised intractable chest pain. A pleural effusion often develops. Dysphagia, hoarseness, Horner's syndrome and superior vena caval obstruction may all arise as a result of the invasion of mediastinal structures.

Pericardial mesothelioma presents with symptoms of constrictive pericarditis or tamponade. Peritoneal disease may present in a similar way to advanced ovarian cancer with ascites and abdominal masses.

Most cases of mesothelioma are advanced at the time of diagnosis. Treatment with curative intent is only rarely possible. Chemotherapy and radiotherapy are sometimes used, but beneficial effects are usually short lived. Symptom control measures and specialist palliative care input are very important. Financial compensation is available to those whose mesothelioma is industrially acquired. The June Hancock Mesothelioma Research Fund (Chapter 58) provides information and support for patients and their families.

CARCINOMA OF THE PENIS

In general, carcinoma of the penis is a rare disease of elderly men. It is associated with phimosis, poor hygiene and HPV infection. Circumcision affords a very high level of protection against this disease. It usually arises on the inner aspect of the foreskin, or on the glans penis in the coronal sulcus. They may appear as an ulcer, nodule or verruca which invades underlying tissue. Histologically, these cancers are usually squamous cell carcinomas (SCCs). Spread is initially to the inguinal lymph nodes.

Treatment methods include surgery and radiotherapy. Chemoradiotherapy may also have a role. Very early stage cancers may be treated with conservation surgery. For more advanced, localised tumours, radiotherapy is usually recommended as first-line treatment in an attempt to conserve the penis. Both external beam radiotherapy and brachytherapy may have a place. The alternative is partial or complete penile amputation. Radical surgery may be essential in patients who present with very advanced cancers with invasion of the corpora, or if there is lymph node involvement. Postoperative radiotherapy or chemoradiotherapy may be recommended.

Results of treatment are, of course, dependent on the stage of disease at the time of diagnosis. The majority of patients will be cured. Careful follow-up is necessary, especially after conservation treatment as local relapses may be identified at a stage when salvage surgery can be curative.

THYMOMA

The thymus gland is situated in the anterior mediastinum, and can be the seat of several types of malignant disease. Hodgkin's disease, non-Hodgkin's lymphomas (NHLs), germ cell tumours, carcinoid tumours and primary carcinomas may all involve this organ, and these must be distinguished from true thymoma, which accounts for about one in five of all mediastinal tumours.

Thymoma is a slowly growing malignant tumour which tends to infiltrate adjacent structures. Thymomas diagnosed early before local invasion used to be regarded as benign, but this is unwise as all true thymomas have the potential to behave in a malignant fashion. Distant spread is rare. Thymomas may present with local symptoms, such as cough, dyspnoea, chest pain stridor or superior vena cava compression. Thymomas may present with one of two unusual non-metastatic manifestations. Myasthenia gravis has been observed in about one-third of patients with thymoma, and all patients presenting with myasthenia gravis should be screened for a thymoma, which will be found in about 10% of cases. Pure red cell aplasia which is diagnosed in the investigation of anaemia is seen in about 1 in 20 thymoma patients, and a thymoma is discovered in about 40% of patients with pure red cell aplasia.

When a thymoma is diagnosed, the principal treatment is with surgery. For early stage disease, complete surgery is all that is required. Postoperative radiotherapy is often given for more advanced tumours, and where there is doubt about the adequacy of excision. It will reduce the incidence of recurrence. Chemotherapy, usually a cisplatin-based regimen, is effective in producing responses in recurrent or inoperable disease, but its place in the management of operable disease has yet to be established.

Following complete surgery, about four out of five will be alive without disease recurrence at 5 years, compared with only about half of those with more advanced disease treated with incomplete resection and radiotherapy. The disease has a long natural history, and there is a significant possibility of recurrence after the 5-year timepoint.

Cancers at different ages

SECTION CONTENTS

Cancer in children

Compared with cancer in adults, cancer in children is very rare, with only about 1,500 new cases per year in the UK. The average general practitioner (GP) may, therefore, expect to see only one or two new patients in a lifetime's practice. Nonetheless, it is important as it is second only to accidents as a cause of death in children in this country. In addition, because the majority of patients are cured, and approximately 1 in 1,000 young adults is a survivor of childhood cancer, every GP may expect to care for one or two patients who are cured of their disease, but who may have continuing health care needs as a result of the treatment they have received. Parents and other relatives of children with cancer are amongst the best informed, often due to long hours spent trawling the internet in search of finding better treatments than those on offer. It is, therefore, helpful for a GP to have a source of basic information about these rare conditions and their management.

PAEDIATRIC ONCOLOGY CENTRES AND SHARED-CARE HOSPITALS

Due to the rarity of cancer in children, and the fact that successful outcome is critically dependent upon expert management, care of such children is always undertaken in specialist children's cancer centres which are equipped with a critical mass of expertise not just in paediatric oncology but also in the specialist areas of imaging, pathology, surgery and allied medical disciplines. In the UK and Ireland there are 22 such centres, principally one for each regional teaching hospital city with a cluster in London, which for the last 25 years have been networked through an organisation called the UK Children's Cancer Study Group (UKCCSG). The UKCCSG sets the standards of care for children with cancer in this country, and runs a broad portfolio of clinical and scientific studies covering almost all tumour types. These are often in conjunction with international organisations as many individual tumour types occur too infrequently for trials to be run successfully in one country. The network of paediatric oncologists throughout the country and internationally means that any consultant faced with a difficult clinical problem can readily seek advice from colleagues who may have greater experience or access to the many individual disease databases which exist.

As each paediatric oncology centre serves a large geographical area, much of the care required by a child with cancer can be delivered closer to home in conjunction with a district general hospital-based "shared-care paediatrician" who will have a special interest in the management of children with cancer. The shared-care consultant will not be responsible for determining treatment policy (that is, the job of the paediatric oncology centre), but and will provide continuing supportive care such as haematological monitoring and blood or platelet transfusions, treatment of neutropenic sepsis and other emergencies, linking with local rehabilitation services such as physiotherapists and dieticians, and may also deliver some chemotherapy locally. Liaison between the cancer centre, the shared-care hospital and community services is facilitated by paediatric oncology outreach nurses who may also be involved in some aspects of hands-on care such as care of central venous access lines and symptom control in terminal care.

The third and equally important leg of service provision in the care of children with cancer is the GP. The GP will have known the child and the family before the diagnosis was made, and will be involved both during the acute phase of illness and in the long term if treatment is successful. If it is not, the GP will be of critical importance during the terminal stages and will still continue to be involved with the family during their bereavement and possibly for many years after the death. In either event, the GP will be involved with other members of the family at this stressful time, and may be asked by the parents about many issues such as any possible genetic basis of the cancer and the wisdom of their having further children. Unlike the situation a few decades ago, parents now expect that each of their children will survive into adulthood – death in childhood is now rarely considered by parents.

THE SPECTRUM OF CHILDHOOD CANCER

Of the many different types of cancer seen in children, most are unique to children or children and adolescents. The common adult cancers are virtually never seen in children. The commonest malignancy in children is leukaemia, which accounts for about one-third of all cases. This is most commonly acute lymphoblastic leukaemia (ALL), but one in five patients with childhood leukaemia has another type such as acute myeloid leukaemia which is still about as common as Hodgkin's disease in childhood or rhabdomyosarcoma. After leukaemia, the next most common group of childhood cancers is brain tumours, accounting for about one in five cases. However, each individual type is quite rare. Lymphoma, including both Hodgkin's disease and the non-Hodgkin's lymphomas (NHLs) account for about 10% of cases, and Wilms' tumour, neuroblastoma and soft tissue sarcomas each account for about 7%.

FREQUENCY OF PRINCIPAL CANCER TYPES IN CHILDREN AGED 0–14

◆ *Leukaemia*	33%
ALL	26%
Acute myeloid leukaemia	5%
Other leukaemias	2%
◆ *Lymphoma*	10%
Hodgkin's disease	4%
NHL	6%
◆ *Central nervous system (CNS) tumours*	22%
Gliomas	12%
Medulloblastoma and primitive neuroectodermal tumour (PNET)	5%
◆ *Neuroblastoma*	7%
◆ *Soft tissue sarcoma*	7%
Rhabdomyosarcoma	4%
Non-rhabdomyosarcoma soft tissue sarcoma	3%
◆ *Wilms' tumour*	6%
◆ *Bone sarcomas*	5%
◆ *Retinoblastoma*	3%
◆ *Others*	7%

THE AGE DISTRIBUTION OF CHILDHOOD CANCERS

For each individual childhood cancer, there is often a varying incidence according to age. Retinoblastoma for example, is a disease of infants, and very few cases are seen over the age of 1 year. Similarly, neuroblastoma is most common in the first year of life and becomes less common in each succeeding year. Acute leukaemia and rhabdomyosarcoma may be seen in children of any age, but are most common in the pre-school age group. Malignant bone tumours such as Ewing's sarcoma and osteosarcoma are very rarely seen in young children and are, by and large, diseases of the teenage years (see Chapters 43 and 47).

THE CAUSES OF CHILDHOOD CANCERS

Little is known about the causes of childhood cancers. Unlike the adult situation where environmental carcinogens such as cigarette smoke are well recognised, carcinogens do not seem to be important. The one well-documented exception, now no longer seen, was when oestrogens were given to pregnant women with a history of recurrent miscarriage and vaginal adenocarcinoma developed in their daughters, although usually in adolescence rather than childhood. Acute myeloid leukaemia is one of the more common second malignancies among survivors of cancer treated with chemotherapy.

There is definite evidence that significant radiation exposure *in utero* can predispose to the development of cancer, but now that risk has been recognised it can to a very large extent be avoided. There has been much public speculation about the possible leukaemogenic effect of low-level radiation exposure coming from living near to a nuclear power plant or reprocessing facility, but the evidence to prove this is lacking. Similarly, although there is anxiety in relation to electromagnetic fields in children who live close to overhead power cables, evidence of a causal relationship is not present.

Childhood leukaemia rates are above average in areas, such as new towns, where there has been extensive population mixing. There is a hypothesis that the development of leukaemia could, in some cases, be due to an unusual reaction to a virus spreading into a previously unexposed population as a result of migration of communities, although there is no suggestion that the leukaemia is itself an infectious disease. This hypothesis has also been used to explain some of the clustering of childhood leukaemia cases around nuclear installations.

Some childhood cancers undoubtedly have a genetic basis. Retinoblastoma is the classic example, and it occurs in two forms. About 40% of patients have the genetic form of this disease which is inherited as an autosomal dominant condition with high penetrance. It is caused by an inherited deletion of the tumour suppressor gene called Rb1 on one copy of chromosome 13, coupled with an acquired insult to its opposite number. Children with the familial form of the disease tend to be younger at presentation and are more likely to have multiple tumours or bilateral disease. These patients are also more prone to develop second primary tumours such as osteosarcoma in later life. In the sporadic form of the disease, it is thought that by chance there has been an acquired mutation of both alleles. Other childhood cancers, such as Wilms' tumour, may have a genetic component in their aetiology, although most cases are in fact sporadic.

There are a large number of familial genetic diseases in which tumours in affected children and adults may be part of the syndrome. These include neurofibromatosis, tuberose sclerosis, and ataxia telangiectasia. However, such conditions are associated with only a small proportion of childhood cancer cases. Some chromosomal conditions, most notably Down syndrome, is associated with an increased risk of leukaemia in childhood, although again only a small proportion of leukaemic patients have an underlying chromosomal abnormality of this type.

ACUTE LYMPHOBLASTIC LEUKAEMIA (26%)

Mature lymphoid cells can be divided into B-cell and T-cell subtypes. Most cases of ALL are derived from immature B-cell precursors which lack B-cell markers, so-called pre-B or common ALL. T-cell ALL is uncommon and true B-cell ALL is very rare.

Many children with ALL present to the GP with what at first appears to be a viral infection. They may be tired and lethargic because of anaemia, they may have fever and a sore throat, due to neutropenia and lymphadenopathy and hepatosplenomegaly. These symptoms may suggest glandular fever. Bone pain is not uncommon. A high index of suspicion is required if a child returns to the GP after a "viral" presentation with no improvement in symptoms. Purpura and bruising due to thrombocytopenia may raise the possibility of non-accidental injury. Although the full blood count is usually abnormal with anaemia, thrombocytopenia, and a high white cell count with blasts visible on the film, a normal count does not exclude the diagnosis.

THE PHASES OF TREATMENT OF ALL

- ◆ Induction treatment
- ◆ Intensification blocks
- ◆ CNS directed therapy
- ◆ Continuing therapy

The standard pattern of treatment involves four components: induction, intensification, CNS directed therapy and continuing treatment. The induction phase of intensive chemotherapy based on vincristine, steroids (dexamethasone) and asparaginase lasts for 4 weeks and is given with the aim of producing a remission that is clearing detectable disease from the bone marrow. Three further blocks of intensive chemotherapy are given at intervals, so-called consolidation or intensification treatments aimed at eradicating subclinical disease. Because there is otherwise a substantial risk of CNS relapse, some form of CNS directed therapy is essential. Nowadays, intrathecal chemotherapy with methotrexate is given by lumbar puncture and intravenous high-dose methotrexate is given. Cranial radiotherapy was formerly used in this setting but is now reserved for the treatment of established CNS disease at presentation or CNS

relapse. Great care must be taken at the time of lumbar puncture to ensure that the correct drugs are administered. The accidental intrathecal injection of vincristine is fatal, and manslaughter charges can result. Continuing or maintenance therapy is given between the blocks of intensive treatment and carries on until 2 years have elapsed since presentation. This comprises daily oral medication with mercaptopurine or thioguanine, weekly oral methotrexate and monthly injections. The doses of continuing chemotherapy are titrated against the white count.

ALL is one of the great success stories of modern medicine. The prognosis for the average child is now good with cure rates in excess of 70%, whereas a generation ago virtually none survived long term.

ADVERSE PROGNOSTIC FACTORS IN ALL

- ◆ High presenting white count
- ◆ Chromosomal abnormalities in the leukaemia cells
- ◆ CNS involvement
- ◆ Age less than 1 year
- ◆ Male sex
- ◆ Failure to go into remission on time
- ◆ Relapse on treatment

If relapse does occur, further treatment can be offered. This will include further chemotherapy and possibly radiotherapy and bone marrow transplantation. This is from a related donor if possible or failing that a matched unrelated donor transplant might be considered, although it is associated with greater toxicity. Prognosis is poor for patients who relapse while still on treatment. Outlook is most favourable with later relapses, and for isolated testicular relapse.

For the most part, once induction treatment has been completed satisfactorily, children with ALL will be healthy and able to participate in a near normal lifestyle during their continuing treatment.

ACUTE MYELOID LEUKAEMIA (5%)

Children with acute myeloid leukaemia require very intensive treatment which carries a substantial chance of serious morbidity. Patients with poor prognosis disease may well benefit from a transplant. Nonetheless, survival rates have improved very considerably over recent years, and cure can be expected in the majority of patients.

NON-HODGKIN'S LYMPHOMA IN CHILDHOOD (6%)

NHLs in childhood are very different from those seen in adult life. NHL in children is almost always rapidly progressive and high grade in nature, extra-nodal disease predominates and there is a high incidence of both CNS and bone marrow involvement. Whatever classification system is used, there are three principal types. High-grade small cell undifferentiated B-cell lymphoma histologically resembles Burkitt's lymphoma, but in the West most children will present with an abdominal mass rather than with the classical jaw swelling first described by Burkitt in black African children. Lymphoblastic lymphoma has cells which are indistinguishable from those of ALL, but the T-cell disease accounts for 90% of lymphoma cases but only 10% of leukaemia cases. T-cell lymphoblastic lymphoma often presents with a large mediastinal mass, and is arbitrarily distinguished from leukaemia if fewer than 25% of bone marrow cells are malignant. The third group comprises the uncommon large cell lymphomas which can be of B-cell, T-cell or indeterminate immunophenotype.

> **TYPES OF CHILDHOOD NON-HODGKIN'S LYMPHOMA**
>
> ◆ Small non-cleaved cell undifferentiated B-cell lymphoma
> ◆ Lymphoblastic lymphoma (usually T-cell)
> ◆ Large cell lymphoma (T or B or neither)

Children with NHL are grouped into four stages. The majority of children at presentation will be found to have advanced mediastinal or abdominal disease (Stage III) or CNS or bone marrow involvement (Stage IV disease).

Treatment of NHL in childhood is with intensive chemotherapy. B-cell disease requires a relatively short course of treatment. T-cell disease requires prolonged, leukaemia style treatment. Radiotherapy has no place in the initial management of NHL. Surgery can sometimes be needed for abdominal disease, for example, if a perforation develops as a response to treatment. On the whole, results are good with the majority of patients being cured. However, if the disease relapses the prognosis becomes very poor.

CHILDHOOD HODGKIN'S DISEASE (4%)

Most children with Hodgkin's disease are over the age of 10, and the presentation pathology and staging is the same as in adults (see Chapter 41). Treatment protocols are guided by the desire to avoid late effects, and so chemotherapy is the mainstay of treatment, and radiotherapy is only used as the initial treatment in a proportion of patients with Stage I disease. Unlike the case with NHL, patients whose disease relapses after initial treatment are often retreated successfully. The overall outcome is very good, with approximately 90% of patients being cured.

CENTRAL NERVOUS SYSTEM TUMOURS IN CHILDHOOD (22%)
Symptoms and signs

The presenting symptoms and signs of brain tumours in childhood are varied, and depend on the age of the child and the location and speed of growth of the tumour. Most childhood brain tumours are situated in the posterior fossa, and so one of the most common constellation of symptoms in the older child is headache, characteristically present on waking in the morning, vomiting which often occurs in the absence of nausea, and visual disturbance.

> **SYMPTOMS OF RAISED INTRACRANIAL PRESSURE**
>
> ◆ Headache
> ◆ Vomiting
> ◆ Visual impairment

This is caused by the posterior fossa tumour compressing the fourth ventricle leading to hydrocephalus and raised intracranial pressure. Symptoms such as neck tilt and clumsiness and difficulty in walking may also be present. On examination, tremor, truncal ataxia, poor limb co-ordination and nystagmus may be seen. Such posterior fossa symptoms and signs can be found in the absence of features suggesting raised intracranial pressure if the normal cerebrospinal fluid (CSF) flow has not yet become obstructed. In babies and younger children the symptoms may be less clear cut. Irritability, poor feeding and developmental delay may be noted and enlargement of the head circumference may possibly be found if the sutures have not yet fused. With the development of the child health surveillance (CHS) programme in the UK, occipito-frontal circumference (OFC) will have been measured on several occasions since birth and the results plotted in the parents' "handbook" and in the GP notes. Any sudden deviation from the child's original pattern of OFC growth can therefore be seen at a glance.

> **CEREBELLAR SIGNS**
>
> ◆ Tremor
> ◆ Truncal ataxia
> ◆ Poor limb co-ordination
> ◆ Nystagmus
> ◆ Dysarthria

Brain stem tumours may present with cranial nerve palsies resulting in impaired eye movements, facial weakness, dysarthria, dysphagia and choking; and long tract problems such as difficulty in walking or hand movement, with or without symptoms of raised pressure. Various tumours arise in the midline in the pituitary and hypothalamic area. They include optic pathway gliomas, craniopharyngiomas and intracranial germ cell tumours. These too may cause hydrocephalus by obstructing the third ventricle, but more often they cause impaired vision, endocrine dysfunction, most often growth hormone insufficiency causing short stature or delayed or precocious puberty, behavioural disturbances and eating disorders. Most often the latter takes the form of obesity, but sometimes children later found to have a brain tumour in this area may initially be misdiagnosed as having anorexia nervosa.

ENDOCRINE PRESENTATIONS OF BRAIN TUMOURS

- Short stature or failure to grow normally (growth hormone insufficiency)
- Polyuria and polydipsia (diabetes insipidus)
- Altered timing of puberty (precocious or delayed)
- Altered eating patterns (obesity or anorexia)

Tumours in the cerebral hemispheres may present with focal or grand mal convulsions (which usually suggest a slowly growing, low-grade tumour), raised intracranial pressure, or focal neurological deficit, such as hemiparesis depending on location.

Investigation and classification

Any child suspected by their GP to have a brain tumour should be seen that day by a paediatrician for investigation. Nowadays, some form of neuroimaging, usually computed tomography (CT) but increasingly often magnetic resonance imaging (MRI), will be undertaken locally to confirm the presence of a brain tumour and the child will then be referred on to a regional paediatric neurosurgical centre for definitive diagnosis and treatment in conjunction with the paediatric neuro-oncology multidisciplinary team.

There are three principal indications for neurosurgical intervention, to obtain tissue for a histological diagnosis, to relieve symptoms such as hydrocephalus, and of course either to remove the tumour completely with the aim of cure (if this can be done without risking major neurological damage) or to remove as much of the bulk as is safely possible if this will make non-surgical treatments, such as radiotherapy or chemotherapy more effective.

Classification of brain tumours in children is by anatomical site (supratentorial or posterior fossa) and by histology in most cases. For some tumours the characteristic imaging appearances and the potential hazards of biopsy mean that no histological confirmation is obtained before treatment with radiotherapy.

PRINCIPAL SITES AND TYPES OF BRAIN TUMOURS IN CHILDREN

Posterior cranial fossa
- Cerebellum
  - Low-grade (pilocytic) astrocytoma
  - Medulloblastoma or PNET
  - Ependymoma
- Brainstem
  - Diffuse intrinsic pontine glioma
  - Midbrain tumour
  - Cervicomedullary tumour

Supratentorial compartment
- Suprasellar region
  - Optic pathway glioma
  - Craniopharyngioma
  - Germ cell tumour
- Pineal region
  - Germ cell tumour
  - Pineoblastoma (PNET)
  - Glioma
- Thalamus and basal structures
  - Glioma
- Cerebral hemispheres
  - Glioma
  - Ependymoma
  - Choroid plexus tumour
  - PNET

Treatment and prognosis

Cerebellar pilocytic astrocytomas
These are the most common tumours, accounting for about 15% of cases. They are relatively benign. The majority will be managed by surgery alone, and the outlook is exceptionally favourable. In some cases, complete resection may not be possible, but a watch and wait policy can usually be followed, reserving further surgery or radiotherapy for regrowth which is not inevitable. Most patients will have normal or near normal neurological function at the end of the day.

Primitive neuroectodermal tumours
Medulloblastoma is the most common type of PNET. It is a malignant brain tumour arising in the cerebellum. Tumours of identical histological appearance and behaviour in the supratentorial compartment were formerly known by a variety of names, depending on their exact location, but they are now all grouped together as PNETs. The standard treatment for these tumours is surgical resection, followed by chemotherapy and radiotherapy to the whole brain and spine because they have a tendency to spread through the CSF pathways. Chemotherapy is indicated in very young children with

the aim of delaying the need for radiotherapy. Across the board survival rates are of the order of 60%. The minority of patients who have definite metastatic disease at presentation, a tumour which is not completely resectable, or a primary tumour outside the cerebellum and very young children tend to fare worse: the survival rates are only about 25%. Conversely, survival rates greater than 70% may be expected in patients with completely resected, non-metastatic cerebellar medulloblastoma. Unfortunately, survival may often be at the cost of significant late effects which are described below.

Ependymoma

Ependymoma usually arises from within the ventricles of the brain, most commonly the fourth ventricle. It is a malignant tumour which has a tendency to infiltrate and grow into adjacent brain tissue, to recur locally after surgery, and sometimes to metastasise through the CSF pathways. Treatment is with complete surgical excision wherever possible. Postoperative radiotherapy to the tumour bed is often given, but whole brain and spine radiotherapy is not nowadays used in the absence of disseminated disease as the hazards outweigh the likely benefit. Chemotherapy has no established role as an adjuvant treatment, but may be used in very young children with the aim of delaying the need for radiotherapy.

Brainstem tumours

Unfortunately, most brainstem tumours are diffuse infiltrating high-grade pontine giomas. There is often considerable neurodisability at presentation with squint, facial weakness, dysarthria, dysphagia and choking due to lower cranial nerve palsies and a hemiparesis due to long tract involvement. The clinical and imaging findings are usually sufficiently characteristic to make a diagnosis without a biopsy which could be hazardous. Steroids often improve symptoms in the short term, but should not be continued indefinitely. Treatment is with "radical" radiotherapy, but it is, in truth, essentially palliative. The tumour in some patients will progress and cause death even before treatment is complete, but in the majority there will be some improvement. At best, there will in some patients be a complete clinical and radiological response, but the natural history of this type of tumour is for almost inevitable tumour recurrence and death. The median survival is less than a year. Many chemotherapy regimens and other treatments have been tried experimentally without success. A minority of brain stem tumours have more favourable characteristics. Those arising higher up in the midbrain tend to be low grade, and radiotherapy is often effective. Surgery is indicated for the rare cervico-medullary low-grade tumours at the lower end of the brainstem, in cases where there is a predominant cystic element or in the case of dorsal exophytic tumours which grow out from the brainstem into the fourth ventricle. In these cases, postoperative radiotherapy will usually be given, and prolonged survival may be achieved. Surgery may also be needed to control obstructive hydrocephalus.

Optic pathway tumours

These low-grade tumours tend to occur in pre-school children. A significant minority will have a family history of neurofibromatosis type 1. They may be situated anywhere along the optic pathway from the optic nerve in the orbit to the optic tracts extending backwards towards the occipital cortex. They most commonly involve the optic chiasm, where the tumour can grow to some size. They may present with proptosis, visual failure, hydrocephalus and endocrine or hypothalamic disturbance. Radical surgery is not often indicated but biopsy is recommended as other tumour types can occur at these sites. An initial policy of observation may be followed, especially in the younger child if there are no pressing symptoms. If there is evidence of tumour progression on close follow-up, treatment with chemotherapy may be started. Radiotherapy is indicated if there is progression on chemotherapy or as the first-line treatment in older children. The disease is not usually rapidly life threatening and may have a very long natural history. Many children will have considerable difficulties at school as a result of visual handicap, behavioural disturbance and poor intellectual abilities, coupled with the need for endocrine treatments such as growth hormone replacement, and so require considerable community support.

Craniopharyngioma

Craniopharyngiomas are slowly growing solid and/or cystic tumours which are always situated in the pituitary fossa or suprasellar region. They may present with visual failure, endocrine problems or as a result of tumour mass effect and hydrocephalus. Although histologically "benign", their potential for causing death and disability is considerable. The initial treatment is usually surgical and "complete" resection should be performed if possible, although in many cases resection is really subtotal. Surgery is usually followed by radiotherapy, but in some cases observation with further surgery and/or radiotherapy at the time of relapse may avoid the late consequences of radiotherapy in a young child. Ill-judged attempts at complete removal of advanced tumours can cause a lot of damage. In some cases it is wise for the surgeon to make the tumour mass smaller by decompression of the cysts and then to use radiotherapy as the principle treatment. In the majority of cases the tumour is controlled long term, but in others repeated recurrences may occur over many years. Survivors are often handicapped by visual impairment, cognitive and behavioural disorders as well as having endocrine dysfunction. Long-term support of the patient and the family in the community will be necessary.

Intracranial germ cell tumours

There are many similarities between germ cell tumours occurring in the brain and those in the testis and at other extracranial sites. The most common sites in the brain are the suprasellar and pineal regions, and sometimes tumours are found at both sites. Germinoma is the equivalent of seminoma in the testis or dysgerminoma in the ovary. It is most common in teenagers, and radiotherapy (which is to the whole brain and spine because of the tendency for dissemination through the CSF pathways) is usually curative. Secreting germ cell tumours produce the tumour markers AFP and/or βhCG, which can be measured in blood or CSF. They are malignant, and intensive chemotherapy is the first line of treatment. Surgery may be indicated for residual disease after chemotherapy, and radiotherapy is needed. Despite combined modality therapy results are less good than for testicular tumours with only about 70% survival rates. Rarely benign teratomas may be encountered in very young children, and these are usually managed surgically.

Other gliomas

Gliomas form a very diverse group, both in terms of anatomical location and histological grade and natural history. Brain stem, cerebellar and optic pathway gliomas have already been mentioned. The remaining gliomas are supratentorial and may be either low grade or high grade. They may occur in accessible sites in the cerebral hemispheres or deep within the central part of the brain, for example, in the basal ganglia. Accessible tumours should be resected as fully as possible, without risking additional neurodisability. Most deeply seated tumours will not be considered operable and a biopsy only will be performed. Completely excised low-grade gliomas, including pilocytic astrocytomas and variants such as ganglioglioma, pleomorphic xanthoastrocytoma and oligodendroglioma will not need any further treatment, although anticonvulsants may be necessary, particularly if the presentation was with fits. Survival rates are relatively good. Unresectable tumours and high-grade (Grade III anaplastic astrocytoma and Grade IV glioblastoma multiforme) tumours will require radiotherapy. Chemotherapy has been used for high-grade gliomas but its benefit is not clear. The outlook is much worse with high-grade tumours, and only about one in three children will survive. Nonetheless, a child with glioblastoma multiforme does have a chance of survival, whereas virtually all adults with the same histology will succumb.

NEUROBLASTOMA (7%)

A spectrum of tumours arise from the sympathetic nervous system. Neuroblastoma is an undifferentiated malignant tumour, ganglioneuroma is its benign counterpart and ganglioneuroblastoma is intermediate. Most cases are retroperitoneal, often arising from the adrenal gland. Others have their origins elsewhere along the sympathetic chain and the primary tumour may be in the neck or the posterior mediastinum. Although, it may occur in children of any age, it is principally a disease of young children, being most common in the first year of life. It can be congenital and may even be diagnosed antenatally.

Presentation is with symptoms specific to the primary site, for example, abdominal pain and a palpable mass or spinal cord compression if the tumour extends through an intervertebral foramen, with symptoms of distant metastases, such as bone pain, with irritability and hypertension related to catecholamine production or other non-specific symptoms. Sometimes children who present with advanced disease involving the bones of the skull and have anaemia and thrombocytopenia as a result of bone marrow replacement may have swellings on their head and bruising around the eyes and be mistaken for victims of non-accidental injury.

Tumours may be localised and resectable (Stage 1) or localised but not completely resected (Stage 2) or locally advanced (Stage 3) or with distant metastases most commonly in bone, bone marrow and liver (Stage 4). There is a peculiar variant of neuroblastoma found in babies with a small primary neuroblastoma tumour where there are distant metastases most often in the liver, sometimes in the skin and often to a limited extent in the bone marrow although never in cortical bone. This is called Stage 4S disease where the S stands for special. Often only minimal treatment, sometimes even no treatment at all, is called for as the disease may well regress spontaneously.

Neuroblastoma is a contrary disease, and the behaviour can vary from essentially benign to highly malignant. The principal adverse prognostic factors are older age, advanced stage and a number of biological factors such as amplification of the *MycN* oncogene which is now used to guide treatment.

Patients with Stage 1 or 2 disease will usually require surgery only. Patients with more advanced disease will require chemotherapy, and there is now evidence that very intensive chemotherapy produces better long-term results in Stage 4 disease, as does high-dose chemotherapy with bone marrow or peripheral blood stem cell support. After apparently successful therapy for Stage 4 disease, there is still a significant risk of relapse which can be reduced by adjuvant oral *cis*-retinoic acid which causes differentiation of any residual immature neuroblasts. Some patients with neuroblastoma are given radionuclide therapy with ^{131}I-labelled *meta*-iodobenzylguanidine (mIBG). This is a radiopharmaceutical which concentrates in cells of neuroendocrine origin and can be used both for diagnostic scanning and treatment.

SOFT TISSUE SARCOMA (7%)

Rhabdomyosarcoma is the most common type of soft tissue sarcoma occurring in childhood. It can occur in the head and neck region (40%), the genito-urinary system (20%), limbs (20%) and many other sites. The head and neck group may be divided into orbital tumours which have a very favourable prognosis, non-parameningeal tumours, such as those in the oral cavity and larynx which have an intermediate prognosis, and parameningeal tumours, such as those in the nasopharynx or ethmoid sinuses which abut the skull base and have a worse prognosis because of their propensity for intracranial extension. Similarly, the genito-urinary primary sites are divided into bladder and prostate tumours which fare less well than those at other sites such as the vagina, uterus and paratesticular region.

There are various histological types. Embryonal rhabdomyosarcoma has the most favourable outlook and fortunately is relatively common. Only the minority of patients have the highly malignant alveolar rhabdomyosarcoma. The majority of patients will be found to have localised (Stage I) disease at presentation. Distant metastases (Stage IV) disease is more commonly found in patients who have limb or "other" primary tumours. The treatment plan is based on site, histology and stage. Radical surgery is rarely called for as initial treatment, the one exception being paratesticular rhabdomyosarcoma where an inguinal orchidectomy is performed. Chemotherapy is the mainstay of curative treatment these days. Relatively, gentle short-course treatment is given to those with the best outlook with intensive chemotherapy used for more advanced disease. Subsequently, if there is any evidence of residual disease, local therapy with surgery or radiotherapy or both will be considered.

Cure rates of the order of 90% can be expected for orbital disease with most patients retaining their eye. Over 80% of patients with genito-urinary primary tumours will be cured, and most will retain normal bladder function. About 70% of non-parameningeal patients will be cured, whereas the survival rates for patients with tumours at parameningeal, limb or other sites are only of the order of 60%. Site by site outcome figures disguise the fact that patients with metastatic disease fare badly whatever the primary site. Only about a quarter of patients with Stage IV disease will become survivors.

WILMS' TUMOUR (6%)

Childhood renal tumours are most common in the pre-school age group and usually present as an abdominal mass. There are several different histological types, but fortunately favourable histology Wilms' tumour predominates and has a good outcome, with survival rates approaching 90%. Patients with anaplastic Wilms' tumour,

the bone-metastasising renal tumour of childhood (clear cell sarcoma) and malignant rhabdoid tumour require more intensive treatment and fare worse. Adult type renal cell carcinoma occasionally occurs in teenagers.

In addition to histological type, stage, not surprisingly, has an important effect on outcome. Localised, completely resected tumours (Stages I and II) do better than incompletely resected tumours (Stage III) or cases with distant metastases, usually found in the lungs (Stage IV). When both kidneys are affected it is called Stage V disease, but it would perhaps be better to call it bilateral Wilms' tumour as the prognosis is almost as good as that of Stage II disease, not worse than Stage IV disease.

The main treatments are chemotherapy, which is of greater intensity with more advanced disease, and surgery to remove the affected kidney. Radiotherapy to the flank, abdomen or lungs is indicated in a miniority of patients with more advanced disease.

RETINOBLASTOMA (3%)

Retinoblastoma is a cancer of the eye which occurs in infants. If there is a family history, children should be screened, and most tumours will be detected before they become symptomatic. However, most cases are sporadic, and often parents will notice eye signs and receive false reassurance from their GPs before the diagnosis is made. Babies who develop a white light reflex or a squint or unilateral painful red eye or any evidence of visual loss should be examined carefully and referred for an urgent ophthalmological opinion if there is any doubt. Management should only be undertaken in specialised centres. A variety of surgical treatments, combined with chemotherapy and radiotherapy in carefully selected cases will result in cure rates of over 90%, with most patients retaining their eyes.

LATE EFFECTS OF TREATMENT

Children differ from adults in many ways, but two are especially important when it comes to considering the late effects of successful cancer therapy. Firstly, the tissues of children are immature, and these growing tissues are much more susceptible to damage by chemotherapy and radiotherapy than the corresponding tissues in adult life. Secondly, a child who survives their cancer has hopefully six or seven decades of life ahead of them, and that is a long time to live with any structural or functional disability, and a long time for very late effects such as the development of second malignant neoplasms to become apparent. Finally, there are the psycho-social consequences of having to go through treatment for cancer, including time missing from school, and of having to put up with surveillance, functional and cosmetic disabilities and continuing treatment of endocrine dysfunction. It is perhaps surprising that the majority of survivors are so well adjusted.

LATE EFFECTS OF TREATMENT
- Bone and soft tissue effects
- Endocrine sequelae
- Neuropsychological function
- Cardiac function
- Lung function
- Renal function
- Fertility
- Second malignant neoplasms

Bone and soft tissue effects

Surgery and radiotherapy can both have localised effects on bone and soft tissue structure and function. A limb amputation for a bone sarcoma is a constant and clearly visible reminder of the disease, and of course, impairs function. Paradoxically, however, some patients who have undergone limb-sparing treatment with surgery and radiotherapy and who have consequent limb weakness, joint stiffness and shortening or deformity may have more functional disability than an amputee. Paraspinal surgery for a neuroblastoma may lead to scoliosis, and flank radiotherapy to the flank of a young child for a Wilms' tumour may lead to asymmetry of muscular development around the waist. Radiotherapy to the spine for medulloblastoma will lead to shortness of stature even if any associated growth hormone insufficiency is corrected. Thoracic irradiation may lead to failure of breast development during puberty, and neck irradiation for Hodgkin's disease may cause the neck to appear very thin and scrawny in adult life. Radiotherapy for sarcomas in the head and neck may lead to failure of facial development with consequent asymmetry and cosmetic problems.

Endocrine sequelae

The hypothalamus and pituitary gland are unavoidably irradiated during the treatment of many brain tumours and some other cancer types such as parameningeal rhabdomyosarcomas and during total body irradiation prior to bone marrow transplantation. All patients at risk should be followed up until adult life by a paediatric endocrinologist specialising in the management of late effects. Growth hormone is the most sensitive hormone, but deficiency does not usually become apparent until 18 months to 2 years have elapsed. If there is any evidence of loss of growth velocity on serial height measurements, then blood tests for pituitary function should be undertaken. Growth hormone replacement is

safe now that biosynthetic hormone is available, and parents should be reassured about this as they may be very mindful of the tragedy when a number of survivors of cancer in childhood succumbed to Creutzfeld-Jacob disease following administration of infected human cadaveric growth hormone. There is no evidence that use of growth hormone leads to relapse of brain tumours. Growth can also be impaired by spinal irradiation, hypothyroidism and precocious puberty. Hypothyroidism is more likely to be caused by a direct effect on the thyroid gland, resulting in primary hypothyroidism with elevated TSH levels than it is by irradiation of the pituitary of hypothalamus.

Neuropsychological function

Intellectual and neurological dysfunction in children treated for brain tumours can be caused directly by the primary tumour, by the indirect effects of hydrocephalus, by surgery and by chemotherapy, but radiotherapy is often the only modality blamed. Certainly radiotherapy does have important adverse effects on brain function, and the extent of this depends on factors such as the dose used, the volume and location of brain tissue treated and critically on the age of the child at the time. This is because the brains of very young children are rapidly growing, and neural tissues are most vulnerable to radiation damage at this time. Care is taken to minimise all these factors wherever possible, and in fact most very young children will now have their brain tumours treated with chemotherapy in preference to radiotherapy for this reason. A child who has had cranial irradiation may manifest no disability at the end of treatment, but close surveillance by an experienced neuropsychologist and educational psychologist will reveal at an early stage special educational needs which can then be most appropriately met, hopefully with the child remaining in mainstream schooling. If the likely neurocognitive deficit is not recognised early, remedial measures may be less beneficial.

Cardiac function

The growing heart is sensitive not only to radiation but also to drugs such as the anthracycline doxorubicin. All patients should have cardiac function monitored prior to and during treatment. The cumulative dose of any cardiotoxic drug is limited, and lower maximum doses are tolerated if thoracic irradiation has been necessary. These measures are usually sufficient to prevent severe damage, but occasionally a patient has an idiosyncratic reaction and develops intractable heart failure. Sometimes cardiac transplantation is indicated if one can be confident that the tumour has been cured. Puberty and subsequent pregnancy can put additional stresses on a heart with diminished functional reserve, and patients may require additional monitoring at these times. It is not yet known whether patients who have received cardiotoxic treatment, but who are apparently well from a cardiac point of view, may incur a cardiovascular risk in adult life.

Lung function

Some drugs such as Bleomycin, used in the treatment of Hodgkin's disease, are recognised as causing pneumonitis and pulmonary fibrosis. This effect can be exacerbated by the concomitant use of radiotherapy to the thorax. This can result in chronic loss of respiratory functional reserve. Subsequent anaesthesia can be dangerous if high concentrations of oxygen are used. Atypical infections in the immunocompromised patient after bone marrow transplantation, particularly after total body irradiation, may give rise to pneumonitis.

Renal function

Drugs such as cisplatin and ifosfamide can reduce the glomerular filtration rate and cause renal tubular damage. They may require long-term supplementation of magnesium and potassium to make up for renal losses. Radiotherapy can also have an effect on the kidneys, and patients who have needed renal irradiation are at risk from developing hypertension, which can of course damage renal function further.

Fertility

Many drugs, particularly alkylating agents, and radiotherapy (as well as some operations) may destroy future fertility or at least put it at risk. Treatment strategies are selected to minimise the risk of infertility, but sometimes it is unavoidable if the child is to be cured of the tumour.

In the adult or adolescent male, semen can be collected prior to treatment for cryopreservation, but this is not possible in prepubertal boys. There has been much in the press about the possibility of saving and cryopreserving testicular or ovarian tissue in children at risk. There is, however, no evidence that these tissues can subsequently be used to restore fertility. As well as the ethical issues surrounding fertility, there is also a very strict legal framework in place, and many potential treatments are at present forbidden by the Human Fertilisation and Embryology Authority.

Second malignant neoplasms

Many of the treatments we use for cancer may be carcinogenic. Radiation and cytotoxic drugs, especially alkylating agents, such as cyclophosphamide and ifosfamide and the epipodophyllotoxins, such as etoposide, are both implicated. Added to this is the fact that many childhood cancers may arise on a background of genetic abnormalities which themselves may predispose the individual to a second cancer. Secondary leukaemias, usually AML, tend to appear earlier than other tumours, after an average interval of 3–4 years. Sarcomas, the most common second cancers appear after an average of 11 years, but the latent interval can be much longer. Benign nodules commonly occur after irradiation of the thyroid gland, well-differentiated papillary carcinomas are less frequent. Prolonged stimulation by TSH may be a factor here, so patients who develop compensated primary hypothyroidism (an elevated TSH with a normal T4) should be started on thyroxine replacement without waiting until clinical hypothyroidism with a low T4 level develops. Having had one cancer does not immunise the survivor against the carcinogenic effects of tobacco, which may in fact be synergistic with the effects of previous radiotherapy and chemotherapy. Advice against smoking is, therefore, an important part of the secondary prevention strategy in childhood cancer survivors.

Cancer in adolescents

Adolescence – often synonymous with the teenage years from 13 to 19 – is a time of turmoil for most individuals and their families. It is a time of struggle to leave behind the dependency of childhood and enter adult life. It is a time when there is often a conflict between the unparalleled pressure to conform to the peer group norm and the need to continue to respect parental standards and aspirations. It is a time when the body undergoes the physical changes of puberty and the soul may wrestle with the emotional stresses of early sexual relationships. It is often during this difficult period that the importance of continued study to the achievement of career aims and social and economic independence becomes apparent.

> **CANCER IN ADOLESCENTS IS DIFFICULT TO MANAGE BECAUSE OF THE**
>
> ♦ psychological and social stresses of adolescence
> ♦ complexity of treatment needed for the cancer types occurring in the teenage years

Imagine then the effect of cancer on an adolescent. It comes uninvited, unexpected and unexplained. It is seen by the patient as an end to life when most consider themselves immortal. It may threaten mutilation when body image is more important than at any other time. Fertility may be lost on the threshold of reproductive life. As soon as independence is perceived as a realistic prospect it is snatched away. Study is interrupted and education and career goals may need to be deferred or redefined. A lifetime of regular attendance at hospital clinics looms.

As if those psychological and social factors do not make medical management of the seriously ill adolescent difficult enough, the tumour types occurring in the teenage years are among the most complex to treat. Pre-treatment staging investigations may be lengthy and distressing. Intensive therapy with prolonged spells of hospitalisation – often a long way from home – is frequently necessary. Rigorous compliance is essential for successful therapy when more factors conspire against this than at any other time.

EPIDEMIOLOGY OF CANCER IN ADOLESCENCE

Cancer in adolescents is rare. The incidence rate in the 13–20-year-age group is about 1 per 100,000 population per year – meaning that there are about 600 cases per year in the UK. Looked at another way, a group practice with 10,000 patients registered may expect to see a new adolescent cancer patient every 10 years.

> **COMMONEST TUMOUR TYPES IN ADOLESCENCE:**
>
> ♦ Acute leukaemias
> ♦ The lymphomas
> ♦ Central nervous system (CNS) tumours
> ♦ Bone and soft tissue sarcomas

Cancer is slightly more common in males than females in this age group overall, but the sex ratio varies between the tumour types. In males, the incidence rates of bone tumours, leukaemia and lymphoma is higher than in females. Females, however, are more prone to get thyroid cancer and melanoma.

The types of cancer seen in adolescence are different both qualitatively and quantitatively from those seen in childhood and adult life. The characteristic embryonal childhood tumours, such as neuroblastoma, medulloblastoma and Wilms' tumour, are seldom seen. Similarly, the common epithelial cancers of adults namely, cancers of the breast, colon, lung and stomach, for example, are very rare. Leukaemia and lymphoma, brain tumours and sarcomas predominate.

Over a quarter of cancers in 15–19-year-old males are lymphoma – more often Hodgkin's disease (18%) than non-Hodgkin's lymphoma (NHL) (9%). Leukaemia accounts for 16%, brain tumours for 13%, and testicular cancer (most often non-seminomatous germ cell tumours) for 12%. Bone tumours – osteosarcoma and Ewing's sarcoma – comprise 9%. Malignant melanoma and thyroid cancer, the commonest epithelial malignancies in this age group, account for 3% and 2%, respectively.

SEX DIFFERENCES IN ADOLESCENT TUMOUR TYPES

	Males (%)	Females (%)
◆ *Common in both*		
Hodgkin's disease	18	22
NHL	9	7
Leukaemia	16	12
Brain	13	9
Other	18	21
◆ *More common in males*		
Bone sarcoma	9	6
Testis cancer	12	–
◆ *More common in females*		
Thyroid cancer	3	11
Malignant melanoma	2	7
Ovarian cancer	–	5

In females aged 15–19 years leukaemia and lymphoma account for more than one-third of cases: Hodgkin's disease (22%), NHL (7%) and leukaemia (12%). Thyroid cancer (11%) and malignant melanoma (7%) are more common than in males. Brain, bone and ovarian tumours account for 9%, 6% and 5%, respectively.

The cause of cancer in most adolescents remains unknown. Many environmental causes – from nuclear power stations to pesticides – have been postulated as causes for cancer but few are proven. A clear genetic basis is apparent in a few, for example brain tumours in patients with neurofibromatosis and sarcomas in Li Fraumeni families. Sadly, some cases may be iatrogenic – such as vaginal adenocarcinoma in girls who were exposed *in utero* to diethylstilboestrol, lymphoproliferative disorders in organ transplant recipients, and thyroid cancer following irradiation in childhood – previously commonly used for a variety of benign disorders before the risks were appreciated.

Second malignant neoplasms occurring in survivors of childhood cancer are particularly tragic. These may be caused by treatment – especially if alkylating agents or radiation have been used – but it is difficult to distinguish effects of treatment from a possible genetic susceptibility. The osteosarcomas often seen in survivors of retinoblastoma treated in infancy are probably multifactorial in origin.

THE ADOLESCENT CANCER UNIT

Teenagers sit ill at ease amongst the soft toys and Disney posters in children's hospitals – and are no better placed in adult cancer wards with their clientele of often geriatric dying patients. A dedicated adolescent cancer unit is, therefore, ideally suited for the unique constellation of both psycho-social and medical features of cancer in adolescents. Gradually, more regional cancer centres are developing special facilities.

These units should be able to offer skilled multidisciplinary medical teams with expertise in the management of the types of cancer encountered in the teenage years, and experience of family dynamics and psychological difficulties in this age group. The success of this medical team is critically underpinned by experienced and sympathetic nurses, social workers, psychologists, teachers, dieticians and other staff.

The physical environment of the adolescent unit is designed to be more appealing to teenagers than the standard hospital ward, and daily routine is typically more relaxed. Clustering of adolescent patients together makes social interaction easier, allowing the sense of isolation often felt by ill teenagers to be alleviated.

Cancer in the elderly

The types of cancer, which arise in the elderly are, by and large, the same types that occur in middle age. Cancers of the breast, lung, prostate and gastro-intestinal tract predominate. For a variety of reasons, they often present at a more advanced stage than in younger patients. For example, patients may ignore early symptoms because they are unaware of their significance. Alternatively, they may recognise the possible significance, but be too frightened of the illness or its treatment to come forward for help, or they may believe that cancer is not only incurable but also untreatable. Also, elderly people often come to have an expectation of ill health, or may be too preoccupied with other matters to attend to the new symptoms. In addition, the screening programmes, which detect cancer earlier in younger age groups are not offered to the elderly.

WHO ARE THE ELDERLY?

It is perhaps helpful at this stage to consider what is meant by the term "elderly". An arbitrary age limit of say 65 years as the threshold to being elderly is convenient. On the other hand, people over the age of 65 years form a very disparate group. Some are very fit and may still be working, but others have multiple medical problems and are frail. The social background also varies. Some have a large, willingly supportive network of family and friends nearby, others live in isolation. Some very elderly patients may seem fit in that they have no major health problems and they may also live alone with minimal support. Yet these people's balance between successful independence and failure to cope may be very fine, so that any new or additional stress can push them from health to illness with dependency, possibly even requiring short- or long-term inpatient care.

When an elderly patient presents to their general practitioner with a symptom which might represent cancer, or when a sign, such as a breast lump, is discovered in an asymptomatic patient, the question of further investigations or referral to hospital arise. Investigations in this setting are for three reasons: to confirm or refute the diagnosis, to assess the tumour to see what treatments may be possible and to assess the patient to see what treatments they might tolerate. Younger, fitter patients should always be referred and fully investigated, if a treatable malignancy is in the differential diagnosis. Frailer patients, and those whose clinical features indicate an advanced problem should receive more limited investigation, sufficient to confirm the diagnosis and institute appropriate palliative and supportive care.

PROBLEMS WITH CANCER TREATMENT IN THE ELDERLY

- Advanced disease at presentation
- Co-existent illness
  - Physical
  - Mental
- Limited functional organ reserve
- Lack of social support
- Pressure of other responsibilities
- Difficulties in attending for treatment

The principal problem of treating elderly patients with cancer is that of co-existing illness. Even in the absence of another condition, cancer is often more difficult to treat because older patients are, in general, frailer, and lack of reserve in organ function means that the toxicity of treatment is often greater. Many elderly patients find attending hospital for treatment daunting and decline treatment simply because of its inconvenience or fear. For some patients, the duty of care they owe to their partner, who probably will also be elderly and may be in poor health, or even their pet dog, which cannot be left alone, may make them decline treatment, which will make them feel ill or take them away from home for a period.

Thus, it is frequently the case that only palliative treatment can be offered, even though the tumour may be localised and technically amenable to radical treatment. For some localised tumours, for example early cancers of the oesophagus, cervix and rectum, both surgery and radiotherapy can be used as potentially curative treatments in fit patients. In the elderly, many surgeons will refer a patient with an operable tumour for radical radiotherapy on the grounds of their age and frailty. However, a patient who is unfit for major surgery may well be unable to withstand the demands a course of radical radiotherapy makes.

Elderly patients often have mobility problems, such as arthritis, dizziness or deteriorating vision. These factors, compounded by non-medical problems, such as having given up driving and the high cost of taxis make clinic attendance difficult. Even if daily transport from home to hospital can be provided for a 6-week course of radiotherapy, the daily reminder of cancer and the increasing fatigue is often too much to tolerate.

Psychological factors including pre-existing depression or anxiety and expectations of ill health in old age may also mitigate against radical treatment of the elderly. Older patients may refuse offers of treatment because "I've got to die of something", "it's not causing any pain", "I don't want an operation – I wouldn't come through the anaesthetic" or simply because "I'm too old".

RADICAL TREATMENT IN ELDERLY PATIENTS

Whether or not an elderly patient is suitable for radical treatment depends on just how old and how fit that person is, and what the treatment entails. For example, a fit and active 80-year-old woman with early breast cancer, probably, merits radical treatment with surgery and radiotherapy and adjuvant tamoxifen. Her life expectancy without cancer is 8.4 years, and her prospect of "cure" may be 70%, whereas the prospect of control of the disease by tamoxifen alone for the next 8 years is much less. On the other hand, a 65-year-old woman with Alzheimers disease or severe congestive cardiac failure may best be treated in the first instance with hormone therapy only. Even at 95, a fit person with a skin cancer may be suitable for radical treatment.

Very often the aggressive multimodality treatment used to maximise the chances of cure in a younger patient is inappropriate in the older patient. That does not, however, mean that they cannot be treated radically with an expectation of cure. A younger woman with early breast cancer may receive surgery, radiotherapy and adjuvant chemotherapy. In an older patient with identically staged

disease, it may be wiser to offer just surgery and tamoxifen, leaving out chemotherapy and radiotherapy. This treatment is simpler and more easily tolerable, but still offers a significant chance of cure, even though the recurrence rates may be higher than with more radical treatment. Similarly, high-grade non-Hodgkin's lymphoma in a 65-year old may be suitable for an attempt at cure with relatively gentle outpatient chemotherapy, but high-dose chemotherapy with bone marrow support would be too toxic. Moderately, intensive short-course chemotherapy regimens with limited toxicity have been devised for use in the elderly – they last only about 12 weeks and are well tolerated. Again, prospects of cure with these regimens in older patients may be less than with more complex treatments, but this difference is offset by the greater acceptability of therapy and diminished treatment-related mortality.

Table of life expectancy (years) in the elderly

Age	Males	Females
65	14.3	18.1
70	11.2	14.5
75	8.6	11.2
80	6.4	8.4
85	4.8	6.1

It is important to recognise that fit old people often have a significant life expectancy, and patients should not be denied treatment just because they are old. Fit patients with asymptomatic or minimally symptomatic disease, which can be treated radically should, where possible, be offered treatment before more severe problems occur.

BEST SUPPORTIVE CARE

For those patients in whom radical treatment is precluded by their general condition or the stage of the tumour, it does not automatically follow that they require active anti-cancer treatment for palliation. The side-effects of palliative chemotherapy, and sometimes of radiotherapy can be significant, and the likelihood of benefit may be small. For patients with few symptoms, and in those patients whose symptoms can be controlled in other ways, such as with appropriate analgesia, best supportive care without any active anti-cancer treatment may be the best policy.

SECTION CONTENTS

CHAPTER 49

Looking after patients with metastatic disease

It is one of the great success stories of modern oncology that there are diseases in which the presence of distant metastases at the time of diagnosis, or developing subsequently, is not an automatic death sentence. Patients with metastatic testicular cancer (Chapter 38), for example, and many Stage IV childhood cancers (Chapter 46), may be cured with systemic treatments, such as chemotherapy.

For patients with the common solid tumours, such as lung, breast, colon and stomach cancer, however, the development of metastatic disease, for all practical purposes, indicates incurability. Often, as has been indicated in the various chapters about each cancer type, disease specific palliative treatment with chemotherapy or endocrine manipulation may cause at least partial regression of the disease, diminish symptoms and improve well-being and extend life expectancy.

This chapter is concerned with the palliative management of symptoms related to metastases affecting specific sites, such as the brain, liver, lungs and skeleton, regardless of the primary site of the tumour. The symptomatic management of other problems, which may occur in patients, such as pain, psychological distress and constipation, is covered in Chapter 50.

The management of patients with metastatic disease represents a large part of the workload of anyone involved in cancer treatment. Their proper care represents one of the greatest challenges in oncology. It is a paradigm of teamwork, involving the general practitioner (GP) and community services, the oncologist and hospital-based services and the specialist palliative care physician and hospice services working together in partnership with the patient and the family. Palliative care is more than just the essential rapid and effective control of symptoms caused by the disease and of side-effects due to various treatments. Patients need emotional, psychological and spiritual support as well, coupled with practical measures to facilitate their care, delivered in the most appropriate environment.

It has been said that high-quality palliative care is not just the rightful expectation of every patient with advanced cancer, but also the obligation of every responsible health care professional. While this does not mean that every oncologist or GP needs to know all the answers to every palliative care problem, it does mean that they cannot absolve themselves of all responsibility and leave everything to the palliative care physician. All involved

must recognise that the patient has needs, and be willing and able to listen and to deal well with the simple problems, calling in expert help from the palliative medicine specialist or indeed another member of the primary care team for more complex matters.

BONE METASTASES

Bone metastases are common in patients with breast, prostate and lung cancer. They are a less common feature of advanced colorectal and upper gastro-intestinal cancer, but they are seen sufficiently often to be borne in mind. There should, therefore, be a constant high index of suspicion of bone metastases, if patients with any type of cancer develop bone pain. While the usual symptom is pain, they may also cause pathological fracture and hypercalcaemia. Patients found to have bone metastases require careful evaluation.

ASSESSMENT OF PATIENTS WITH BONE METASTASES

- ◆ History and examination to characterise pain
- ◆ Exclusion of fracture, cord compression and hypercalcaemia
- ◆ Bone scan
- ◆ Plain radiographs
- ◆ Other investigations, such as computed tomography (CT), magentic resonance imaging (MRI) or biopsy, if doubt

---

Careful questioning will reveal the site, nature and amount of pain being experienced. It must be borne in mind that the patient may have other causes of pain, which need to be treated separately. Other symptoms, such as difficulty in moving need to be considered carefully. Is it just back pain, which is limiting mobility, or has the patient developed spinal cord compression? Is the inability to walk just due to a painful hip, or has the patient developed a pathological fracture of the femur through a metastatic deposit? Questions such as these needs to pass through the mind of the GP and other doctors not just when bone metastases are newly diagnosed, but at every consultation when there has been a change in symptoms.

Investigations such as a bone scan will be very helpful in confirming the diagnosis of metastatic bone disease and in defining the extent. While often bone scan appearances leave no room for doubting this diagnosis, bone scans merely show areas of increased osteoblastic activity, and there is a lengthy differential diagnosis for hot spots on bone scans. This list includes trauma, osteoporosis, osteomalacia and bone infarcts. Care must be exercised before attributing bone scan abnormalities to the presence of bone metastases, especially if they are solitary or unexpected in the context of the patient's disease. Sometimes, other investigations, such as CT, MRI or positron emission tomography scans or even a bone biopsy may be necessary to confirm or exclude the diagnosis of bone metastases.

Plain radiographs of weight-bearing bones, such as the femur are advised, if a bone scan shows bone metastases. There is a risk of pathological fracture developing, if more than half the cortex of the bone is eroded. If this is the case, referral to an orthopaedic surgeon for an opinion about the value of prophylactic surgical fixation is helpful. It is clear that patients are much more likely to be successfully rehabilitated after an elective procedure to prevent a pathological fracture developing than they are following treatment of an established fracture. Such a surgical procedure is often followed by radiotherapy with the aim of allowing more effective bone healing at that site.

TREATMENTS FOR BONE METASTASES

- Analgesia
- Surgical fixation
- Palliative radiotherapy
- Strontium
- Bisphosphonates
- Systemic treatment (hormones, chemotherapy) for the primary tumour

---

When patients have a clearly localised pain in relation to a site of bone metastasis, palliative radiotherapy can be beneficial in terms of pain relief. A single treatment or a short course of radiotherapy is as effective in this regard as a more protracted schedule. Planning palliative radiotherapy is less easy when the patient has widespread metastases and the pain seems to be "all over the place". Sometimes, wide field radiotherapy can be helpful in such cases. Upper half body irradiation covers from the level of the umbilicus upwards to the neck, including the thorax and arms. The head is usually omitted from this field unless there are definite sites of disease in the skull, which need to be treated. Lower half body irradiation covers from the umbilicus to the knees, unless there are symptomatic deposits at a lower level than this. It thus covers the pelvis, hips and femora. Sequential upper and lower half body treatments may be given, but it is wise to allow a gap of at least 6 weeks between the two treatments.

Systemic radionuclide treatment is an option for the treatment of patients with diffuse skeletal involvement by a predominantly osteoblastic tumour producing sclerotic metastases. The most common example of this type is prostate cancer. Strontium is the most frequently employed radionuclide, but others are being investigated. Strontium has been shown in some clinical trials to provide more effective pain control than external beam radiotherapy.

In recent years, the value of bisphosphonates in the management of patients with bone metastases (Chapter 14) has become more apparent. They are useful in treating both established hypercalcaemia of malignancy and bone pain. They can also be of value in patients without symptoms for preventing pain, hypercalcaemia and pathological fracture.

Finally, of course, patients with painful bone metastases require effective analgesic medication. Successful treatment of pain requires careful attention to detail and is described in Chapter 50.

BRAIN METASTASES

Central nervous system metastases are relatively uncommon in newly diagnosed patients, even if there are metastases at other sites. They are more often a feature of advanced disease.

POSSIBLE PRESENTING FEATURES OF BRAIN METASTASES

- Headache
- Nausea and vomiting
- Confusion or personality change
- Weakness of one or more limbs, ataxia and falls
- Grand mal convulsions or other seizures
- Impaired eye movement (III and VI nerve palsies)
- Loss of visual acuity or visual field defects

The presenting features of brain metastases depend on the site and number of deposits. They may cause focal neurological signs, such as a hemiparesis or cranial nerve palsy. Cerebellar deposits may cause ataxia. If the normal flow of cerebrospinal fluid is interrupted, there may be symptoms of obstructive hydrocephalus, such as headaches, vomiting and visual impairment. Similar symptoms may be caused by raised intracranial pressure due to the mass effect of the deposits along with surrounding oedema in the absence of hydrocephalus. Convulsions are uncommon.

Often, especially in the elderly and if there is no eyewitness account, the presenting features of brain metastases may be vague and non-specific, for example falls, dizziness, headache and confusion. These symptoms could well be caused by a wide variety of other causes, both benign and malignant. Examples include hypercalcaemia, renal failure, cerebrovascular disease and drug toxicity. Clearly, patients with these symptoms need careful investigation, which will include a biochemical profile and, usually, a CT or MRI scan of the brain.

Sometimes, cerebral metastases may be diagnosed on the imaging findings of multiple intracranial tumours in the absence of a known primary tumour. Usually, a careful history, examination and selected investigations will reveal the primary site. Sometimes, a neurosurgical biopsy may be needed to distinguish between metastases on a multifocal primary brain tumour (Chapter 39). Less often, a patient with no other clinical features will undergo neurosurgery for what is believed preoperatively to be a primary brain tumour only for the histology to reveal the true diagnosis to be a solitary metastasis. It should not be forgotten that the development of an intracranial lesion in a patient previously treated for cancer may be an unrelated condition.

Diffuse meningeal disease, or carcinomatous meningitis, is characterised by signs of meningeal irritation including headache, vomiting, neck stiffness and cranial nerve palsies. The suspected diagnosis is confirmed by demonstration of malignant cells in the CSF at lumbar puncture, but this is only performed after the brain has been scanned to ensure that there are no deposits within the brain, which might lead to the fatal complication of coning, if a lumbar puncture is attempted.

Once diagnosed, the treatment of brain metastases depends on a number of factors, such as the number and location of metastases, age of the patient, nature of the primary tumour, level of fitness and neurodisability and extent of any extracranial disease.

FACTORS AFFECTING THE TREATMENT OF BRAIN METASTASES

- Relating to the intracranial disease
  - Number of lesions
  - Location of lesions
- Relating to extracranial disease
  - Type of primary cancer
  - Extent of extracranial disease
  - Prior therapy and remaining options for systemic therapy
- Relating to the patient
  - Age and co-morbidity
  - Extent of neurodisability
  - Performance status

The first line of treatment is usually steroid therapy. Most often this is dexamethasone at a dose of 8–16 mg daily in divided doses. Sometimes, especially if there is

extensive oedema around the metastases, there may be a very dramatic response. On most occasions, there may be a lesser but still worthwhile improvement in symptoms and only rarely there is no benefit. Care must be exercised when using steroids, as unpleasant side-effects including Cushingoid appearance, diabetes, proximal myopathy, weight gain and psychological changes may develop very rapidly.

TREATMENTS FOR BRAIN METASTASES

- Steroids
- Neurosurgery
- Radiotherapy
- Systemic therapy (chemotherapy and endocrine therapy)
- Physiotherapy
- Radiotherapy
- Specialist palliative care input

Consideration should be given to neurosurgical involvement, especially if the diagnosis is not entirely clear cut, or the patient is young and fit with a solitary lesion in an accessible place. Neurosurgical intervention is more likely in those cases where the brain lesion is the only known site of disease, and where there is effective systemic therapy available for extracranial disease. In some circumstances, such as in patients with metastatic testicular tumours, chemotherapy is very effective, and neurosurgery should be performed prior to chemotherapy to prevent the possibility of chemotherapy-induced haemorrhage into necrotic tumour in the brain.

Radiotherapy is most effective, if there has been a good response to steroids. One of the principal benefits of radiotherapy for brain metastases is to enable the steroid dose to be reduced and stopped. In this way, the patient is spared the adverse effects of weeks of dexamethasone, which can greatly reduce the quality of life. Many patients with brain metastases have a poor life expectancy. Just two whole brain radiotherapy treatments are as effective as longer courses. Some patients, however, for example those with hormone responsive breast cancer, may live for a number of years after the development of brain metastases. For these patients with a better prognosis, it is probably wiser to use a longer course, for example 10 fractions over 2 weeks. No great advantage has been shown for giving a stereotactic boost to the individual metastases after whole brain radiotherapy.

The treatment of carcinomatous meningitis is difficult. Steroids will be used, and palliative cranial or craniospinal radiotherapy is often given. This may be combined with regular lumbar punctures to administer intrathecal chemotherapy. Sometimes, responses are seen, but these are commonly short lived and this diagnosis usually carries a dismal prognosis.

Handbook of Community Cancer Care

Physiotherapy is important in helping to rehabilitate patients with neurodisability from brain metastases. Similarly, an occupational therapy assessment of the patient, preferably performed in their own home, may be very valuable. It may lead to appropriate aids being made available and adaptions of the home environment, which make it possible for the patient to return home and live independently.

The care of patients with brain metastases can be very demanding for family members. Of course, carers are faced with the prospect of the gradual physical decline of their relative and are anticipating bereavement. In addition, memory problems or personality changes caused by the tumour or by steroids can be very distressing for loved ones. The GP should be familiar with the various drugs available for dealing with a terminally ill patient with, for example, agitation or aggression. The GP might indeed consider requesting a domiciliary visit from the local psychiatric team. The physical care of an incapacitated patient who may be paralysed to some extent, or who has developed a proximal myopathy on steroids, is difficult at the best of times, and is much worse, if the carer is elderly or frail. Specialist palliative care involvement can, therefore, be tremendously valuable, both directly for the patient, and indirectly through the support given to the family.

SPINAL CORD COMPRESSION

SYMPTOMS ASSOCIATED WITH SPINAL CORD COMPRESSION

- Weakness or paralysis of both legs
- Falls and immobility
- Back pain
- Urinary retention
- Urinary and faecal incontinence
- Altered sensation below a particular level (depending on the site of disease)

Spinal symptoms, such as weakness of the legs, associated with bladder and bowel dysfunction and perhaps a sensory level, are more commonly caused by spinal cord compression associated with extra-axial deposits, such as bone metastases in the thoracic spine than to metastases within the spinal cord itself. Back pain is a common, but not universal feature.

In the same way that symptoms suggesting brain metastases can be caused by a wide variety of other conditions, other factors can produce a constellation of symptoms mimicking cord compression. For example, an elderly man with bone metastases from prostate cancer, who is, of course, at risk from developing spinal cord compression, may complain of weakness, impaired mobility, back pain,

constipation and urinary retention or incontinence. These symptoms, caused by a combination of his primary and metastatic tumour compounded by side-effects from opiates and steroids, may bring to mind the important possibility of spinal cord compression.

Often a carefully taken history and detailed neurological examination may reveal the true cause allowing conservative management. Nonetheless, suspected spinal cord compression should be investigated and treated as an emergency, if any neurological function is to be restored. Plain X-rays of the spine may show bone destruction, a paravertebral mass or vertebral collapse. An MRI scan is, however, the definitive investigation. This will show the whole length of the spinal cord, and accurately identify the vertebral level or levels involved. Often, at this time, the disease may be found to be much more extensive than clinically suspected.

As with brain metastases, steroids are often the initial treatment. Neurosurgery may be contemplated, if there is doubt about the diagnosis, or if there is compression at a single level in the absence of widespread disease. Neurosurgeons are reluctant to intervene, if there are multiple levels of vertebral involvement, or if the prognosis is poor because of widespread disease elsewhere in the body.

Radiotherapy is administered urgently as the principal treatment if surgery is not performed, or is given postoperatively. Treatment, whether surgery or radiotherapy, is more likely to be successful if the onset of symptoms has been gradual, and the degree of neurological disability is not complete at the time of surgery. A very sudden onset may indicate that a spinal artery has become blocked infarcting the cord, and so relief of pressure will not result in recovery of function. Complete paraplegia with bladder and bowel involvement, which has been present for more than 48 hours is rarely reversible. In this case, radiotherapy may still be beneficial for pain control.

LIVER METASTASES

Asymptomatic liver metastases may be diagnosed at presentation on routine staging investigations or at laparotomy, or subsequently on follow-up imaging investigations. More commonly, liver metastases present with symptoms. These may be non-specific, such as tiredness, weight loss, anorexia, nausea and vomiting, or a localising symptom, such as right upper quadrant pain due to distension of the liver capsule. Jaundice, bruising, ascites and leg oedema are usually late features.

Patients with a solitary liver deposit from a locally controlled colorectal primary tumour may be candidates for a potentially curative liver resection, which is usually performed in conjunction with chemotherapy. Interstitial, imaging guided treatments, such as radiofrequency ablation, laser destruction or alcohol injection, may be appropriate for a small number of suitably located deposits, which do not exceed a particular size. Units performing this type of treatment may vary in the criteria used for selection of suitable patients, but no more than five lesions and none more than 5 cm diameter is an example. Again, interstitial treatments are often preceded by or followed by chemotherapy to improve results. These are promising new approaches, but the long-term results are not known.

For the most part, patients with liver metastases have disease, which is too extensive or otherwise unsuitable for consideration of such approaches. Palliative anti-cancer treatment with chemotherapy or endocrine therapy in the case of breast cancer may be possible.

Patients whose disease is not suitable for chemotherapy, or which has recurred after earlier treatment will require palliative interventions depending on their symptoms. Simple anti-emetics, such as metoclopramide or cyclizine can be tried in the first instance to help nausea and vomiting. Failing this, steroids may be helpful. They may reduce nausea and vomiting and stimulate the appetite. For pain, analgesics may be required, starting with simple ones, such as paracetamol at the bottom of the ladder. Steroids may also help to reduce the pain caused by capsular distension. If stronger analgesics become necessary, it must not be forgotten that the metabolism of opiates is reduced in hepatic failure. If morphine is required, low starting doses should be used. It should be remembered that opiates often cause nausea and constipation, and anti-emetics and laxatives may need to be prescribed as well.

Jaundice associated with liver metastases, although there is often an obstructive component in its aetiology, is not usually amenable to the mechanical forms of relief, which may be beneficial in pancreatic or bile duct cancer. The pruritis associated with jaundice may be mediated by histamine and serotonin, and so the use of antihistamines (H1 receptor antagonists), such as chlorpheniramine and serotonin blockers (5HT-3 receptor antagonists), such as granesetron may be helpful.

The ascites associated with liver metastases is not usually severe enough to require intervention. If tense ascites does cause discomfort, this can be relieved by abdominal paracentesis. However, ascites often reaccumulates quickly, and there will be considerable loss of protein, which may exacerbate peripheral oedema. Rarely, consideration may be given to the insertion of a shunt, which allows ascitic fluid to drain back into the venous system.

Most patients with advanced liver metastases have a limited life expectancy once they start to show signs of liver failure, such as jaundice and ascites. They rapidly become weaker and cachectic, and gradually slip into coma. Clearly, the help of specialist palliative care nurses is appropriate, and often hospice care may be called for.

PULMONARY METASTASES

DIFFERENTIAL DIAGNOSIS OF DYSPNOEA IN CANCER PATIENTS

- Pulmonary metastases
- Pleural effusion
- Lymphangitis carcinomatosa
- Endoluminal bronchial obstruction by tumour
- External bronchial compression by nodal disease
- Superior vena cava obstruction
- Pericardial effusion
- Anaemia
- Heart failure
- Pulmonary embolism

Not surprisingly, dyspnoea is the most common symptom in patients with lung disease due to metastatic cancer. Cough is another common symptom. The type of lung involvement can, however, take a variety of forms, so it is important to assess the nature of the problem before deciding on treatment.

Pleural effusions are a common oncological problem; interstitial lung involvement or lymphangitis carcinomatosa is rarer and more difficult to treat. Lumpy lung disease, or parenchymal pulmonary metastases, is often asymptomatic finding on chest X-ray. Mediastinal nodes can cause dyspnoea through compression of the trachea or bronchi, or superior vena cava obstruction.

Other complications of cancer, such as anaemia and pulmonary thromboembolic disease can also cause dyspnoea. Finally, it must not be forgotten that people with cancer can often be dyspnoeic as a result of pre-existing or intercurrent acute or chronic conditions, such as asthma, congestive cardiac failure and chronic bronchitis and emphysema. Any of the conditions listed above may, of course, co-exist.

Following a history and examination, a chest X-ray is the most commonly requested investigation in patients with dyspnoea. Other investigations, such as full blood count, spirometry, ECG, CT scan of the thorax or an echocardiogram may also be helpful in certain circumstances.

Pleural effusions in patients with cancer are usually exudates caused by pleural involvement by tumour, most commonly breast and lung cancer. These can often be very substantial when they are recognised, and cause a complete white-out on the affected side on a chest radiography. Pleural effusions may also be associated with pneumonia, hypoalbuminaemia, heart failure and pulmonary emboli.

Large effusions should be aspirated, or drained. Care must be taken not to remove too much fluid too quickly or pulmonary oedema may occur. If nothing more than drainage is performed, malignant effusions have a tendency to recur fairly quickly. So when a malignant effusion has been drained to dryness, a chemical pleurodesis is commonly performed to prevent recurrence. Various sclerosant drugs, such as tetracycline and bleomycin, are irritant to the pleura and cause adhesions to develop. This may be completely successful, but sometimes loculated recurrent effusions develop. These can be difficult to aspirate or drain unless imaging is used to guide the insertion point of the drain. With troublesome recurrent effusions, a thoracic surgeon may be able to help by stripping the pleura or by performing an open or thoracoscopic pleurodesis with talc.

Pulmonary metastases are usually treated with chemotherapy in the case of chemosensitive tumours. Occasionally, such as in osteosarcoma, a thoracotomy and resection of individual metastases may result in extended survival or even cure. Radiotherapy has very little role in the treatment of pulmonary metastases.

While pulmonary metastases may lead to a strikingly abnormal appearance on chest X-ray, patients with lymphangitis may have extreme dyspnoea with a virtually normal chest X-ray. CT scanning may be a more sensitive investigation to confirm the diagnosis. Treatment is often difficult, and the prognosis is correspondingly poor. Steroids may provide some symptomatic relief, and chemotherapy can be used if the underlying cancer is known to be chemosensitive. Opiates may be helpful for treating cough and dyspnoea in the terminal phase of life.

SUPERIOR VENA CAVA OBSTRUCTION

The syndrome of superior vena cava obstruction is characterised by swelling of the face and upper torso, with distension of the veins and venules across the chest, upper arms and neck. Dyspnoea, pain, cough, orthopnoea and hoarseness are common features. Dizziness, headache, lethargy and syncope are less common. Most commonly, it is due to lung cancer, but other malignant causes, such as mediastinal lymphoma or secondary involvement of mediastinal lymph node by a variety of other cancers occur. Rarely, the cause may be benign. Nowadays, with the increasing use of central venous catheters for cancer patients and in the management of other diseases, catheter-associated thrombosis is a more frequent cause.

As with other causes of dyspnoea, it is important to make an accurate diagnosis. Initial symptomatic management involves sitting the patient up, and giving oxygen and steroids. Then the underlying cause can be treated. Clearly, if the cause is a potentially curable tumour, such as a lymphoma, this is treated appropriately. Most commonly, however, the cause is an incurable lung cancer, and palliative radiotherapy to the mediastinum can lead to prolonged symptom control. If this does not help, or the symptoms later recur, consideration can be given to stenting the compressed vessels.

BONE MARROW DISEASE

It is important to distinguish bone metastases and bone marrow infiltration by cancer. Although the two may co-exist and may, in fact, be opposite ends of one spectrum, they present differently and are managed differently. Patients may have widespread skeletal involvement, yet have no signs of bone marrow infiltration or failure, while others may have profound myelosuppression due to marrow involvement with no detectable cortical bone metastases apparent on a bone scan or on X-ray.

Anaemia and thrombocytopenia are the principal symptoms of diffuse bone marrow infiltration by tumour. Neutropenia is less commonly caused by marrow involvement. Care should be taken before assuming that marrow infiltration is the cause, as there are many other causes of anaemia including bleeding, haemolysis and chemotherapy. Bruising and haemorrhage may be caused by liver failure as well as thrombocytopaenia. Suspected bone marrow infiltration may be confirmed by marrow aspirate and trephine biopsy, and is usually a very grave development. In the previously untreated patient, chemotherapy may be appropriate for some tumour types. Endocrine therapy may also be possible for patients with breast or prostate cancer. Otherwise, supportive care with blood and platelet transfusions may be all that can be offered. Growth factors, such as epoietin and G-CSF, may help treatment-related anaemia and neutropaenia, but are unlikely to be of value in marrow failure caused by infiltration by cancer cells.

Management of specific symptoms

This chapter covers the management of those symptoms commonly encountered in those with advanced cancer, which often have multiple causes. The first principle is to assess the patient carefully, considering the underlying differential diagnosis, in order to identify treatable causes of the symptom in question. To a large extent this approach will be governed by the phase and pace of the patient's illness.

For example, the development of breathlessness in a relatively fit, active and independent woman with metastatic breast cancer may be due to anaemia, pleural effusion or lymphangitis carcinomatosa, amongst other things. Each of these will require different treatment; and, in addition, there may still be scope for further disease modifying therapy, such as further chemotherapy or additional endocrine therapy.

On the other hand, symptomatic breathlessness in a bed-bound terminally ill patient with a life expectancy measured in days might be better treated with morphine rather than a blood transfusion or pleural drainage, even if anaemia or an effusion is the cause.

Hence, careful evaluation of the patient with a symptom means more than accurate diagnosis of the cause of the symptom. It also means the development of an understanding of the point the patient is now at in their disease trajectory. It is also important to assess the impact of the symptom on the patient's quality of life, and to discuss with the patient, and any carers as appropriate, their fears and aspirations, and their degree of understanding and acceptance.

Together, these pieces of information will enable formulation of a management plan which is individualised and appropriate for the symptom, and appropriate for the patient at that time. The plan must be discussed with, and agreed by, the patient and carers. Sometimes, careful negotiation is necessary; for example, to overcome the beliefs or fears a patient might have about morphine. The patient needs to understand and agree with the plan, otherwise compliance will be poor and the treatment will be ineffective. Careful monitoring is required as doses may need to be adjusted and side-effects may need alleviating or new symptoms may have arisen. Attention to detail is an essential component of good quality palliative care.

> ## PRINCIPLES OF SYMPTOM CARE
>
> - Take a history to discover all symptoms and their impact
> - Accurately diagnose the cause of the symptoms
> - Ascertain the patient's stage in their illness
> - Explore the patient's fears and hopes
> - Negotiate an individualised management plan and explain it carefully
> - Review progress regularly

PAIN

Pain is among the most feared of symptoms. "Will I be in pain?" is top of the list of frequently asked questions, when patients first learn that their disease is incurable, and that the intent of treatment is changing from potentially curative to palliative. The most honest answer is that nowadays, with good medical and nursing care, prolonged severe pain is most unusual. Most patients with cancer will develop pain of some sort, but usually it is possible for it to be treated swiftly and effectively.

Pain, of course, is a subjective experience. Unlike blood pressure or haemoglobin, it cannot be measured by a machine. Pain is what the patient says it is. The doctor has to listen to what the patient is saying, both in words and non-verbally. Expression of pain varies according to age, gender, educational level, emotional state, spiritual beliefs and cultural values, and according to the level of understanding of its significance. The pain a patient feels is a complex amalgam of physical, psychological, spiritual and social components. Pain can be exacerbated by fatigue, anxiety, depression, ignorance and isolation. Conversely, sleep, understanding, hope and companionship may relieve pain.

The doctor or nurse assessing a patient with pain needs to get a full description of the pain and understand the non-physical factors which are affecting the perception of pain. These features elicited from the history, must be supplemented by what is already known about the illness, physical examination and possibly some additional investigations. Then it should be possible to work out from a differential diagnosis of the possible causes of the pain, namely, what the actual cause is and the physiological mechanism through which it is mediated.

PAIN ASSESSMENT

Description of pain

- *Anatomy*: site or sites, radiation
- *Quality*: dull, sharp, aching, throbbing, burning
- *Time factors*: time of onset and subsequent course – acute, intermittent or chronic
- *Concomitant features*: sweating, breathlessness, increased pulse rate, insomnia, anorexia, lethargy, depression, loss of interest in pleasurable things
- *Modifying factors*: things which make the pain better or worse
- *Severity*: mild, moderate, severe, intolerable

History, examination and investigations

- Knowledge of the cancer and its treatment and co-morbidity
- Careful and complete physical examination to establish cause of pain
- Selected investigations, such as X-ray or ultrasound, which may help

Non-physical factors

- Psychological
- Social
- Spiritual

Possible causes

- *The cancer itself*: primary tumour or metastatic disease
- *Side-effect* of treatment or general debility caused by the cancer or its treatment
- Separate *problem unrelated* to the cancer

Mechanism

- *Pathological*: nociceptive or neuropathic
- *Functional*: cramp or colic

After full assessment of the pain, it should be possible to decide about how best to treat it, or, still better, how to treat the underlying cause. For example, abdominal pain caused by constipation will resolve as enemas or laxatives take effect; the pain of urinary retention will be eased by catheterisation of the bladder; and the pain caused by a pathological fracture of the femur will be helped by surgical fixation.

Sometimes, even in a patient with advanced cancer, pain can be helped by active anti-cancer treatment, for example chemotherapy, endocrine therapy or radiotherapy. The pain caused by distension of the capsule of the liver by metastatic deposits can be helped by chemotherapy, if the tumour type is known to be responsive. Localised bone pain often responds well to a single radiation treatment,

minimising the need for visits to hospital. Sometimes, the pathological process mediating the pain can be modified, even if the progression of the cancer itself will not be affected; for example, the use of bisphosphonates to ameliorate widespread skeletal pain in patients with bone metastases (Chapter 14).

Lifestyle changes or modification of the patient's environment may affect pain. For example, someone whose mobility is impaired by a pain in the leg may benefit from the use of a walking aid, such as a stick or a frame, or a wheelchair. If movement brings about pain, a sling for the arm or a soft collar for the neck may be helpful. Involvement of a physiotherapist or occupational therapist (Chapter 15) is sometimes recommended.

Physical methods are sometimes helpful in alleviating pain. Many patients find a heat pad or hot-water bottle brings comfort, although care must be taken to avoid burns. Transcutaneous electrical nerve stimulation (TENS) can alter perception of chronic pain. Nerve pathways can also be blocked in certain circumstances. Visceral pain from a pancreatic cancer may be helped by a coeliac plexus block. Chest wall pain from an invasive tumour may be helped by an intercostal nerve block. Rarely, severe chronic pain unresponsive to other treatments may call for the involvement of a neurosurgeon to perform a spinal cordotomy.

Running alongside these physical treatments are emotional and psychological strands to treatment. Probably, the most important component of psychological pain management is taking time to (a) listen carefully to the patients symptoms and worries and (b) give reassurance and to explain, in detail, the pathogenesis of the pain and what is being done to alleviate it. Sometimes, the expression of pain is a proxy for another worry. If that can be uncovered and dealt with, then the pain which was the surrogate presentation may ease. Sometimes, more formal psychological input with cognitive-behavioural therapy, teaching of relaxation methods and psychodynamic therapy may help. A clinical psychologist can, sometimes, be the most valuable member of the pain team.

PAIN MANAGEMENT IN ADVANCED CANCER

- Careful assessment of the pain and the patient (see box above)
- Treat treatable underlying causes of pain
- Carefully selected palliative treatment of the cancer itself
- Lifestyle adaptions
- Physical treatments
- Explanation and empathy
- Psychological treatments
- Analgesic therapy
- Revisit, review and modify treatments as appropriate

ANALGESICS

Of course, painkillers are also important tools in the management of pain. We have, however, not mentioned analgesics until now to emphasise that there is much more to pain management than morphine. Doctors are usually good at the drug treatment of illnesses; but, sometimes, are prone to forgetting about other helpful measures.

Drugs used for the treatment of pain can be divided into three groups: (1) non-opioid drugs (such as paracetamol) and non-steroidal anti-inflammatories; (2) opioids (weak, such as codeine and dextropropoxyphene and strong, such as morphine or fentanyl) and (3) adjuvants (such as corticosteroids, antidepressants, anti-epileptics and so on).

DRUG TREATMENT OF PAIN

- Non-opioid analgesics
- Opioid analgesics
- Adjuvant drugs or co-analgesics

These three classes of drugs should be given, as appropriate, to the circumstances of individual patients "by the mouth, by the clock and by the ladder".

PRINCIPLES OF ANALGESIC ADMINISTRATION

- By the mouth
- By the clock
- By the ladder

Oral medication is usually the preferred route in patients who are able to swallow. Various other routes, such as transdermal, rectal, intramuscular injection, continuous subcutaneous infusion, may be appropriate in selected circumstances, but it is important not to jump into using a "pump" before it is needed.

Analgesia should be administered regularly (and in adequate quantity) in patients with chronic pain. The aim is to keep the patient pain-free by having adequate levels of drug in the system. It is unkind and unhelpful to allow the pain to return before giving the next dose. Of course, in a patient who is having a regular, long-acting opiate as background analgesia, it is good practice to prescribe a fast-acting morphine solution to be taken, if pain does break through. However, if breakthrough analgesia is required more often than occasionally, the dose of the long-acting drug needs to be increased. One exception to this is in the use of methadone, where the next dose is given only when the effects of the previous dose begins to rear off in order to avoid toxic accumulation of the drug.

The concept of the analgesic ladder comes from *Cancer Pain Relief Guidelines* published by the World Health Organisation. These describe three steps: the first being simple (non-opioid) analgesia; the second mild opiates and the third strong opiates.

WHO ANALGESIC LADDER

1 Simple analgesia
2 Weak opioids
3 Strong opioids

The aim of the ladder is to ensure that drugs are used alone or in combination both rationally and appropriately to maximise the benefit and to minimise adverse effects. There is often a rationale for using a combination of drugs which act by different mechanisms, but no logic in using a combination of two drugs from the same class which act in the same way.

Paracetamol and weak opioids

The mainstay of simple analgesia is paracetamol. This is best given regularly at a dose of 1 g four times a day. Its advantages are that side-effects, particularly on the gastric mucosa and platelets, are less than with aspirin and other non-steroidal anti-inflammatory drugs (NSAIDs). Also, it does not cause gout. It is, however, hepatotoxic in overdose. A maximum dose of 4 g daily should not be exceeded in adults. As it is so widely known and available as an over-the-counter medicine, some patients and their relatives, if recommended paracetamol, may think that the doctor or nurse is not being serious about their pain. Careful explanation is, therefore, necessary.

Paracetamol is included with mild opiates in a number of compound analgesics. As the paracetamol content, and the amount of the other drug, may vary, it is important to be aware of the quantities in each preparation (see box). As the maximum amount of paracetamol which may safely be taken each day is 4 g, care must be taken to explain to patients that paracetamol should not be used in conjunction with co-codamol, co-didramol or co-proxamol. Similarly, there are literally dozens of proprietary compound analgesics which also contain paracetamol and may be obtained over-the-counter, so patients should be counselled against taking any such drugs in addition to prescription medication. When a patient moves up the ladder to a strong opioid (such as morphine), mild opioid-containing preparations should be withdrawn, although it may still be a good idea to continue with plain paracetamol.

The weak opioids, codeine, dihydrocodeine and dextro-propoxyphene have been mentioned in association with paracetamol. This is logical, because when weak opioids are introduced, they should be used with non-opioids but not as substitutes for them. If a weak opioid given at optimal dose is inadequate to control the pain, it should be substituted with a strong opioid, there will be no advantage in merely switching to another weak opioid. The main troublesome side-effect of weak opioids is constipation, and laxatives may need to be given regularly. Prescription of a laxative when opioid therapy is commenced is good practice. Nausea and vomiting are not usually a problem.

┌───┐

PARACETAMOL-BASED COMPOUND ANALGESICS

Co-proxamol

◆ 32.5/325	Dextropropoxyphene 32.5 mg	Paracetamol 325 mg

Co-codamol

◆ 8/500	Codeine 8 mg	Paracetamol 500 mg
◆ 30/500	Codeine 30 mg	Paracetamol 500 mg
◆ 60/1000	Codeine 60 mg	Paracetamol 1000 mg

Co-didramol

◆ 10/500	Dihydrocodeine 10 mg	Paracetamol 500 mg
◆ 20/500	Dihydrocodeine 20 mg	Paracetamol 500 mg
◆ 30/500	Dihydrocodeine 30 mg	Paracetamol 500 mg

└───┘

Tramadol is fairly potent for a weak opioid when given by mouth as its oral bioavailability is good. It also acts by enhancement of adrenergic and serotoninergic pathways. It can also be given parenterally.

Non-steroidal anti-inflammatory drugs

NSAIDs are valuable if there is an inflammatory component to the pain. They work by inhibiting the enzyme cyclo-oxygenase (COX) which exists in two forms in the metabolic cascade that leads to the formation of prostaglandins which are powerful inflammatory mediators. The principal adverse effect is gastric mucosal toxicity which varies between different NSAIDs. It is greatest with azapropazone and ketorolac, intermediate with flurbiprofen, naproxen and piroxicam, low with diclofenac and ibuprofen and is least with COX-2 selective agents (such as rofecoxib). Diclofenac is available as a compound preparation with misoprostol which is aimed at reducing gastro-intestinal (GI) intolerance. Some NSAIDs may also induce bronchospasm, precipitate gout and cause renal dysfunction.

NSAIDs are usually given orally. Melt in the mouth preparations of piroxicam are available for patients who find tablets or capsules difficult but can swallow saliva. Diclofenac and ketorolac can be administered by continuous subcutaneous infusion.

Morphine

When weak opioids do not provide adequate pain control, it is time to move on to strong opiates. Although several are available, the most commonly used is morphine. It is important to get the dose right, so that patients have adequate pain control with the minimum side-effects. In the first instance, it is often best to use as an oral, short-acting formulation regularly every 4 hours starting at a dose of 5–10 mg, gradually increasing the dose over 24–48 hours until analgesia is achieved. Then, the patient can be given the same total daily dose of morphine as a modified release preparation in one or two divided doses as background analgesia, reserving the normal release oral morphine solution or tablets for occasional breakthrough pain. If breakthrough analgesia is needed more than occasionally, the dose of modified release morphine needs to be increased. If the pain always returns before the next dose of modified release morphine is due, then the dose of that preparation needs to be increased.

It is very important to explain carefully to the patient and any carers about the purpose of the two different preparations. Sometimes, a patient will take a controlled release preparation for an acute exacerbation of pain, and finding no immediate relief will wrongly conclude that morphine is not an effective drug for his/her pain. It is invaluable for patients with chronic cancer pain at home to have regular input from the community palliative care nurse to supervise the analgesic regimen. As patients are sometimes reluctant to ask for help with pain control, it is important for the nurse to be proactive about ensuring that the analgesic regimen is optimal.

Strong opiates, like their weaker counterparts, cause constipation; and a stimulant laxative, such as co-danthramer or co-danthrusate, will almost always be required. They may also cause nausea or vomiting, and so an anti-emetic should be prescribed so it is available for the patient, if necessary. Respiratory depression is very rarely encountered as a result of strong opiate use in palliative care. This is because (a) pain is a powerful respiratory stimulant, (b) the dose is increased gradually and (c) few patients are opiate naïve when commenced on morphine, most will have been taking a weak opioid. It should be explained gently to patients and their relatives, if they express anxiety about the addictive effects of opioids, that their worries are unfounded with appropriate therapeutic use.

Other side-effects of morphine may include sedation, delirium with hallucinations, myoclonus, hyper-excitability and histamine release causing pruritis and bronchoconstriction. Nonetheless, morphine is tolerated well by most patients, and it remains the strong opioid of first choice in most situations.

Common reasons for morphine not being successful in controlling opioid responsive pain are inadequate absorption because of vomiting, inadequate dosing and poor compliance by the patient. Sometimes, when these factors have been excluded as a cause of inadequate analgesia, it seems that the patient has a pain which is truly unresponsive to morphine. Co-analgesics may be helpful, and a change to another strong opioid may be beneficial. The concept of "opioid rotation" is based on the fact that there are various opioid receptors, which differ in their response to different opioid drugs. Optimal management of opioid rotation may require input from a specialist palliative care physician.

Fentanyl

Fentanyl is another strong opioid. When given intravenously it has a short duration of action, making it suitable for anaesthetic use. Administered transdermally, fentanyl has found a place in palliative care. It is prescribed as the amount which is absorbed each hour from a patch. Four strengths of patch are available, delivering 25, 50, 75 or 100 micrograms of fentanyl per hour. Multiple patches can be used to deliver doses greater than 100 micrograms per hour. Each transdermal patch lasts for 3 days, and replacement patches should be put onto a different area of skin. As the speed of absorption of fentanyl from patches may be speeded up by heat, care should be taken if patients develop a fever, and patients should be warned not to use hot-water bottles or heat pads over the site of the patch.

When initiating fentanyl patch therapy, it takes a while for circulating concentrations to build up. Previous analgesic therapy should be reduced gradually over a day, and assessment of efficacy should not be performed until at least 24 hours have elapsed. Patients who have not been on morphine or other strong opioids should be started on the lowest dose, 25 micrograms per hour. For patients who have been on morphine, the starting fentanyl dose should be related to the previous morphine dose. A daily dose of about 100 mg morphine is approximately equivalent to 25 micrograms per hour of transdermal fentanyl. Fentanyl is less constipating than morphine, so the dose of laxatives may need to be reduced when changing from one to the other.

Dose adjustments should be in increments of 25 micrograms per hour at the time of patch change every 3 days. If patients are being changed from fentanyl patch therapy to another analgesic, the starting dose of the new drug should be low and increased only gradually over the first day, as it may take a day after the removal of a patch for the plasma fentanyl concentration to reduce by a half.

Hydromorphone

Hydromorphone is another strong opiate which may be used as an alternative to morphine. It is only available for oral administration. The standard preparation needs administration 4 hourly, or there is a modified release preparation which may be used 12 hourly. It is more potent than morphine, 1 mg of hydromorphone equates

to 7.5 mg of morphine. Approximately equivalent doses are shown in the box.

PREPARATIONS OF HYDROMORPHONE, AND CORRESPONDING MORPHINE DOSES	
Hydromorphone capsules (mg)	Morphine equivalent (mg)
◆ 1.3	10
◆ 2.6	20
Modified release hydromorphone (mg)	Morphine equivalent (mg)
◆ 2	15
◆ 4	30
◆ 8	60
◆ 16	90
◆ 24	120

Methadone

Methadone is best known as a substitute opioid in the treatment of addiction. It can be successfully used for that indication, because its long half-life tends to reduce the rapid highs and sudden withdrawal which occurs with morphine. As the half-life is long and unpredictable, the use of methadone in palliative care breaks the "by-the-clock" rule, as regular dosing may lead to its excessive when the patient feels that the effects of the previous dose are beginning to wear off. The principal indications for the use of methadone are in patients who have had poor pain relief and troublesome adverse effects, such as delirium and agitation, with morphine combined with a non-opioid. A relatively small dose of methadone may well provide good analgesia with fewer side-effects. Methadone is less constipating than morphine. Methadone can also be used safely in patients with renal failure, who tend to accumulate toxic metabolites of morphine.

Diamorphine

Diamorphine, widely known as heroin, is the opiate of choice for subcutaneous administration, as it is much more soluble than morphine, and so the volume of fluid to be injected for a given analgesic effect is much less. When changing from oral morphine to subcutaneous diamorphine, the starting dose in milligrams per 24 hours

CONVERSION FROM ORAL MORPHINE TO SUBCUTANEOUS DIAMORPHINE
◆ The starting dose of diamorphine (in milligrams per 24 hours) should be one-third the daily total morphine dose (including both modified release and breakthrough preparations)

Handbook of Community Cancer Care

should be one-third the daily total morphine dose (including both modified release and breakthrough preparations).

Other opioids

Some opioids valuable in the treatment of acute pain, for example postoperatively or in labour, are not recommended for use in the palliative care setting. Buprenorphine and pentazocine are both partial antagonists as well as agonists, and may precipitate withdrawal symptoms, including pain, in patients who are already on other opioids. Pentazocine causes hallucinations and thought disorder. Pethidine and dextromoramide are short acting and less potent than morphine. Dipipanone is available only in combination with the anti-emetic cyclizine, which means that there is no flexibility in dosing.

Co-analgesics

Co-analgesics or adjuvant analgesics are a group of agents with miscellaneous actions which can be used with conventional analgesics to help alleviate pain in specific circumstances.

> ### CO-ANALGESICS
>
> ◆ Steroids
> ◆ Antidepressants
> ◆ Anticonvulsants
> ◆ Antispasmodics
> ◆ Muscle relaxants

Corticosteroids, such as dexamethasone or prednisolone, are widely used in palliative care for a number of indications. They are helpful in reducing pain caused by inflammatory swelling, such as distension of the liver capsule by metastases, the headache of raised intracranial pressure, and pain caused by pressure of a tumour mass on a nerve. As with any drug treatment, steroid therapy should not be prescribed lightly. A careful risk benefit analysis is important. As steroids may not work, they should be prescribed initially for a short period and stopped if there is no benefit. The acute and long-term side-effects of steroids, such as gastric perforation, proximal myopathy, mood fluctuation and Cushingoid appearance, are well known, and may detract from the benefits of treatment. Enteric-coated preparations or co-prescription of, for example, ranitidine may be beneficial, especially in patients with a history of peptic ulceration. Although it may be thought that any "long-term" side-effects are irrelevant in the palliative care setting, they often appear remarkably quickly, and so do need to be considered in anyone whose life expectancy is longer than a few weeks.

Antidepressant drugs can be helpful for nerve pain, including chronic pain associated with surgical scars, post-herpetic neuralgia, burning pain, dysaesthetic pain and sudden lightening pains. Drugs such as amitriptyline, are often more effective than selective serotonin re-uptake inhibitors (SSRIs). Amitriptyline may be effective more quickly and in lower doses for nerve pain than is the case with depression. It is wise to start at a low dose, for example 10 or 25 mg at night, and if no benefit is seen gradually increasing the dose by 10– 25 mg every few days to 75 mg. At these low doses, anticholinergic and other side-effects are less common, but patients should be monitored for drowsiness, dry mouth and confusion. Various forms of artificial saliva can be used to help a dry mouth, including Glandosane, Luborant and Oralbalance.

Anticonvulsant drugs have a valuable place in neuropathic pain, and carbamazepine, sodium valproate and gabapentin are the most widely used. Recommended doses vary, but it is a good practice to start at a low dose and gradually titrate the dose in small increments, stopping with the minimum effective dose. Sometimes, patients may lose patience with this approach and decide that a particular drug is of no benefit, but it is the best way to minimise adverse effects. Careful explanation and close monitoring are the key to gaining patients' understanding, trust and compliance. The input of experienced palliative care nurses is invaluable.

Antispasmodics are used to treat the colicky visceral pain, such as intestinal cramps associated with obstructing lesions, when surgery is not appropriate. The antimuscarinic drug hyoscine butylbromide is the drug of choice, as it is more effective than mebeverine and dicycloverine. It can be given orally, as a subcutaneous bolus or put into a continuous subcutaneous infusion pump. Care must be taken not to confuse hyoscine butylbromide where doses of 20–60 mg daily are used with the more sedating hyoscine hydrobromide used for nausea and vomiting, sedation and to dry excessive respiratory secretions, where doses up to only 2.4 mg daily are used.

Muscle spasms can be troublesome. Non-drug treatments, such as local heat and massage and relaxation therapy may be valuable. Sometimes, if there is a trigger point, injection of a local anaesthetic may alleviate the symptom. Muscle relaxants may, however, be indicated where skeletal muscle spasms are problematic. Benzodiazepines, such as diazepam 5–10 mg daily (or midazolam at a starting dose of 20 mg per day in a continuous subcutaneous infusion) are often helpful. Alternatively, baclofen, 5–10 mg three times a day may be beneficial.

ANOREXIA, NAUSEA AND VOMITING

Anorexia, nausea, retching and vomiting are distinct but related symptoms which occur commonly in patients with advanced cancer. As with pain, the first thing the doctor must do when faced with any of these symptoms is to assess the cause and put right the remediable. Symptom-directed therapy without prior careful evaluation is likely to be counter-productive.

Anorexia often occurs as a symptom by itself in advanced cancer. Alternatively, it may occur in conjunction with cachexia or excessive weight loss, fatigue and muscle wasting; early satiety or the feeling of being "full-up" soon after starting to eat; or with nausea and vomiting.

Anorexia may be caused: by the underlying cancer, for example anorexia is common in people with liver metastases; by metabolic disturbance related to the cancer, such as hypercalcaemia or hyponatraemia; anti-cancer treatments such as chemotherapy and radiotherapy; physical impediments such as a painful sore mouth; and psychological factors such as depression or anxiety.

CAUSES OF ANOREXIA

- Malignant disease (e.g. primary lung cancer, ascites caused by ovarian cancer or liver metastases)
- Metabolic disturbance (e.g. uraemia or hypercalcaemia)
- Anti-cancer treatments (e.g. chemotherapy or radiotherapy)
- Physical factors (e.g. dysphagia or mouth ulcers)
- Psychological factors (e.g. anxiety or depression)

The other important factor to take into account when assessing the patient with a poor appetite, is the stage in the illness, and both the patient's and the family's attitude. Some degree of anorexia is to be expected in patients who are terminally ill with cancer. Often patients, even if they are aware of their limited appetite, are not worried by it. Relatives may worry unduly, perhaps through an unreal expectation of the prognosis at that stage. They may fear that, if not properly fed, their loved one may die of starvation rather than cancer. They may feel that they are failing in their role as carer, if they cannot persuade their loved one to eat. Here, the general practitioner (GP) or community nurse can play an important role by discussing, with the patient's agreement, the stage of the illness and realistic expectations for eating with the relatives. Emotional support of carers at this time is every bit as valuable as the physical care of the patient.

As with pain, non-drug treatments should be given equal or greater emphasis than pharmacological remedies when treating anorexia. The first thing is to make food attractive and palatable to the patient. Small portions of simple food are often better than large elaborate meals. Softer food, such as mashed potato and milk puddings, may be easier to eat than fried steak and crunchy vegetables. An apple or orange may be more easy to eat if it has been peeled and divided into segments, than it is offered whole. Patients with anorexia will cope better with small snacks offered frequently. Any uneaten food should be removed immediately without comment. Patients, if they are able to dress and sit at a table, are likely to fare better than if presented with food in bed. Nutritional supplements, for example Maxijul, Fortisip, Ensure or Jevity, can be offered instead of, or in addition to, ordinary drinks.

Anorexia is not easily treated with drugs. In the short term, steroids (such as prednisolone up to 30 mg daily or dexamethasone up to 4 mg) daily may boost the appetite in some patients, but the benefit may be short lived and, as always when steroids are prescribed, care has to be taken that the possible adverse effects do not outweigh the benefits. Progestogens, such as megestrol acetate starting at a dose of 160 mg daily, may stimulate appetite and lead to weight gain. This, however, happens only slowly, and they are probably not appropriate for use in patients whose life expectancy is measured only in weeks.

Nausea and vomiting, like pain, have many possible causes. Accurate elucidation of the cause of the pain is the first step in successful therapy.

CAUSES OF NAUSEA AND VOMITING IN PATIENTS WITH CANCER

Directly related to the cancer
- Gastroparesis
- Liver metastases or hepatomegaly
- Brain metastases or raised intracranial pressure
- Ascites
- Bowel obstruction or gastric outflow obstruction
- Hypercalcaemia or renal failure
- Upper GI bleeding

Related to cancer treatment
- Chemotherapy or radiotherapy
- Opioid analgesia and NSAIDs
- Steroid gastritis

Indirectly related to the cancer
- Constipation and faecal impaction
- Infection

The principle causes are directly related to the cancer (such as liver or brain metastases), or its treatment (such as chemotherapy or opioid analgesia), or indirectly related (such as faecal impaction caused by constipation). An open mind should, however, be kept about the possibility of unrelated factors playing a role.

Hence, in the assessment of nausea or vomiting, as in the assessment of pain, it is important to have a full knowledge of the state of the illness, its treatment and its possible natural history. Maybe the new symptom of vomiting in a previously well woman with breast cancer is the first sign of cerebral metastases or of hypercalcaemia? Maybe the vomiting has been caused by a change in the patient's medication, such as the introduction of opioid analgesia? Consider whether it may be worthwhile arranging for a blood test to check the urea or calcium level.

Following the assessment, the treatable should be treated; for example, constipation may call for enemas and laxatives; hypercalcaemia for rehydration and bisphosphonates.

Symptomatic treatment will depend largely on what other symptomatic remedies may have been tried before. As with every other aspect of shared care, communication between the hospital and the community, as well as between the community and the hospital, is vitally important. Patients often forget what medication they have been prescribed, and do not realise that one shared-care partner (e.g. the hospital oncologist) will not know what the other shared-care partner (e.g. the GP) has prescribed, unless this information is explicitly communicated. A patient may have severe vomiting after her first course of chemotherapy, for which the hospital prescribed prophylactic anti-emetics are ineffective. She may call on her GP for help, but rational prescribing is impossible, if the GP does not know which anti-emetics have been used so far. This can be rather frustrating. Equally, it is not helpful when the patient, attending for the second course of chemotherapy, says "those anti-sickness tablets you gave me last time were not much use, I was sick for days, but my doctor gave me something which was really good. Would you give me some more of it please?", but does not know what it was. Problems are avoided, patients are treated better, and time is saved for all, if everyone troubles to communicate well.

Prokinetic anti-emetics, such as metoclopramide or domperidone are often effective as first-line therapy. Clearly, oral anti-emetics may not be much good, if the patient is actually vomiting, and parenteral injection or suppositories may be called for.

Major tranquillisers, such as haloperidol, levomepromazine or prochlorperazine, are effective anti-emetics, and can be used in syringe drivers if necessary. It must be remembered that some drugs, such as prochlorperazine and metoclopramide, can sometimes cause dystonic reactions.

The antihistamine cyclizine is also useful where metoclopramide or domperidone have failed. It can be given parenterally as well as orally.

The antimuscarinic drug hyoscine hydrobromide is a useful alternative anti-emetic. It has the advantage of being available in a transdermal patch formulation. Antimuscarinics should not be used in conjunction with metoclopramide or domperidone as they are antagonists.

In recent years, the 5-hydroxytryptamine-3 (5HT-3) receptor antagonists, such as granisetron and ondansetron, have completely revolutionised the management of acute chemotherapy- and radiotherapy-related emesis. They are, however, less effective at treating the delayed nausea which may follow chemotherapy.

Anticipatory vomiting may occur in patients attending for chemotherapy, although it is less common now that severe chemotherapy-related emesis is unusual. Due to anxiety and fear of chemotherapy-associated vomiting, patients start to feel sick, or actually vomit, when they arrive at the hospital or see familiar staff whom they associate with the treatment. The use of a minor tranquilliser, such as the benzodiazepines, lorazepam and diazepam, the night before or the morning of treatment is an effective anxiolytic, and substantially reduces the likelihood of anticipatory vomiting.

Steroids, notably dexamethasone, are valuable when used in conjunction with other anti-emetics, such as metoclopramide or granisetron. The mechanism for this is, however, unclear. Steroids are particularly useful, in conjunction with domperidone or metoclopramide, for treatment of delayed nausea and vomiting where 5HT-3 antagonists are less helpful.

COMMONLY USED ANTI-EMETIC DRUGS AND POSSIBLE ROUTES OF ADMINISTRATION

Prokinetic agents
- Metoclopramide — po, im, iv, csci
- Domperidone — po, pr

5HT-3 antagonists
- Granisetron — po, iv
- Ondansetron — po, pr, im, iv

Minor tranquillisers
- Lorazepam — po, iv, im
- Midazolam — iv, im, csci

Antimuscarinies
- Hyoscine hydrobromide — po, sc, im, td, csci

Antihistamines
- Cyclizine — po, im, iv, csci

Major tranquillisers
- Haloperidol — po, im, iv, csci
- Levomepromazine — po, im, iv, csci
- Prochlorperazine — po, pr, im, buccal

Corticosteroids
- Dexamethasone — po, iv, csci

po	by mouth as tablet or liquid and swallowed
pr	by suppository
iv	by intravenous injection or infusion
im	by intramuscular injection
td	by transdermal patch
buccal	by mouth, tablet to be left between lip and gum for transmucosal absorption
csci	by continuous subcutaneous infusion

As with painkillers, there is often logic in combining different agents with distinct modes of action, such as metoclopramide and dexamethasone, but no value in combining two or more agents of the same group, such as haloperidol am levomepromazine.

As with painkillers, anti-emetic medication should be reviewed regularly, changed if ineffective or causing adverse effects, or stopped if no longer than necessary.

CONSTIPATION AND DIARRHOEA

Constipation is a common symptom in patients with advanced cancer. Opioid analgesia is possibly the most common cause, but other factors (such as diminished appetite and mobility, intestinal obstruction, dehydration) and metabolic disturbances (such as hypercalcaemia) may contribute or be the principal cause.

As with the management of all symptoms in palliative care, the first principle is careful assessment of the patient to identify the cause and consider the stage of the patient's illness, with the aim of putting right remediable problems before offering symptomatic treatments. Assessment will usually include a rectal examination to identify co-existing faecal impaction which may need to be cleared before other measures are introduced. If an intervention, such as the prescription of opioid analgesia, is being considered which is likely to cause constipation, the patient should be warned and appropriate medication, to be used prophylactically, should be co-prescribed.

Different laxatives act by various mechanisms. The main categories are: osmotic or small bowel laxatives (such as lactulose), stimulant or large bowel laxatives (such as bisacodyl and dantron) and stool softeners or stool-wetting agents (such as polaxamer and docusate sodium). Bulk-forming laxatives, such as ispaghula, stercualia and methylcellulose, have little to offer in the palliative care environment and may make matters worse.

CATEGORIES OF LAXATIVES MOST COMMONLY USED IN PALLIATIVE CARE

Stimulant laxatives
- Dantron
- Bisacodyl
- Senna
- Sodium picosulphate

Stool softeners
- Docusate sodium
- Polaxamer

Osmotic laxatives
- Lactulose

As with the analgesic ladder, there is a series of logical steps which may be taken in the management of constipation. The first step is to facilitate regular defaecation by general measures according to the patient's overall condition, which may include some of the following: Firstly, encouraging a good diet with plenty of fluid, particularly fruit juice, and if possible fruits (such as prunes, apricots and figs), mobilising the patient, responding promptly to a patient's request for toileting and offering a commode rather than a bedpan. Secondly, a stimulant laxative by itself may be used. Choices include senna: two 7.5 mg tablets at night initially, increasing if necessary to two

tablets twice daily; and bisacodyl initially 5 mg at night increasing if necessary up to 20 mg. Dantron is only licensed for use in terminally ill patients because of its possible carcinogenicity. After that, a compound preparation of stool softener and stimulant (such as co-danthrusate or co-danthramer) may be tried, titrating the dose upwards as necessary. If problems persist, the next step is to add in an osmotic laxative. Finally, a minority of patients will need local rectal measures, such as an enema, manual evacuation or stimulant suppositories in addition to oral laxatives.

Just as there are different preparations of co-codamol containing different proportions of the two active ingredients, there are also different preparations of co-danthramer. It is important not to get these confused, and it can be helpful, when asking a patient about what laxatives are being taken, to inspect the preparation just to be sure.

For a given dose of opioid medication, different patients laxative requirements vary considerably. In general, however, one co-danthramer 25/200 capsule daily is an appropriate starting dose for someone not on opioids, whereas two co-danthramer 25/200 capsules twice daily are likely to be needed for the patient on opioids.

COMPOUND PREPARATIONS OF A STIMULANT AND A SOFTENER

Co-danthramer capsules
- Co-danthramer 25/200 (dantron 25 mg, polaxamer "188" 200 mg).
- Strong co-danthramer 37.7/500 (dantron 37.5 mg, polaxamer "188" 500 mg)

Co-danthramer suspension
- Co-danthramer 25/200 in 5 ml (dantron 25 mg, polaxamer "188" 200 mg in 5 ml)
- Strong co-danthramer 75/1000 in 5 ml (dantron 75 mg, polaxamer "188" lg in 5 ml)

Note: Co-danthramer suspension of 5 ml is equivalent to one co-danthramer capsule, but 5 ml strong co-danthramer suspension is equivalent to two strong co-danthramer capsules.

Co-danthrusate capsules
- Co-danthrusate 50/60 (dantron 50 mg, docusate sodium 60 mg)

Co-danthrusate suspension
- Co-danthrusate 50/60 (dantron 50 mg, docusate sodium 60 mg in 5 ml)

Diarrhoea is not as common as constipation in the patient with advanced cancer. The first aim in the assessment of a patient who complains of diarrhoea is to make sure that the diarrhoea is real. Spurious diarrhoea occurs in constipated patients, and is the passage of loose or liquid stool around faecal impaction. A rectal examination will reliably distinguish between genuine diarrhoea, when the rectum is usually empty, and spurious diarrhoea when the rectum is loaded with hard, impacted faeces. This is important in, for example, the patient who is constipated due to opioid analgesia. The patient may decide to stop taking laxatives in the belief that the "diarrhoea" is due to an excessive laxative dose. In fact, faecal impaction and spurious diarrhoea have developed and require an enema, suppositories or manual evacuation followed by increased regular laxatives to prevent the situation from recurring.

Rectal examination will also distinguish other abnormalities, such as malaena, due to an upper GI haemorrhage, and steatorrhoea, caused by cancer of the pancreas, from ordinary diarrhoea.

COMMON CAUSES OF DIARRHOEA IN PATIENTS WITH ADVANCED CANCER

- Chemotherapy (e.g. fluorouracil, irinotecan)
- Antibiotics
- Excessive laxatives
- Infections including gastro-enteritis and pseudomembranous colitis
- Dietary indiscretion
- Abdominal radiotherapy
- Prior bowel surgery or fistula formation
- Partial bowel obstruction
- Carcinoid syndrome

Hence with diarrhoea, as with other symptoms, careful evaluation of the nature and cause of the problem is essential before initiating treatment. A detailed history, including a review of the diet, drugs and other treatments used, combined with examination will make the cause clear in many cases. If an infective cause is suspected, stool culture or tests for *Clostridium difficile* toxin may confirm the diagnosis.

Treatment of diarrhoea starts with ensuring an adequate fluid intake. If a patient has become seriously dehydrated, it may be important to check the urea and electrolytes and consider intravenous rehydration. If a specific cause for the diarrhoea has been identified, it may be possible to consider a specific remedy. For example, some infections, such as pseudomembranous colitis, require specific antibiotic treatment. If there is steatorrhoea due to obstructive jaundice which cannot be relieved or pancreatic insufficiency, pancreatin supplements may be helpful. Carcinoid syndrome diarrhoea can be controlled with octreotide or lanreotide. Loose stool associated with a shortened bowel, for example in patients with an ileostomy, may be helped by the regular use of a fibre supplement (such as ispaghula or stercualia).

Otherwise, symptomatic control of diarrhoea can be achieved with codeine or loperamide. It is helpful, particularly with acute diarrhoea, to titrate the dose of loperamide to the response. For example, start with a 4 mg immediate dose (two capsules) and give a further capsule (2 mg) after each loose bowel movement, with a maximum daily dose of eight capsules (16 mg). In that way, if the diarrhoea stops, no further treatment is given.

Although most cases of diarrhoea can be satisfactorily managed in the community setting, remember that there are circumstances where urgent hospital admission may be indicated; for example, in the patient who develops severe diarrhoea when neutropaenic following chemotherapy with irinotecan for colon cancer.

DYSPHAGIA AND MALNUTRITION

STAGES OF SWALLOWING

- Chewing, salivation and preparation of food in the mouth
- Formation of a bolus in the mouth and moving food to the back of the mouth
- Transit of food through the pharynx with closure of the larynx
- Transit of food down the oesophagus into the stomach

Swallowing is a complex phenomenon, which we all take for granted until it goes wrong. In the first phase of eating, food is chewed and moistened with saliva. When a mouthful of food has reached the right consistency, it is formed into a bolus by the tongue and pushed to the back of the throat, then swallowed through the pharynx following closure of the larynx and down into the oesophagus.

Dysphagia, or difficulty in swallowing, which may be painless or associated with discomfort, can be due to structural abnormalities in the mouth, pharynx or throat, with inflammation in these areas, or with functional problems due to neuromuscular problems.

Dysphagia may be continuous or intermittent, and the difficulties may occur with solid food only, or with liquids and solids. It may be associated with coughing or choking due to aspiration of food through the larynx.

Dysphagia or difficulty in swallowing due to intra-luminal narrowing of the throat or gullet is often the presenting symptom of oesophageal and pharyngeal cancers. Dysphagia caused by structural or functional defects in the oral and pharyngeal components of swallowing often results from the treatment of other head and neck cancers; for example, loss of tongue bulk due to surgery or xerostomia related to loss of salivary gland function as a result of radiotherapy. Mechanical obstruction of swallowing may also occur due to extrinsic pressure from bronchial cancers and metastatic disease in lymph nodes in the thorax. Dysphagia with pain may also be caused by mucosal inflammation following thoracic irradiation or due to oesophageal candidiasis or acid reflux from the stomach. Neuromuscular defects, such as lower cranial nerve palsies caused by a brain-stem glioma, base of skull involvement by tumour or carcinomatous meningitis, may produce nasal regurgitation during swallowing due to palatal incompetence, difficulty in formation of a bolus and in initiating the swallowing reflex, or laryngeal aspiration. With obstructive causes of dysphagia, swallowing of liquids is often easier than solids. With neuromuscular causes, soft solid food may be easier to swallow than drinks.

COMMON CAUSES OF DYSPHAGIA IN PATIENTS WITH ADVANCED CANCER

Structural factors
- Tumour within the mouth
- Loss of tongue bulk by surgery
- Palatal fistula
- Presence of pharyngeal tumour
- Oesophageal cancer obstructing lumen
- Pharyngeal or oesophageal stricture following surgery or radiotherapy
- Extrinsic pressure on the oesophagus due to cervical or thoracic mass

Inflammation and pain
- Oral ulcers due to chemotherapy
- Oesophagitis due to mediastinal radiotherapy
- Oropharyngeal or oesophageal candidiasis

Functional factors
- Dry mouth due to salivary gland irradiation
- Neuromuscular difficulty due to lower cranial nerve palsies
- Paraneoplastic neuropathy
- Sensory loss in the lips, mouth or throat

As with the management of all other symptoms in patients with advanced cancer, dysphagia requires careful and expert evaluation before treatment is offered. Here, the speech and language therapist is invaluable. In addition to a detailed history and clinical assessment, investigations, such as videofluoroscopy or functional endoscopic evaluation of swallowing, may be called for. When the cause has been identified, it may be possible to correct it. For example, painful dysphagia caused by candidiasis should respond to treatment with antifungal agents, such as nystatin or fluconazole. Obstruction due to an oesophageal cancer may be treated by surgery, radiotherapy, lasering or intubation.

SOME ADVICE FOR PATIENTS WITH DYSPHAGIA AND THEIR CARERS

- Sit at a table to eat with your head upright
- Avoid distractions to concentrate on eating
- Relax, do not hurry and remain sitting for some time after eating
- Eat small regular snacks, not large meals
- After eating, rinse your mouth and cough to clear your throat
- Make food appetising in line with the patients' known taste
- Eat calorie rich foods to get the most value from small snacks
- Replace tea, water and squash with liquid nutritional supplements
- Always have a drink with food
- Avoid dry foods by having sauces and gravy
- Go for soft food alternatives, such as mashed potatoes rather than chips

---

Often, however, the cause may not be remediable, and hence other measures will be called for. The speech and language therapist is well placed to give advise on the management of dysphagia as well as help in its investigation. The dietician will also be able to provide valuable dietary advice to the patient and to any carers responsible for helping with preparation of food.

If dysphagia is complete or near complete, and cannot be dealt with by simple measures, thought may need to be given to tube feeding. Nasogastric tubes are not pleasant for patients, physically or emotionally owing to their visibility, and they can be difficult to pass in patients with swallowing difficulties. These days, gastrostomy tubes are routinely inserted percutaneously either by gastroenterologists using endoscopic guidance (which may be hazardous, if there are structural abnormalities which may make passing of an endoscope difficult) or by the interventional radiologist using ultrasound guidance. Of course, insertion of a tube for feeding is not appropriate for all patients, especially those who are moribund. Nonetheless, they can greatly enhance quality of life for the ambulant patient whose life expectancy may be measured in months or more.

RESTLESSNESS AND AGITATION

Restlessness and agitation are common in patients in the terminal stages of cancer. Moribund patients cannot express their feelings easily, and it is important to look out for common problems which may manifest themselves as restlessness or agitation rather than in the usual way. Does the patient need to pass urine or defaecate? Is pain a problem? If remediable causes are found, these should,

Handbook of Community Cancer Care

of course, be put right. Some drugs, such as steroids, can also cause these symptoms. Metabolic disturbances, such as hypoxia, hypercalcaemia and uraemia, may contribute. If the patient is recognised to be near to death, active correction of such abnormalities may be inappropriate, and a more symptom-orientated approach will be called for. Haloperidol and levomepromazine are often effective, and both can be used in syringe drivers for continuous sub-cutaneous infusion.

ANXIETY AND DEPRESSION

Anxiety and depression are two separate but often inter-twined emotional responses which are commonly seen both in patients with cancer and their carers. Sometimes, patients may have features of both disorders.

Anxiety is often a combination of psychological symptoms (such as worry, indecisiveness, tension, irritability, and an inability to relax, sleep or concentrate) and physical symptoms (such as tremor, sweating, tachycardia and anorexia). Anxiety may be acute, for example while waiting for test results to come back, or more prolonged.

Depression is characterised by sadness and depressed mood, fatigue, loss of interest or pleasure in most activities, weight loss (or weight gain), sleep disturbance particularly early waking, impaired concentration, loss of feelings of self-worth, which may, for example, manifest as loss of interest in personal appearance or family and non-compliance with treatment, guilt, development of phys-ically unexplained somatic symptoms and suicidal ideation. Up to one in five patients with cancer develops a patho-logical depressive state requiring specific treatment.

As some degree of anxiety and some features of depres-sion are an almost universal response to the initial diag-nosis of cancer, and later if the disease recurs, and when the patient or the carers realise that the disease will prove fatal, it can be difficult to separate out patho-logical depression and anxiety from a typical reactive mental state.

There are several psychological tools, such as the Hospital Anxiety and Depression (HAD) questionnaire, which can be used to screen patients for the presence of features of anxiety and depression. These instruments cannot be used all the time, and an abnormal result is not, by itself, diagnostic. The GP should keep the possi-bility of pathological anxiety and depression in mind, and, if any pointers are apparent, asks specific questions to define the patient's mental state.

If a definite diagnosis is made, precipitating factors, other than the obvious fact that the patient has cancer, should be looked for. Physical risk factors include unre-lieved pain, biochemical and endocrine disturbances, cere-bral tumours including metastases and treatments, such as steroids. Psychological risk factors include a past his-tory of endogenous depression, bereavement and social isolation. Causes of anxiety include fear of the cancer and its possible consequences, such as disfigurement, infertility, disability, loss of independence and death, fear of possible treatments and their side-effects, financial worries, and steroids.

As with other troublesome symptoms, a cause may be identified which can be dealt with. For example, a patient with a good prognosis may imagine, having heard the word "cancer", that a slow painful death is inev-itable. In this (fortunately uncommon) case, an honest reassurance that the majority of patients with that par-ticular malignancy are cured with appropriate treatment may reduce the fear. A patient may be terrified of chemotherapy-related vomiting, having witnessed her mother's sickness years ago before the introduction of 5HT-3 antagonists and other effective anti-emetics. Again, honest reassurance may be sufficient to allay anxiety.

Non-drug treatments including attendance at hospice day care centres, counselling and psychotherapy may be beneficial for patients with both anxiety and depression.

Drug treatments may also be required. Benzodi-azepines, such as diazepam, are often sufficient for mild anxiety. Occasionally, it may be necessary to consider the use of antidepressants or major tranquillisers, such as haloperidol. For depression, many different drugs are available, and the choice may depend on local practice and experience, and the desire to avoid side-effects. The more modern SSRIs, such as fluoxetine and citalopram, tend to be favoured these days over the tricyclic anti-depressants, such as amitriptyline and imipramine, because they are less sedating, less cardiotoxic and have fewer antimuscarinic side-effects. SSRIs, however, may cause nausea and vomiting, anxiety and other troublesome side-effects, so cannot be regarded as a panacea.

Patients with serious depression, especially those in whom the prognosis with regard to the cancer is good, or those thought to be at risk of suicide, may benefit from a psychiatric opinion, and supervision by the com-munity psychiatric services.

CONFUSION

Confusion can be a difficult symptom to manage in the terminally ill patient. It is certainly distressing for loved ones and carers, and if the patients have insight into their own confusion they too can find it distressing. Features include disorientation in time, place and person, hallucinations and delusions, sometimes with paranoid features, sleep disorder, loss of memory, and incompre-hensible speech.

Common causes include infection, especially pneumo-nia with fever, dehydration and hypoxia or urinary tract infections; medication, such as steroids, opiates, and anti-muscarinics; metabolic disturbances, such as renal or hep-atic failure, hypercalcaemia and hyponatraemia; primary brain tumour or cerebral metastases; faecal impaction and urinary retention; and tobacco, alcohol or drug (e.g. opiate, benzodiazepine or phenothiazine) withdrawal. Often more than one causative factor will be implicated; for example, a patient with cerebral and bone metastases from carcinoma of the breast may have hypercalcaemia and be on steroids.

Management of confusion has to be placed in the context of the patient's current position in the course of their illness. If a patient is moribund with advanced malignancy, it might be considered meddlesome to treat pneumonia if this is likely to be the terminal event. On the other hand if a previously relatively fit patient with a good life expectancy from their cancer suddenly becomes confused, then it is important to identify and treat the underlying cause. It follows, therefore, that the confused patient requires a thorough and detailed assessment, so that any easily reversible causes of confusion may be put right.

Day–night reversal, where the patient catnaps or sleeps for most of the day then is awake at night is not easily put right. It is worthwhile reviewing the medication, giving steroids as a single dose first thing in the morning, and by ensuring that night-time analgesia is adequate. Sometimes, a little night sedation may be helpful. It is important to provide gentle social stimulation during the day and ensure a restful, quiet, dark environment at night.

If no underlying cause for confusion is found, it may be possible to manage the patient with constant gentle reassurance and explanation. It is important that carers understand that this situation is not uncommon and is not their fault. It may be possible to help them cope better with the patient, if there is greater community professional input for support and reassurance. Sometimes, especially if the patient is distressed, it may be necessary to use a psychotropic drug, such as haloperidol.

DRY AND SORE MOUTH

The causes of a dry and sore mouth in patients with advanced cancer include oral candidiasis, bacterial parotitis, chemotherapy-related mucositis and ulceration, radiotherapy-related acute mucositis and chronic xerostomia after salivary gland irradiation, antimuscarinic drugs, mouth breathing, dehydration and hypercalcaemia.

Management of the dry or sore mouth begins with a careful assessment to identify the cause. Sometimes, this may be obvious, as in the case of the patient receiving radiotherapy for an oral cavity cancer, but care must be taken not to overlook other factors, such as candidal infection, which may co-exist. Where possible, the cause should be remedied, for example a patient who develops a troublesome dry mouth on amitriptyline should be considered for another drug without anticholinergic side-effects.

Symptomatically, a dry mouth can be helped by the use of artificial salivas, of which there are several proprietary

preparations available. Patients should be advised to carry a small water bottle around with them, and also always to have a drink with each meal or snack. The cholinergic drug, pilocarpine, can stimulate salivary flow in a proportion of patients with a dry mouth, but its side-effects including sweatiness may put some patients off.

Mouth care is very important in patients undergoing many different types of chemotherapy, and undergoing radiotherapy for head and neck cancer. As the development of mucositis can, to some extent, be predicted, it is possible to recommend mouth care regimens which will minimise discomfort. Regular saline mouthwashes are as good at keeping the mouth clean as more exotic preparations. Teeth should be cleaned with a soft brush which will not abrade the gums. The mouth should be inspected regularly, and antifungal medication should be given if there is any suspicion of candidal infection. Benzydamine oral rinse has an anti-inflammatory effect which may reduce pain. The pain from oral mucositis can be severe and analgesia, often liquid morphine, will be called for.

Dental care is important in patients with head and neck cancer who may develop permanent xerostomia as a result of salivary gland irradiation. Ideally, patients will have seen a dentist before treatment. If advanced caries is present, a full dental extraction may be indicated, but in most cases conservation of teeth should be possible. Following treatment, advice on oral hygiene, dental surveillance and prompt treatment of any problems is called for, as accelerated dental caries may develop with xerostomia. Regular use of fluoride mouthwash and toothpaste may help to maintain dental integrity. The health authority or primary care trust may have a list of dentists who will visit the patient at home under the NHS Domiciliary scheme, if the patient's usual dentist does not do so.

In very sick or terminally ill patients, who are unable to do their own mouth care, oral hygiene is still very important for comfort. The mouth should be cleansed regularly with mouthwash using lollipop sponge sticks. Chewing fruit, such as pawpaw or pineapple, is a pleasant way of keeping the mouth fresh, but fruit acid may cause pain, if there is mucosal ulceration. Patients should be helped to keep their mouths moist. If they are not able to drink easily, they may be able to suck small lumps of ice. Thrush is very common in the moribund, and patients will almost always benefit from its treatment.

COUGH

Cough is a troublesome symptom, and may cause vomiting, or pain if there is pleurisy or a rib fracture. Coughing may be considered physiological, when it is a natural response to clear the airways of excessive secretions (wet cough), or pathological, when it is a useless response to an irritant stimulus (dry cough).

Cough may be caused by various things including irritation from a primary bronchial carcinoma, aspiration due to a poorly protected airway or a tracheo-oesophageal fistula, infections, such as bronchitis and pneumonia, dry atmosphere, and occasionally as an adverse drug reaction, for example, to angiotensin-converting enzyme (ACE) inhibitors, such as captopril and enalapril. Many patients with a pre-existing, often smoking-related cough, such as those with chronic bronchitis, subsequently develop cancer. If this occurs, it is important to distinguish any new cough caused by the cancer from the old cough.

In the case of a productive or wet cough, if a cause (such as acute infective bronchitis) has been identified, it may be possible to do something specific about it, such as give antibiotics. If the patient is aspirating food or fluid into the upper airway, input from a speech and language therapist may be valuable. Symptomatically, productive coughs may be helped by steam or friar's balsam inhalations and physiotherapy to clear the secretions and, encourage good posture and proper breathing. Mucolytic drugs, such as squill or carbocisteine, may help coughing by making the secretions less tenacious. It is better to avoid antitussives with a wet cough, although these may be indicated at night to enable sleep and reduce daytime exhaustion.

Similarly, if an avoidable cause of a dry cough is identified, this should be avoided. For example, the cough caused by ACE inhibitors can be circumvented by changing to an angiotensin-II receptor antagonist, such as losartan or valsartan.

Antitussive treatment is possible when no remediable cause has been identified. Moisturisation of the air can be a simple and practical way of diminishing the symptom. Opioids are often effective, if the cough remains troublesome. If the patient is not already requiring strong analgesia, codeine or pholcodeine linctus may be helpful. Otherwise, oral morphine can be used. The usual caveats about side-effects, such as constipation, are still pertinent when opioids are prescribed for this indication. Methadone is an effective antitussive agent, but it is probably better avoided as its long half-life can make safe dosing difficult.

BREATHLESSNESS

The same general rules apply for the management of breathlessness for other symptoms, such as pain, vomiting or dysphagia. Firstly, there needs to be a thorough assessment of the patient, with the aim of identifying the cause or causes of the symptom and also the stage the patient is at, in the course of the illness. This will involve reviewing the history and clinical examination, and, perhaps, selected investigations also.

Then, if appropriate, for the patient in the light of the prognosis and other factors, that is to say if the risk benefit balance is in the patient's favour, remediable causes should be put right. For example, if a fairly fit and ambulant patient develops dyspnoea because of the development of a large malignant pleural effusion, pleural aspiration or drainage and pleurodesis will be indicated. Similarly, shortness of breath on exertion which is found to be due to anaemia will merit a blood transfusion. On the other hand, the development of an effusion or anaemia in someone who is bed-bound and moribund may be better managed in less interventional ways.

Non-drug treatments and lifestyle modifications can, then, be used to ameliorate or limit the effect of the symptom. Finally, drugs may be helpful. There then follows a process of regular review and adjustment of medication in the light of the changing situation.

**MANAGEMENT OF BREATHLESSNESS
IN THE PATIENT WITH ADVANCED CANCER**

- Assessment of the patient (history, examination, investigations) to
  - identify the cause and severity of breathlessness
  - the point in the patient's illness trajectory
- Correct the correctable causes of dyspnoea, if appropriate
- Non-drug treatments and lifestyle modifications
- Drug treatment

Breathlessness in the patient with cancer has many causes. It is with this symptom, perhaps, more than some others where careful clinical assessment and is critical to successful treatment.

**POSSIBLE CAUSES OF BREATHLESSNESS
IN THE PATIENT WITH ADVANCED CANCER**

- Pleural effusion
- Pulmonary emboli
- Pericardial effusion
- Cardiac failure
- Lymphangitis carcinomatosa
- Pulmonary metastases
- Superior vena caval obstruction
- Laryngeal, tracheal or bronchial obstruction by tumour or extrinsic compression
- Anaemia
- Pneumonia
- Anxiety
- Gross abdominal distension (e.g. ascites)
- Metabolic disturbance
- Tetraplegia
- Treatment effects: pneumonectomy or pulmonary fibrosis
- Intercurrent disease
- Combinations of the above

Of course, these causes do not necessarily occur in isolation, for example a woman with advanced ovarian cancer may have ascites, be anaemic and develop pulmonary emboli. Also, it must be remembered that many patients have pre-existing lung disease which has led to a reduced respiratory reserve, even if not symptomatic dyspnoea, before they develop cancer. Most patients with lung cancer have, of course, been smokers, and chronic bronchitis and emphysema are common.

MANAGEMENT OF MALIGNANT PLEURAL EFFUSIONS

- Small effusions without symptoms may not need treatment
- Aspiration of up to 1 l is a simple outpatient procedure, providing rapid, but often short-lived improvement. It may be all that is required in someone with a short-life expectancy; it can be a valuable initial approach providing diagnostic information
- Pleural drainage requires inpatient care, but can be followed by a chemical pleurodesis which may provide better long-term control in those with a better prognosis; following repeated procedures, the effusion may become loculated and difficult to drain without imaging guidance
- Thoracoscopic talc pleurodesis, surgical pleurodesis or pleurectomy can be very effective in good prognosis patients, but requires a thoracic surgeon to be involved

Having identified the cause or causes, attention turns to treating the treatable, if the patient's condition and their point in the illness, including previous treatments, allow it. Sometimes, the principal cause is directly related to the presence of cancer, for example a malignant pleural effusion in a woman with breast cancer or superior vena caval compression in a patient with lung cancer. In such cases, specific anti-cancer treatment with chemotherapy, radiotherapy or endocrine therapy may be indicated. These can be given in conjunction with treatments aimed at overcoming the physiological problems causing dyspnoea. For example, draining the pleural effusion or stenting the superior vena cava.

Non-drug treatments for dyspnoea are aimed at making the patient more comfortable. Posture is important. Many patients find dyspnoea more troublesome, if they are lying flat or are semi-recumbent, their distress can be eased by sitting them upright. Allowing patients to hold a table may enable them to fix their shoulder girdles and use the accessory muscles of respiration more easily. Physiotherapy may be valuable in clearing the airways of secretions, and in helping patients to breathe more deeply and more effectively.

LYMPHANGITIS CARCINOMATOSA

- Caused by diffuse infiltration of pulmonary lymphatics by cancer cells
- Clinically characterised by marked breathlessness, sometimes cough and cyanosis
- Chest X-ray may be normal or just show peri-hilar streakiness
- Lung function tests show a restrictive rather than obstructive pattern
- Spiral computed tomography (CT) is the best investigation to confirm the diagnosis
- Prognosis is generally very poor
- Treatment with chemotherapy or endocrine therapy, if possible
- Steroids may be beneficial
- Oxygen, morphine or benzodiazepines may be indicated

Oxygen may be very beneficial in hypoxic patients, but care needs to be exercised. Patients who have pre-existing chronic obstructive pulmonary disease and are carbon dioxide retainers may be dependent on hypoxia for their respiratory drive.

Patients who have been treated with bleomycin may develop severe lung toxicity following over-oxygenation. Sometimes, just the availability of oxygen will have a profound placebo effect for a dyspnoeic patient.

Dyspnoea is often a feature of, or may be compounded by anxiety or psychological distress. Similarly, dyspnoea with a clear-cut pathological cause is often accompanied by anxiety. It can be difficult to disentangle the cause and effect relationship between anxiety and dyspnoea, unless the patient is thoroughly assessed for physical causes of dyspnoea, and time is taken to explore the emotional aspects of care in some detail. It may, then, be possible to institute some anxiety management strategies which will help to ameliorate anxiety whether as a cause or consequence of the dyspnoea.

Not, infrequently, one is left with a patient with advanced cancer and symptomatic dyspnoea for which the cause cannot be directly treated, and only symptom care remedies are possible. Benzodiazepines can be helpful, especially, if an anxiolytic effect is required. Opioids can also be helpful, especially if there is an associated non-productive cough. In the terminally ill patient, a syringe driver with a mixture of diamorphine and midazolam or levomepromazine may be helpful.

In the dying patient, breathlessness associated with noisy loose upper airway secretions, sometimes known as the death rattle, may occur. This can be more distressing for the family than for the patient who by this stage is often unaware. Hyoscine hydrobromide, which can be administered either by a continuous subcutaneous infusion or with a transdermal patch, can be effective at drying secretions. Glycopyrronium is an alternative. Suctioning should be avoided in the conscious patient as it is very distressing. It may be helpful, if the patient is comatose.

SUPERIOR VENA CAVA OBSTRUCTION

- Characterised by dyspnoea, headache, dizziness and stridor in association with distended veins in the neck and arms, and venules over the chest, and also oedema or puffiness of the face and arms
- Chest X-ray usually abnormal with a widened mediastinum and often a hilar mass
- May be the initial presentation of malignant disease or occur later in the illness
- Most commonly caused by lung cancer, but malignant mediastinal lymphadenopathy due to lymphoma or metastatic cancers and benign causes are also possible
- Thrombosis in association with central venous catheters is now fairly common
- It is essential to be sure of the underlying cause: bronchoscopy or mediastinoscopy may be indicated
- Specific anti-cancer treatment, if appropriate, should be given first
- Steroids, oxygen and radiotherapy may be beneficial
- Consider anticoagulation, if there is associated thrombosis
- Vascular stenting may be indicated, if the syndrome recurs after initial therapy

---

BLEEDING

Bleeding is a common symptom in patients with advanced cancer. As with all symptoms encountered in palliative care, it must be remembered that there are several possible causes, and that treatment will depend not only on the cause, but also on the patient's point in their illness.

In addition, it should not be forgotten that the patient with advanced cancer can develop a symptom which is not directly due to the cancer, and which merits full investigation and treatment. For example, haematemesis or malaena may be due to peptic ulceration which may be remediable, if the patient has a reasonable prognosis.

Similarly, patients who have been treated effectively for cancer may develop bleeding as a consequence of treatment. This requires investigation and appropriate treatment. For example, patients treated with tamoxifen for breast cancer may develop dysfunctional uterine bleeding. Most commonly, this will be benign endometrial

hyperplasia, but sometimes endometrial carcinoma occurs. Another example of treatment-related bleeding is radiation proctitis causing rectal bleeding after radical radiotherapy for cervical or prostate cancer.

A major external haemorrhage may be the terminal event, for example carotid artery blow-out in a patient with uncontrolled head and neck cancer, massive haemoptysis in a patient with lung cancer which has eroded a major thoracic blood vessel or profuse haematemesis from an oesophageal carcinoma which has eroded into the aorta. Such cases can be very sudden, and are tremendously distressing for the patient and bystanders. Very little can be done in such a terminal situation other than the administration of intravenous diamorphine, if venous access can be achieved.

Bleeding may be associated with abnormalities in blood clotting including thrombocytopenia, clotting factor deficiencies (as in patients with a degree of liver failure) and disseminated intravascular coagulation (DIC) which is not uncommon in patients with advanced malignancy. Bleeding may be due to cancers eroding tissues with ulceration or inflammation in the presence of normal blood clotting.

If the cause of the bleeding is not obvious, it may well be worth checking a full blood count including platelets, and a clotting screen including the prothrombin time or International Normalised Ratio (INR) and fibrin-degradation products (FDP). If the patient has lost a lot of blood, transfusion may be required.

THROMBOCYTOPENIA

- Defined as a platelet count less than $150 \times 10^9 \, l^{-1}$
- Rarely symptomatic unless the count is less than $20 \times 10^9 \, l^{-1}$
- Manifests usually as purpura, bruising and bleeding from the gums
- Causes include chemotherapy, marrow infiltration by tumour, sequestration in a large spleen, immune destruction and DIC
- Platelet function may be affected by drugs, such as aspirin
- Platelet transfusion indicated, if count is less than $12 \times 10^9 \, l^{-1}$ or there is bleeding

---

If the bleeding is due to the presence of tumour which cannot be cured, radiotherapy may provide good palliation. External beam treatment is most commonly used, but sometimes brachytherapy may be a better choice. This applies to cervical and endometrial cancers causing vaginal bleeding, carcinoma of the rectum causing rectal bleeding, lung cancer causing haemoptysis, bladder cancer causing haematuria and so on.

Other measures can be used in specific situations, as outlined in the boxes below.

HAEMATURIA

- Causes include cancers of the bladder or upper urinary tract; infections, such as cystitis and pyelonephritis; cancer treatments, such as haemorrhagic cystitis following cyclophosphamide and chronic radiation cystitis following pelvic radiotherapy
- Assessment usually involves cystoscopy
- Haemorrhage from tumour can be treated endoscopically with diathermy or transurethral resection; chemotherapy or radiotherapy; tranexamic acid; alum instillations
- If haemorrhage is heavy and clots are formed, the patient may need bladder irrigation with a special catheter, and blood transfusion may be required

HAEMATEMESIS AND MALAENA

- Upper GI tract bleeding in the patient with advanced cancer is more likely to be due to "benign" causes than the cancer itself
- "Benign" causes include stress ulcers in the stomach, corticosteroid therapy, NSAIDs, oesophageal varices
- Cancers of the oesophagus, or stomach may bleed, either as a gentle ooze leading to malaena and anaemia, or less commonly as a catastrophic terminal event
- Major surgery is unlikely to be appropriate, but, depending on the condition of the patient, transfusion may be required and endoscopy may be helpful
- Radiotherapy may aid haemostasis from a tumour which is oozing gently

URINARY DIFFICULTIES

Patients with advanced cancer may develop a variety of urinary problems in addition to haematuria (see above). It is important to ascertain clearly the cause, as emergency treatment may be appropriate for some scenarios.

URINARY PROBLEMS IN PATIENTS WITH ADVANCED CANCER

- Haematuria
- Urinary tract infection
- Development of a recto-vesical or vesico-vaginal fistula
- Retention of urine due to bladder outflow obstruction
- Anuria due to compression of the ureters
- Incontinence or urinary retention due to spinal cord compression

Having determined the cause, one can then think about how to treat it in the light of the patient's situation. Except in the moribund, spinal cord compression should always be treated actively; otherwise, the patient will be doomed to be paraplegic for whatever span of life may remain (see below).

Major surgical intervention is not usually appropriate when a fistula develops, but quality of life can be maintained by an indwelling urinary catheter and sometimes by formation of a defunctioning colostomy.

Retention of urine due to bladder outflow obstruction can be managed by catheterisation in the first instance. An urologist can be consulted as urethral stenting or transurethral resection may be indicated, depending on the general condition and prognosis.

Dealing with anuria caused by ureteric compression requires careful thought. Causes include extensive cervical carcinoma and retroperitoneal lymph node metastases. Nowadays, interventional radiologists and urologists are very capable at dealing with this with nephrostomy tubes and ureteric stents which may be antegrade (inserted from above through the nephrostomy) or retrograde (inserted from below at cystoscopy). However, interventions of this type are not always indicated. If the patient's tumour is untreated, and there is a reasonable chance of improving the situation with active treatment, then one may be reasonably aggressive and substantially prolong life expectancy. On the other hand, if the patient has very extensive disease, and there is no reasonable prospect of further active anti-cancer treatment being beneficial, then it may be kinder to allow nature to take its course.

Decisions, such as these, are amongst the most difficult in the field of oncology, and it can be helpful when the issues are discussed openly with patients and their families, and with all relevant doctors and nurses, and a collectively agreeable decision is made.

WEAKNESS AND WALKING DIFFICULTY

Patients with advanced cancer may go "off their legs" for a variety of reasons. Treatment will only be possible, if an accurate assessment of the problem is made, and the diagnosis is considered carefully in the light of the patient's general condition and prognosis.

People will stop walking, if movement hurts. They may not initially mention pain, but just say they cannot walk or are too weak to walk. If there is pain, for example due to bone metastases, mobility may be restored by the use of adequate analgesia or radiotherapy. The management of bone metastases has been covered in more detail in Chapter 49. Pathological fractures, particularly of the femur, are not uncommon in patients who have suddenly become unable to walk. Orthopaedic intervention with open reduction and internal fixation, followed by an active programme of rehabilitation will be indicated in previously fairly fit patients whose prognosis is measured in weeks or months. In patients who are already bed-bound or are almost so by virtue of extensive cancer, and who may only have days to live, are not suitable for such active management. Traction and analgesia may be all that is required.

CAUSES OF WEAKNESS AND WALKING DIFFICULTY IN PATIENTS WITH ADVANCED CANCER

- Pain or pathological fracture
- Proximal myopathy due to steroid therapy
- General debility, anorexia and cachexia, including anaemia and sepsis
- Metabolic disturbance, such as hypercalcaemia and hypomagnesaemia
- Spinal cord compression
- Brain tumour
- Paraneoplastic syndromes

Proximal myopathy can be one of the most distressing side-effects of steroid therapy. It is usually insidious in onset. Patients initially find it difficult to rise from a sitting position, particularly if the chair is low, and gradually climbing stairs and even walking itself becomes difficult. The treatment is withdrawal of the steroids if possible, but this may be difficult and even if it can be achieved, recovery is slow. Problems do not necessarily occur in isolation, and it is common for people who have been on long-term steroids to have other side-effects which may compromise mobility, such as painful osteoporotic vertebral collapse.

Proximal myopathy may be a prominent feature of the paraneoplastic Cushing's syndrome sometimes seen in people with ectopic adrenocorticotropic hormone (ACTH) secretion caused by lung cancer. Steroid synthesis inhibitors, such as metyrapone or trilostane, used in conjunction with replacement doses of hydrocortisone, may help. The syndrome may also improve if there is effective treatment of the underlying cancer. Other paraneoplastic syndromes which can be related to tumours include myasthenia gravis in association with thymoma, and the Eaton–Lambert myasthenic syndrome related to lung cancer, and cerebellar degeneration also most commonly seen in patients with lung cancer. Ataxia related to cerebellar degeneration must be distinguished from ataxia resulting from secondary deposits in the cerebellum.

Spinal cord compression and nerve root compression must be recognised early, if treatment is to be beneficial. Most commonly, it affects the thoracic spine. Features include lower limb weakness, which need not be symmetrical; back pain; disturbance of bladder function which may vary from hesitancy through retention to incontinence; disturbance of bowel function which may be "constipation" or incontinence; and numbness of the legs and lower part of the body with a sensory level. The onset may be gradual or sudden. If the cervical spine is affected, there may also be upper limb symptoms, and breathing may be compromised. If the compression is at a lower level than the bottom of the spinal cord (which finishes around the L2 vertebral level), the spinal nerve roots in the cauda equina will be affected. There may be sphincter disturbance, and the sensory impairment may only affect the sacral dermatomes around the buttock and anus and be missed unless a careful examination is made.

SYMPTOMS OF SPINAL CORD COMPRESSION

- Weakness of the lower limbs (and upper limbs if the cervical cord is affected)
- Disturbance of bladder function
- Disturbance of bowel function
- Back pain
- Altered sensation in the limbs with a sensory level usually on the trunk

---

Suspected spinal cord compression can be investigated with plain X-rays which may show spinal metastases and vertebral collapse. MRI is the definitive investigation, and will accurately identify the level of spinal cord compression. It will often be shown that multiple levels are affected.

MANAGEMENT OF SPINAL CORD COMPRESSION

- Urgent investigation
- Steroids
- Neurosurgical decompression
- Emergency radiotherapy
- Conservative management in the moribund

Treatment is with steroids in the first instance. Neurosurgical decompression is indicated in a previously fit patient with a reasonable prognosis and a solitary lesion. Radiotherapy may also be beneficial. A successful outcome is most likely in a good performance status patient who gradually develops a paraparesis, and is rapidly investigated and treated. A poor outcome is likely, if the onset is sudden and the paraplegia is complete. In moribund patients, spinal cord compression may be a pre-terminal event best manages conservatively.

Managing intercurrent illness in the patient with cancer

Cancer is easiest to manage if it occurs in isolation in a previously fit and healthy person. Unfortunately, life is not always that simple.

RELATIONSHIPS BETWEEN CANCER AND OTHER CONDITIONS

- Underlying disease predisposes to development of malignancy
  - Hepatocellular carcinoma developing in a cirrhotic liver
  - Colon cancer arising in a patient with ulcerative colitis
  - Lymphoma in a renal transplant recipient
- Cancer and another condition caused by a common cause
  - Oral cancer and alcoholic cardiomyopathy
  - Bladder cancer and peripheral vascular disease caused by smoking
- Coincidental conditions, illness and malignancy
  - Pregnancy
  - Cardiac disease
  - Renal failure
  - Thromboembolic disease

There are occasions when a cancer and another medical problem are in some way related. Sometimes, patients have a condition, which predisposes to the development of malignancy. Examples include immunodeficiency caused by a disease like AIDS or by immunosupressive drugs used following a renal or heart transplant, and genetic disorders such as ataxia telangiectasia. Sometimes, patients have some form of functional organ impairment and a cancer with a common aetiology. Examples include cirrhosis of the liver and cancer of the hypopharynx related to alcohol, and chronic obstructive airways disease and lung cancer related to tobacco smoking.

Sometimes, cancer treatment leads to organ impairment, which may make subsequent treatment difficult, for example congestive cardiac failure following anthracyclines, or renal impairment caused by cisplatin. In other cases, a medical condition like diabetes or a physiological state such as pregnancy are unrelated to the subsequent diagnosis of cancer, but complicate its management.

For these reasons, it is important for the general practitioner (GP) to include full details of the patient's past medical history and current drug treatment when referring a patient to hospital for the investigation of suspected malignancy. Similarly, the oncologist needs to take a comprehensive history, including past illnesses and operations, medication and family history, and be alert to the possibility of pregnancy in all women of childbearing age.

When cancer is found in a patient with another condition, or an illness is detected which may complicate cancer management, several questions arise:

- Can the cancer, considered on its own merits, be treated radically?
- What is the severity and prognosis of the co-morbidity?
- Will the concurrent illness make cancer treatment more difficult or impossible?
- Will the cancer treatment make the other illness worse?

There then follows a difficult balancing act to work out what is the best approach for that individual patient. Compromises may be necessary, for example, a less than optimal radical treatment for the cancer may be all that can be offered.

Consider a patient with a relatively early lung cancer, which would be technically operable by lobectomy, but who may be unable to withstand that operation because of poor lung function caused by chronic obstructive airways disease. Radical radiotherapy may remain an option, but one where the likelihood of a successful outcome is less than with surgery.

Alternatively, think of a woman with oestrogen receptor negative, node positive breast cancer who may not be able to receive an anthracycline-containing adjuvant chemotherapy regimen because of pre-existing heart disease. She may still be cured by local therapy alone, or in conjunction with a less toxic regimen of adjuvant chemotherapy, but her chances will be less good.

Sometimes, the presence of another illness may make a life or death difference: it may be appropriate to offer palliative treatment only for a cancer which, if it occurred in a fitter patient, would be considered potentially curable.

For example, a patient with cor pulmonale due to severe emphysema may not be fit enough to withstand a laparotomy for bowel cancer, and it may be decided to use supportive care and symptom control measures only for the cancer. A patient with diabetic retinopathy and peripheral vascular disease and renal failure may not be fit enough to receive intensive and potentially curative chemotherapy with a cisplatin-based regimen for a metastatic germ cell tumour.

In cases such as these, the prognosis of the "benign" disease may be as bad as or worse than that of the "malignant" disease. This may mean that the development of the cancer has no real impact on the timing of an already inevitable death, or merely hastens it by a short period.

To a health care professional, these judgements can seem medically quite straightforward. However, patients and their families sometimes see things in a very different light. Patients may have lived with gradually progressing disability from cardiac disease or diabetes, for example, for many years, and may not realise that their life expectancy is already very limited. They may feel that a diagnosis of cancer poses an immediate threat to life which is very much greater than any problems related to their chronic underlying illness. They may have an unrealistic idea of how effective cancer therapy might be, and no understanding of the toxicities and dangers related to cancer treatment. Therefore, it is not surprising if they react angrily if they feel that they or their loved ones are being denied curative therapy.

It therefore goes without saying that discussions about treatment possibilities and treatment intent must be discussed very sensitively. The GP may have looked after the patient in the context of their family for years, and will understand their feelings and aspirations very well. It can, therefore, be very helpful if the GP is able to discuss the factors relating to the illness, and the problems surrounding cancer treatment, with the oncologist prior to discussions with the family. This sort of communication will greatly facilitate both the immediate discussions with the patient and family, and care in the community at the end of life.

It is not possible to cover every possible scenario, but the rest of this chapter considers a number of fairly common situations, and describes some of the problems relating to decision-making and treatment of cancer in patients with unrelated conditions.

HEART DISEASE

Heart disease is common in the community and may take many forms. Some of these may directly affect a patient's suitability for cancer treatments of different types, and some cancer treatments may affect cardiac function.

Heart disease may affect a patient's fitness for anaesthesia for major cancer surgery. Sometimes, it may be possible to undertake the procedure under local or spinal anaesthesia. Sometimes, it is felt justifiable to operate,

if the patient understands that the co-existing disease will be associated with a greater than average degree of risk.

Heart disease rarely affects the ability of a patient to receive radiotherapy. Occasionally, it is necessary to treat a patient with severe orthopnoea who may be unable to lie flat. Simple palliative treatments can often be given to patients in the sitting position, but complex radical treatments, which depend on CT planning and very accurate patient positioning may be impossible. Radiotherapy does not cause acute cardiac problems, but irradiation of the heart may lower tolerance to the effects of cardiotoxic drugs, such as the anthracyclines. There is now accumulating evidence that radiotherapy to the heart, for example, mantle treatment of Hodgkin's disease and breast radiotherapy, especially when left sided, may lead to an increased incidence of coronary artery disease decades later. The long-term effects of the increasing use of anthracyclines in conjunction with radiotherapy for early breast cancer are not yet known.

Chemotherapy drugs may affect the heart. Anthracyclines may cause arrhythmias in the acute phase, and lead to the later development of a cardiomyopathy causing congestive cardiac failure. The likelihood of this is related to the cumulative dose, and it is more commonly seen in those with pre-existing cardiac disease. fluorouracil can cause coronary artery spasm and angina. The monoclonal antibody trastuzamab used for breast cancer may also cause heart failure. If potentially cardiotoxic drugs are to be used in a patient with known heart disease, or if cardiac complications develop in a previously healthy person, the opinion of a cardiologist will be valuable.

RESPIRATORY DISEASE

Lung disease, like cardiac disease is both common and variable in its cause and severity. Poor respiratory reserve is a common contraindication to radical surgery for lung cancer, and impaired lung function may also compromise fitness for anaesthesia for other operations. Sometimes in these circumstances, early input from a respiratory physician may improve a patient's fitness to withstand a major procedure.

Patients with bad respiratory disease may find lying flat impossible, and this, like cardiac failure, may make radical radiotherapy difficult. Radiotherapy to the lungs may be associated with an acute syndrome characterised by cough and dyspnoea. This is referred to as radiation pneumonitis, although other factors, such as infection and chemotherapeutic agents, may also play a role in its causation. This condition is self-limiting, but steroids and antibiotics are usually given to limit its duration. Pulmonary fibrosis is a late effect of radiation to the lungs. If only a limited volume of lung tissue is affected, this is usually of no significance. In a patient with borderline pulmonary function to start with, great care needs to be given to limiting the volume of lung treated, to prevent the patient's exercise tolerance or dyspnoea from worsening.

Some chemotherapy drugs, for example, bleomycin and busulfan, can lead to pulmonary fibrosis, and caution should be exercised particularly in patients with pre-existing respiratory problems. Toxicity is often dose related and radiotherapy and renal failure may make it more likely. The use of high inhaled oxygen concentrations, for example, during general anaesthesia, can lead to potentially fatal respiratory failure in patients who have previously received bleomycin. This can happen months after the exposure to the drug, and so it is helpful the GP can alert the surgeon when a patient who has received bleomycin is subsequently referred for elective surgery for an unrelated condition. Patients with pleural effusions, or other fluid collections, such as ascites, should not receive methotrexate as it accumulates in the fluid and is only gradually released into the circulation, leading to enhanced toxicity.

LIVER DISEASE

Hepatic resection is indicated for some patients with liver metastases or primary liver cancers. Normal liver tissue has an amazing capacity for regeneration, but if there is an underlying liver disease, such as cirrhosis, surgery of this type may not be possible.

Doses of drugs, which are excreted into the bile, such as anthracyclines, should be reduced in the presence of an elevated bilirubin, and should not be used if there is severe obstructive jaundice. Other drugs, such as methotrexate, which can be hepatotoxic, should be used with caution in liver disease.

DIABETES MELLITUS

Patients with diabetes may have any number of complications including peripheral vascular disease, coronary artery disease, renal failure, retinopathy, neuropathy and so on. General fitness issues and performance status may limit the suitability of the patient for some cancer treatments. Diabetics with gangrenous feet may need surgery to remove septic foci before chemotherapy, which will render them neutropenic.

Care is needed even in fit diabetics, as steroids are widely used and may upset sugar control or even lead to coma. For example, steroids are often used in lymphoma and leukaemia chemotherapy, for raised intracranial pressure in association with brain tumours, as anti-emetics, to reduce the likelihood of allergic reactions to taxanes, and commonly in the palliative care setting to improve appetite and quality of life.

PREGNANCY

Pregnancy and fertility issues need to be considered in any younger woman who is to receive cancer treatment. It is bad enough dealing with cancer in a woman who is known to be pregnant, but it is much worse discovering a pregnancy in a woman who has already started cancer treatment. The issues regarding preservation of fertility have been covered in Chapter 13. The most common diseases where pregnancy and cancer co-exist are cervical cancer, breast cancer and Hodgkin's disease. The management of the pregnancy and the cancer need to be individualised depending on the stage of the pregnancy and the patient's wishes for a child, and the nature and stage of the cancer. In general, however, first-trimester pregnancies can be aborted to allow the patient to receive life-saving treatment for the cancer. In the second trimester it may be safe to treat the cancer without undue risk to the foetus, and in the third trimester it is usual to delay the cancer treatment until the foetus is sufficiently mature to permit safe delivery.

RENAL FAILURE

Patients may have renal failure, which is being managed conservatively, or they may be on dialysis or have received a kidney transplant. All modalities of cancer treatment may affect renal function, and impaired renal function may affect the use of some chemotherapeutic agents.

Sometimes, surgery is necessary to remove a renal tumour. Unless the kidney is already non-functional, loss of viable renal tissue in a patient whose renal function is already borderline may push them into requiring renal replacement therapy.

Radiotherapy affects renal function. Wherever possible the kidneys are spared, but if it is necessary to irradiate some or all renal tissue, hypertension and renal failure may develop, depending on the dose and volume of kidney irradiated. For conditions, which are highly curable, such as Wilms' tumour in children, it is occasionally necessary to give a treatment which will unavoidably lead to end-stage renal failure and the need for dialysis or transplantation. Patients with renal disease often have a degree of anaemia. The success of radiotherapy is often dependent on good oxygenation of the tumour for which an adequate haemoglobin level is essential. Blood transfusion or erythropoietin may be needed to support the level of haemoglobin in this patient group.

Some chemotherapy drugs have renal toxicities. For example, cisplatin causes both a reduction in the glomerular filtration rate (GFR), and also a tubular defect, which leads to loss of minerals, such as magnesium. It is necessary to check the GFR before the first treatment and to monitor it between courses. Ifosfamide also leads to renal tubular problems. It is essential to monitor electrolytes including magnesium and calcium both acutely and in the long term, as renal rickets or osteomalacia may be a long-term complication. Some drugs are excreted in the urine, and the dose may need to be adjusted, depending on renal function. An example is carboplatin. In patients with very poor renal function, it can be difficult to predict pharmacokinetics accurately, and monitoring of blood levels during therapy may be necessary. The administration of some nephrotoxic drugs, for example cisplatin and high-dose methotrexate, is complicated by the need to give large amounts of fluids to promote a diuresis. This can be difficult in patients with renal impairment as a fluid load may push them into cardiac failure.

Some tumours, such as high-grade lymphomas, may melt away very rapidly with chemotherapy. The cellular breakdown products including uric acid and potassium can be toxic, causing the tumour lysis syndrome. This can usually be prevented by the use of adequate hydration, allopurinol or a uricozyme, and frequent monitoring of electrolytes. Sometimes, renal support in the form of dialysis or haemofiltration is needed. Clearly, these problems will be more difficult to manage in someone who already has a degree of renal impairment.

Patients receiving immunosupressive therapy following a renal transplant may develop an EBV-mediated lymphoproliferative disease, which may progress to a high-grade non-Hodgkin's lymphoma. Reduction in the level of immunosupression may reduce the lymphoproliferation but may lead to rejection threatening the graft. If chemotherapy is required, graft function may be affected by the direct nephrotoxicity of some drugs, or indirectly by the tumour lysis syndrome.

Domiciliary terminal care

The care of the individual with cancer, from diagnosis through treatment and on towards cure or death, sometimes called the patient's journey, can be varied and complex. The earlier stages, namely diagnosis (Chapter 5), staging (Chapter 8), surgery (Chapter 11), treatment of metastases (Chapter 49) and so on, have already been covered extensively. This chapter and the next cover terminal care in the home, and in the hospice, respectively. The two locations for terminal care are not mutually exclusive. Many patients dying from cancer spend time in both places. The principals of good management are often common to both places, as well as to those who are terminally ill in the acute hospital setting. Similarly, much of what is described as good practice for the terminally ill is also good practice for those at an earlier stage in their illness.

TERMINAL CARE

- The physical, mental, emotional and social care of the patient with advanced cancer for whom no further active anti-cancer treatment directed at cure, or primarily at prolongation of survival, is appropriate.

For the purposes of these chapters, we can define patients with terminal illness as those who have advanced cancer, for whom no further active anti-cancer treatment directed at cure, or primarily at prolongation of survival, is appropriate. A gradual decline in physical health is anticipated, and the life expectancy is likely to be measured in days or weeks, or at most months. The principal aims of treatment are symptom control (Chapter 50) and support of the patient physically, mentally, emotionally and socially in the context of their family. Terminal care is quite consistent with active treatment of cancer with the aim of alleviating a specific symptom.

The point at which terminal care begins is sometimes easy to pinpoint, but often indistinct. While terminal care ends most often in the death of the patient, sometimes the situation stabilises and there are changes for the better. Sometimes, it becomes possible to consider more active, life-prolonging treatment, which was not possible or thought to be appropriate at an earlier stage.

THE DOMICILIARY TERMINAL CARE TEAM

The terminal care team is essentially one, although who plays the major role and who plays the more minor parts may differ depending on the location of the patient. The principal aim of the team is to focus on the individual patient and minister to his or her needs. While some class solutions to particular problems may be appropriate, a "one-size-fits-all" approach is rarely helpful, and the best outcomes are produced when the plan is carefully tailored to the individual patient.

The general practitioner (GP) is at the centre of the domiciliary terminal care team, although most of the day-to-day decision-making may commonly be undertaken by an experienced community palliative care clinical nurse specialist, often a Macmillan or Marie Curie nurse. Although well placed to advise, counsel and liaise, these specialist nurses are not often able to be involved with hands-on nursing care, such as bathing of the patient, and so they will be supported by district nurses attached to the practice. Specialist medical advice regarding symptom control may be sought from the specialist palliative care physician who will usually be based at the local hospice. Sometimes, it is appropriate to get an updated oncological opinion. Usually, this will mean the patient attending the hospital for an outpatient consultation, but rarely it might be appropriate for the GP to request a formal domiciliary visit. The social worker may be important, especially, if there are financial difficulties, or issues relating to the care of dependant family members. It is often helpful to include an appropriate minister of religion if this is in accordance with the patient's wishes.

THE DOMICILIARY TERMINAL CARE TEAM

- **Key members – nearly always involved**
  - GP
  - Community palliative care nurse specialist (Macmillan or Marie Curie)
  - District nurse
  - Specialist palliative care physician
- **Supporting members – available if required**
  - Oncologist
  - Social worker
  - Minister of religion

Sometimes, especially in uncommon tumour types requiring specialist management, for example, in paediatric oncology, the usual team is supplemented by hospital-based clinical nurse specialists who also do community outreach and perform a valuable liaison function with the acute oncological management team.

COMMUNICATION

To be forewarned is to be forearmed, and so excellent communication lies at the heart of good palliative care. Hospital teams should communicate rapidly and effectively with the GP and the community about the patient with cancer, especially when the situation changes and the focus shifts from active anti-cancer treatment to symptom control. However, communication is a two-way process, and if the necessary information is not arriving spontaneously, it can always be sought. If GPs feel "in the dark" they can request written information or, perhaps more usefully in difficult situations, just pick up the phone and speak to an appropriate member of the hospital team. The various members of the community team should also communicate between themselves, both regularly and also in addition if there are any major changes. There needs to be good communication between the domiciliary team and the hospice team if the patient is to be transferred.

It is not just between members of the terminal care team that excellent communication is mandatory. Communication between members of the team and the patient and the family also needs to be impeccable.

This takes time, and repeated visits may be necessary. The patient and his or her loved ones may well need to come to terms with the fact that the disease for which cure might once have been the aim is now considered to be incurable, and that death might not be too far away. It is often found that the patient and individual family members may be at different stages of acceptance. The patient may understand and acknowledge the seriousness of the situation, and may well be relieved that no further active treatment is planned. The spouse may either have unrealistic aspirations for the future, or be angrily demanding second opinions. Acceptance cannot be forced on anyone, either a family member or the patient, and careful explanation, and reiteration of the facts of the course of the illness to date, are important. It is unreasonable to expect anyone to take in everything at once. Time spent at this stage may repay dividends in smoothing the way later.

Sometimes the carer, fearing or knowing the worst, specifically requests that the patient is not told the prognosis or some other key fact. While it is easy to understand the benevolent motivation of the husband who wishes to shield his wife from an unpleasant truth, such a conspiracy of silence can breach trust and make a difficult situation worse. It can be helpful to explain that while you will not gratuitously force bad news on the patient, you are unable to lie if asked a direct question. It is often helpful for sensitive discussions to take place with both the patient and the key family member present together. In this way, each party knows what the other knows, and it reduces the anxiety that secrets are being kept. Then you can ask the patient what they already know, what is their explanation for the pain, and so on. In that way, it often becomes apparent that the patient in fact knows much more than the relative imagines. In other cases, it is the patient who seeks to protect a family member from the truth, fearing that they will not be able to cope.

In difficult circumstances, it may be helpful for more than one health care professional to be there, for example, the Macmillan nurse may be present when the GP visits. This will reduce the possibility of manipulation, or of one professional being played off against the other.

After the first discussion of this nature has taken place, the patient and the relatives have the opportunity to continue discussion of the issues at home in a more open way than before.

SYMPTOM CONTROL

Symptom control has been covered in detail in Chapter 50, but it is worthwhile here emphasising some of the key points:

- Take time to find out what symptoms the patient has and try to explore the significance of these symptoms in the patient's mind. Patient's sometimes have irrational fears and can be reassured by careful explanation.
- If symptoms which you expect the patient to have are not mentioned, specifically ask about them. The patient may feel they have called you to help with pain, and that their troublesome constipation would not be of any interest to you.
- There is a broad range of causes for most symptoms, and for optimum benefit it is essential to ascertain the underlying problem.
- Clarify the patient's point in their journey in your mind – if they are bed-bound and likely to die in a matter of days, treatment options will be different from if they are ambulant and likely to survive for months.
- If possible, treat any treatable underlying cause.
- Remember that non-drug treatments can often be very helpful.
- Explain to the patient and to the family exactly what is being prescribed and why. Ensure that there is agreement that what you wish to prescribe is wanted. In the absence of concordance you cannot expect compliance.
- Promote compliance with drug treatment regimens by keeping them as simple as possible, by giving the

List of medicines for a patient

Name	Purpose	Dose	Timing	Comment
Morphine sulphate slow release tablets (MST Continus) 15 mg – green 30 mg – purple	Painkiller – to provide a constant background of pain control	One green tablet (15 mg) and one purple tablet (30 mg)	Twice daily at 10 am and 10 pm	To be taken regularly
Morphine sulphate oral solution 10 mg in 5 ml	Painkiller – for breakthrough pain	One 5 ml spoon (10 mg)	Every 4 hours if required	To be used if pain is not controlled
Diclofenac tablets 25 mg	Anti-inflammatory and painkiller	One tablet (25 mg)	Three times a day, 6 am or on waking, 2 pm and 10 pm	
Co-danthramer 25/200 capsules	Laxative to prevent constipation	One capsule	At night – 10 pm	Take an extra capsule daily if constipation occurs
Metoclopramide 10 mg tablet	Anti-sickness	One tablet	Every 6 hours if required	

- patient or carer a written list of what, how much, how often and why.
- Dosette boxes with divisions for days of the week and times of the day can be helpful in promoting compliance with regular medication in forgetful patients, especially, if they live alone.
- Repeatedly reassess the effectiveness of what has been prescribed, and adjust medication in the light of changing circumstances. For example, when a patient finds swallowing difficult, it may be necessary to change all medication to a parenteral route.

AS THE END COMES NEARER

Giving an accurate prognosis is one of the most difficult challenges in oncology and palliative medicine. It may be obvious that a patient has very advanced disease and is dying, but two similar patients may survive for very different lengths of time. With increasing experience, some doctors and nurses find giving a prognosis more difficult. There is usually a general deterioration over time, but sudden death may occur for a variety of reasons such as pulmonary embolism, or a haemorrhage.

When a patient changes from being ambulant and able to undertake, even with help, activities, such as getting dressed and toileting, death may be only days away. Patients who are bed-bound because of weakness, unable to eat or drink more than a few sips, unable to take oral medicine, unable to clear upper airway secretions and are unaware of what is going on around them are likely to be moribund.

Nursing care becomes more important to ensure comfort. If a patient cannot drink, keep the mouth fresh with swabs on sticks. If the patient cannot be got up to a commode or use a bedpan or urinal easily, consider a urinary catheter. Remember to change position regularly to ease pressure. If oral medication cannot be taken, give what is essential parenterally, for example, with a continuous subcutaneous infusion. Stop what may no longer be helpful, such as steroids.

Remember to continue to talk to the patient, and explain what is happening. Even if the patient is too weak to speak, they may still have a degree of awareness of their situation and surroundings. Keep relatives and carers informed of progress, and about the likelihood of death. Remember that this may be a frightening as well as a sad time for them. Carers may never before have been with someone at the point of death, or even seen a dead body.

Hospice care

The so-called "Hospice Movement" has revolutionised the care of those dying from cancer, and some other chronic diseases, over the last 40 years in this country and also throughout the world. It grew from a number of disparate strands, which were brought together by a number of workers, most notably by Dame Cicely Saunders whose hospice, St Christopher's, opened in Sydenham in 1967.

FACTORS LEADING TO THE FORMATION OF THE HOSPICE MOVEMENT

Death, and by implication, terminal illness, had long been regarded as taboo subjects for discussion. There was often a conspiracy of silence, in which patients may not have been told the diagnosis, let alone the prognosis. Patient advocates began to encourage a new openness about death and dying, and the concept of "death with dignity" became prevalent.

There was a perception that patients with advanced cancer were being abandoned by conventional medicine when they reached an incurable state. Statements by surgeons such as "there is nothing more I can do" (to cure you of the cancer) were interpreted as "there is nothing more that can be done" (to help you). While in Britain, there may have been concerns about the neglect of dying patients; in some countries, at the same time, there was anxiety about the inappropriate use of futile medical interventions in the terminally ill. It began to be realised that dying people could be actively managed medically with the aim of alleviating discomfort and avoiding the indignity of unnecessary treatments.

Medical teaching on care of the dying, such as there was, began slowly to move away from anecdote to evidence-gathering and research-based practice. A body of knowledge grew up about the symptoms which were to be expected in the terminally ill, and about what could be done to help them.

Ancient barriers, which separated the body from the mind were eroded, and the subtle interplay between physical, emotional and spiritual factors affecting well-being were recognised.

Initially, the Hospice Movement led to the creation of charitably funded hospices as inpatient units independent of the hospital and community aspects of the conventional health service. It was to these hospices that dying patients were transported as havens, where they could have their suffering relieved and die in peace. These hospices often had strong religious overtones.

THE DEVELOPMENT OF MODERN PALLIATIVE CARE SERVICES

Gradually, the concept of palliative care has developed, which now transcends hospices. What currently exists is a much more diverse and comprehensive service provision than perhaps the founders of the Hospice Movement ever dared to envisage. It integrates palliative care with curative medicine and covers hospitals and the community as well as designated hospices.

LOCATION OF PALLIATIVE CARE SERVICES

◆ Hospices
  – Inpatient units
  – Day care units
◆ Community
  – Specialist palliative care physicians and clinical nurse specialists
  – General practitioners (GPs)
◆ Hospitals
  – Ward-based palliative care teams
  – Outpatient clinic-based palliative care teams

Inpatient units still exist in hospices, but these are not all free standing. Some are separate entities within the grounds of hospitals and some are within the hospitals. Inpatient units are not just for the dying, but are also a setting for the investigation of new problems and active symptom control, so that patients can return to their own homes, and to provide respite care for patients, while their usual carers have a break. Hospices provide outpatient clinics and day centres for physical, spiritual and social care.

Training programmes have been developed for specialists in palliative care medicine and clinical nurse specialists. This expertise is not just confined to hospices: there are now palliative care teams based in hospitals to help patients and support ward-based medical and nursing staff in acute specialties; and in the community palliative care teams help patients at home and support GPs.

Although charities (see Chapter 57), such as Marie Curie, Macmillan and countless smaller organisations, raise enormous amounts of money and still provide much specialist palliative care and run hospices, there is now in addition considerable NHS funding. Collectively, the NHS and the charitable sector are able to run an essentially seamless service between hospitals, hospices and the community.

REFERRAL TO A HOSPICE

Nowadays, it is not usual to refer a patient "to a hospice". Rather patients are referred to a palliative care team, which will usually be lead by a consultant palliative care physician, with much of the service delivery undertaken by clinical nurse specialists. An initial assessment will be made of the patient's needs. It is helpful for the referral to contain as much detail as possible about the patient's disease, symptoms, family support, understanding and perceived needs. A single assessment may not be enough; in many cases, it may be necessary to divide the assessment into more than one episode, dealing first with the most urgent matters, coming to other equally important factors in time. For example, if a patient is in severe pain, dealing with this may be the number one priority. When the pain is controlled, the patient may want to discuss how and where he will subsequently be cared for.

The assessment or assessments will look in detail at the patient's physical symptoms and how best they may be helped. It will look at the home circumstances and the level of support the family is able to give. It will explore the patient's and the family's level of knowledge and understanding. It may also evaluate the patient's fears and preconceptions, and wishes with regard to place of care and place of death. Thought will be given as to whether the patient needs any non-medical input, such as from a priest or a solicitor.

After the assessment, a plan can be formulated, stating what needs to be done, and who should be involved and where it will happen. For example, it may be decided to admit the patient to a hospice to establish pain control and deal with breathlessness, thereafter returning the patient home to be looked after by the community nurse specialists in conjunction with the GP.

Many patients wish to die at home. Others may have inadequate support at home, or a desire not to be a burden to their families and seek hospice admission at the end of their illness. Sometimes, a family who had wished to keep their loved one at home, may find that professional nursing is constantly required or that the strains of looking after a dying relative are too much, and request admission. As far as possible, hospice admission should be planned in advance, and not be necessary as an emergency.

ROLE OF A HOSPICE DAYCARE SERVICE

- Regular symptom control assessment and adjustment of medication
- Nutritional and dietetic advice and support
- Care of bowels, stomas, catheters
- Brief respite period for carers
- Management of anaemia and hypercalcaemia by transfusion or bisphosphonates
- Bathing and hair care
- Social interaction with other patients
- Familiarisation of patients and families with the hospice, so that when inpatient care may be needed, it seems like a natural extension of earlier care
- Physiotherapy

It is ideal, if patients and their families have the opportunity to meet the palliative care team early on in the course of the illness, perhaps even during the initial period of oncological treatment with curative intent. The great advantage of an integrated oncology and palliative care service is that patients transfer seamlessly from active oncological management to palliative care at the appropriate time, and do not feel abandoned to palliative care when the oncologists have nothing further to offer.

The dying child

Care of the child who is terminally ill poses challenges over and above those associated with palliative care of adults. The general practitioner (GP) and the rest of the community team must interact not just with the patient, but also with the parents, any siblings, grandparents and other members of the extended family. They must deal effectively with a number of different people whose reactions to the diagnosis, levels of understanding and expectations of care may vary significantly.

Most children's cancers are potentially curable and are treated radically in the first instance. It is rare for a family with a child, newly diagnosed with cancer, to have to face a "hopeless" prognosis. Active treatment with the expectation of cure, therefore, helps parents to adjust to the new fact that their previously fit and healthy normal child now has a life-threatening illness, and that life will never be the same again for the parents or the child. Even when the cancer relapses, a second attempt at cure may be possible. And so when faced with eventual progression of the disease for which symptom care only is possible, many parents will find acceptance very difficult, and some may even feel a sense of betrayal as the initially optimistic prognosis is revised.

Faced with a "hopeless" prognosis, they may pursue various avenues. Nowadays, parents are very well informed. The internet has made available mountains of information, and has made possible immediate and direct contact with other parents and treatment centres worldwide. Parents may seek a second opinion from another centre close to home, or from abroad, in the belief that treatments are possible there which are unavailable locally. Parents may request experimental therapy or seek to try out unconventional treatments.

Requests for second opinions and the desire for participation in *bona fide* clinical trials of new treatment approaches should be respected and facilitated. Sometimes it may be helpful for the GP, following discussion with the hospital team, to offer referral for another NHS opinion. Wise counsel from another specialist may be tremendously helpful for parents, allowing them to move towards acceptance. International pilgrimages, in search of unrealistic cures and unorthodox approaches, should be sympathetically discouraged. The GP may help by pointing out the negative aspects for the child of a long journey with no prospect of cure. The GP and local services, in partnership with the team from the cancer centre, have an important role in guiding families at this most difficult time. Not infrequently, the mother and father or other relatives may be at different stages in the process of acceptance, which can lead to disharmony. At this time, input from the GP, who may just need to listen in an understanding way, rather than to mediate by providing answers, can be immeasurably beneficial in allowing both parties to move closer together. Sudden death from childhood cancers is not common, and usually the end comes fairly predictably after a period of decline, which allows time for the emotional support from the palliative care team to enable reconciliation.

The aims of the GP and the community team at this time should be quite simple. On the physical side, symptom control is important to ensure that the quality of whatever period of life remains is as good as possible. Predictable new symptoms, such as constipation arising from the use of opiates, should be foreseen and prevented. It is helpful to be able to predict the likely nature of physical deterioration and have plans in place to deal with possible difficulties appropriately. An example here would be the possible development of convulsions in a child with a brain tumour. Parents need to be instructed how to use rectal diazepam, if a seizure occurs. In this way, the inappropriate call out of an emergency ambulance may be averted.

AIMS OF PAEDIATRIC PALLIATIVE CARE

- To alleviate established symptoms
- To prevent predictable new problems from emerging
- To have in place a strategy for coping with deterioration
- To support the patient and their family through and beyond the illness
- To facilitate open and honest communication

Secondly, it is important to promote open and honest discussion between parents, the child and siblings, within the limits of their curiosity and understanding. It is counter-productive to lie to seriously ill children with the aim of shielding them from unpleasant truths. Many children have known everything about their illness and its treatment, within the limits of their understanding, from the beginning. They will be very suspicious, if they are suddenly being given less information or evasive answers, particularly by a person they have previously trusted. Similarly, sibling's questions should be answered openly.

SYMPTOM CONTROL IN DYING CHILDREN

The principles of symptom control in dying children are not materially different from those applicable to adults, or from those in children at an earlier stage in their illness.

Sometimes, active treatment will be indicated, for example a ventriculo-peritoneal shunt may be inserted to relieve raised intracranial pressure, palliative radiotherapy may be given for pain relief and gentler schedules of chemotherapy may be used. Blood and platelet transfusions may be needed, if there is anaemia or bleeding. The appropriateness of measures, such as these will be very dependent on an individual patient's symptoms and other circumstances.

Pain can be one of the biggest worries for parents. Pain is a real issue for many children at some point in the final phases of their illness, but with good management, it is unusual for it to be a persisting problem. Many children are, of course, afraid of needles, but fortunately effective analgesia is usually possible with oral, transdermal or rectal administration. Many children will still have a central venous catheter, which can be used to administer analgesics intravenously. Although a syringe driver delivering continuous subcutaneous drugs requires placement of a needle, this is usually not a problem at the stage when it is required. Co-analgesics, such as carbamazepine, amitriptyline and gabapentin are often useful in addition to conventional painkillers, especially if there is a neuropathic element to the pain.

There are various myths about the use of opiates, and many parents will be torn by their desire for effective and sustained pain relief in their children, and anxieties about addiction, respiratory suppression and hastening of death. It is important for the GP and other health care professionals involved to listen sympathetically to parental fears, and to explain gently how their worries about morphine can be circumvented by careful and judicious prescribing and monitoring. To hurriedly dismiss these concerns as being unfounded is not helpful.

Nausea and vomiting are unpleasant for the patient, and vomiting is unpleasant for the carer also. It is important faced with these symptoms, to try and elucidate the cause. Is there raised intracranial pressure or intestinal obstruction, or perhaps are opiates the cause? Sometimes, if the cause can be removed, the symptom will be relieved. If not, there is a wide range of preparations, which may be valuable including cyclizine and levomepromazine (methotrimeprazine) and octreotide. Although steroids are effective in treating the symptoms of raised intracranial pressure, the side-effects, which develop even with relatively short-term use in children, mean that it is often better to avoid their use, if possible.

Convulsions are not uncommon in children with brain tumours, and witnessing seizure activity can be very distressing for families. Patients with established fits may already be on adequate doses of conventional anticonvulsants, but it can be helpful for the family to have available a rectal preparation of diazepam for use in emergencies.

TALKING TO CHILDREN ABOUT DEATH AND DYING

Some teenagers may choose to approach nurses or doctors, rather than their parents, for information about death or dying. It is usually more appropriate for most children, however, that any discussion about these, the most sensitive of issues, is principally with parents rather than health care professionals. Doctors and nurses, nonetheless, have an important role in ensuring that these important discussions take place, and are not avoided because they may be so painful. For most parents, how to start talking about death, and what to say, seems almost impossible, and they may well look to professionals for guidance. Sometimes, it can be helpful for parents to have a health professional, such as a clinical nurse specialist present at the time of discussions of this nature, even if it is the parent or the patient who leads.

The intrinsic human desire to protect loved ones from pain works in both directions. Parents will be reluctant to say anything, which may distress their children. Children themselves may wish to protect their parents, and often feel guilty that they are the cause of the problem. It is, therefore, important for parents to reassure children that what is happening is not their fault, and to let them know that they are loved in an extra special way.

Discussions of this sort are often initiated by the child asking questions. They are rarely single episodes. They are more likely to happen in instalments, sometimes with a different set of characters, so that the child can check for consistency in the story. Sometimes, questions are asked, and the answer is not known. It is usually possible to answer these simply by admitting to the uncertainty, being optimistic within the realms of reality, and giving reassurance where possible, for example by telling them that pain will be treated effectively. Parents should be made aware that it is alright for them to express emotion in front of their children. It is not a sign of weakness that a father cries with his child; it is in fact an expression of love.

Although the natural focus for the family at this time is the dying child, it is important not to neglect other children but to seek to involve them fully, according to their age and understanding. Their participation at this difficult time will lead to fewer regrets later on. Siblings have their own needs for information and for love, which must be met. Sometimes, brothers and sisters may have strange feelings of guilt or of punishment, which may need to be explored.

ACHIEVING AMBITIONS

It is often said that health care professionals should never allow patients and their relatives to lose hope. But what hope can there be when a child is dying? In fact there can be many hopes. The simplest is often that symptoms will be alleviated and that there will be no prolonged suffering. Other aims, both those more positive and unique, and those of a more everyday nature, may still be possible. Children are sociable beings, and usually enjoy the company and the normality which school provides, when possible. Even if a child is too ill to attend school regularly, it may still be a practical proposition to take him or her into school for a special event, and to encourage visits at home from school friends and perhaps the teacher. Children may wish to have a home study plan, monitored by the teacher, rather than stopping learning altogether and just waiting, while their condition deteriorates.

Children should be encouraged to voice their own ambitions and to set their own targets. A number of charitable organisations (Chapter 57) exist simply to meet the wishes of terminally ill children. It is important that wishes should be practicable, taking into account the child's condition. More fun may be obtained from a visit to a theme park close to home, than from having to endure the discomfort of a transatlantic journey and time away from home and friends in order to visit a bigger and better theme park in Florida.

DEATH AND THE FUNERAL

Parents should be encouraged to discuss in advance their wishes about the likely place of death: home, hospital or hospice. Most families will want their child to die at home, but sometimes parents are afraid that they will not be able to cope, and seek the reassurance, which a hospital or hospice admission will give. It is often possible to reassure parents that adequate experienced community care from the GP, local nurses and paediatric oncology outreach nurses will enable their child to be cared for well at home. Of course, specialist backup from the paediatrician at the district general hospital or the paediatric oncologist or palliative care paediatrician at the cancer centre, is always available, if necessary. Often, such support is not needed, but it is always reassuring to know that it is there.

Although before death the family will want to concentrate on their child's remaining life, it is helpful for them to know what happens after their child passes away, for example confirmation of the death, laying out of the body, death certification and funeral planning. For many parents, it will be their first experience of all these things, and most will welcome advice from the community health care team about the practicalities. Some older children may wish to have a say on the sort of funeral service they may have. Even if neither parent is a member of the church, they will probably want a "proper" funeral, and often a hospice chaplain will be a great support. The cultural ritual surrounding death may vary considerably according to the religious background, for example Anglican, Jewish, Islamic or Roman Catholic. It can, therefore, be helpful to ensure that the family have had appropriate spiritual guidance and pastoral care in advance of the death.

The work of the GP and the community health care team does not end with the death of the patient. The family will require support during their bereavement, and the clinical nurse specialist is usually willing to attend the funeral, if that is wished for. Parents may wish for counselling to help them understand and to come to terms with what has happened. They may well seek a further consultation with the specialist principally responsible for their child's care. Genetic counselling may be appropriate, if there is any suggestion that there may have been a familial cause for their child's cancer, and further pregnancies are planned. Anniversaries are always painful, and visit from the GP prior to the first anniversary of the death is often greatly appreciated.

The remaining siblings often have feelings of guilt persisting into adulthood. "Why wasn't it me who died?" It is worth noting the name and the dates of birth and death of the child who died, clearly on the surgery medical notes of the siblings and the parents.

Death at home

Although many patients with advanced cancer still die in hospitals or hospices, most patients wish to be at home in the peace and tranquillity of their own familiar surroundings, with their loved ones at their side, when they die. It is the role of the community nurses and general practitioner (GP) to facilitate patients' wishes and to try, as far as possible, to ensure that death, when it comes, is a "good death".

There are many cultural aspects to death, and so what different communities regard as a "good death" may vary in detail. Nonetheless, there are some aspects which are common. Of course, the process of dying should not be shaped to fit a preconceived model, rather the process should be moulded to the individual's wishes and preferences.

Ideally, when death comes, it should be regarded as a natural phenomenon. The patient and the family should have had time to come to terms with the fact that the end of life is approaching, and so the imminent arrival of death can and should be openly acknowledged and discussed. Hopefully, any family differences or conflicts will have been resolved. More distant family and friends will have been informed and will have been able to call and say their farewells. Personal business will have been tidied up, a will will have been made or updated, and the family will know of the patient's wishes regarding funeral arrangements and disposal. It goes without saying that pain and any other distressing symptoms will have been effectively alleviated.

COMMON FEATURES OF A "GOOD DEATH"

- In a comfortable, familiar and secure environment, usually home
- With recognition and acceptance of imminent death as natural closure
- With family and loved ones around and differences resolved
- With open discussion of the will and funeral wishes
- Free of any distressing symptoms, such as pain or nausea
- A feeling of spiritual or religious comfort

Perhaps, the key features of a "good death" can be summarised as "peace": peace in terms of freedom from symptoms, peace in terms of resolution of any family conflict, peace in recognition that there is no unfinished business.

Of course, not every death can be a good death; perhaps no death is a perfect death in every respect, just as no life is ever completely perfect. There are patients who never reconcile themselves to the prospect of death – those whose anger at being struck down by a cruel illness too young never recedes. There are families whose internecine strife is not even suspended let alone resolved when one of their number is dying. There can be intractable symptoms, which even the most careful medication is not able to ameliorate. Fear may be one of the major factors preventing the establishment of peace. Fear may affect both patients and carers. There can be fear of death itself; but more importantly, there can be fear of the process of dying. Here, the palliative care team can provide valuable input. They can explore the fears, and provide reassurance that the fear is not justified, or that if it is then something can be done to help.

PRINCIPAL FUNCTIONS OF THE PALLIATIVE CARE TEAM AS DEATH IN THE HOME APPROACHES

- Assess and control physical symptoms
- Monitor progress and change medication as necessary
- Talk to patient about fears and wishes
- Talk to family about their expectations and fears
- Educate family about what to expect and what to do
- Act as liaison with other professionals as appropriate

From the point of view of the palliative care team, the GP and community nurses, not only the physical control of unpleasant symptoms, but also, especially, pain, must be regarded as the number one priority. This is covered in Chapter 50. This is because the symptom control is the unique skill of doctors and nurses; no one else can provide this aspect of care. The other practical, communication and social aspects of care leading up to death and beyond are equally important. It often falls to the community palliative care clinical nurse specialist to lead on these issues, in conjunction with the GP. They can draw in other professionals, such as a minister of religion or lawyer and undertaker as appropriate, if the family have not already done so for themselves.

When a patient dies at home, although community nurses and/or doctors may be visiting as often as two or three times a day, there may very well be no professional presence at the time of death. Family members or other carers, who may well have never witnessed a death before, may need to be alerted about what to expect in the run-up to death. For example, the pauses in Cheyne–Stokes respiration can be confusing for a professional, and so it is easy for carers to think that their loved one has passed away only for them to take another gulp of air.

Families will need to have a contact number to call the nurses after death. The nurses will be able to confirm the fact of death, comfort the bereaved and clean and lay out the body, unless there are any religious barriers to them in performing this task. The nurses will call the GP, who will visit as soon as practicable to medically confirm the death, and to issue a death certificate and perhaps fill out the cremation form. The family should then contact the undertakers, who will arrange for removal of the body in accordance with the late patient's wishes, and the minister of religion, if appropriate.

PRINCIPAL FUNCTIONS OF THE PALLIATIVE CARE TEAM AFTER DEATH IN THE HOME

- Confirm the fact of death
- Lay out the body
- Medical certificate of cause of death and cremation form, if necessary
- Support family in their time of grief
- Advise family about undertaker and religious support

CHAPTER 56 Managing bereavement

The oncologist's duty of care usually ends with the death of the patient. Some contact, however, at this difficult time is often greatly appreciated by relatives. Sometimes, it is appropriate to send a note of condolence. Sometimes, a bereaved relative will visit to ask for more information about the illness. Perhaps, a man whose wife has just died from breast cancer may enquire about the risks for his daughters, if he felt unable to ask before. But, apart from these relatively rare examples, the death of the patient, usually, signifies the end of the contact with the family.

The general practitioner (GP), however, is often in a very different position from the hospital specialist when it comes to bereavement. One of the joys and challenges of general practice is that it is family medicine. Usually the GP will have a continuing duty of care to the widow or widower, any children and perhaps a more extended family. The GP's role will, of course, be to comfort the family in their grief. Perhaps, one of the clinical nurse specialists will represent the palliative care team at the funeral service. The role is, however, greater than that.

The surviving spouse and other members will go through the recognised stages of a grief reaction: shock, denial, guilt, anger and acceptance. Just how well-prepared individual family members were for the death, and to what extent it was a "good death" (Chapter 55), may influence how long the various stages of grieving take, and how severely they are felt. However, individuals may not necessarily react as predicted. Even after an apparently "good death", when the survivors had come to accept the inevitability of death at an intellectual level, they may not have been adequately prepared at an emotional level. Sometimes, couples seem to have an undesirable relationship, always sparring with each other and never happy. When one partner dies, the other may find themselves completely bereft of purpose in life, and guilty that they did not do more to express in life the love they felt. Those left, suddenly also have a great deal of lonely time to fill – the immediately preceding weeks or indeed months having been full of frequent hospital or hospice visits and caring for the patient at home. They may wish they had discussed one or two specific issues, often about events, which happened to them sometime previously, and feel cheated that they will never have "just 5 minutes" for discussion.

Of course, sadness is to be expected – what loving relation would not feel sad, even after a "good death"? However, emotions can go beyond normal sadness to pathological depression. The thoughtful GP will be able to explore the survivors affect and look for somatic symptoms of depression, such as loss of interest in appearance, altered appetite, sleep disturbance and loss of the sensation of pleasure in life. Some widows or widowers will need antidepressant medication, while some may need referral to a psychiatrist. Referral to a self-help group like CRUSE may also be of help.

Among survivors of couples who have been married a long time, there is a significant excess death rate during the first year after the bereavement. Often, it seems as if death is due to "a broken heart". Surviving spouses may have postponed seeing their GP with symptoms of their own, either wrongly attributing the symptoms to the stress of their loved one's illness, or merely waiting until they felt they had time to address their own problems.

Children and teenagers who have lost a parent prematurely may manifest psychological upset in other ways, such as poor quality school work or actual school truancy, delinquency and drug misuse. It may be helpful to mark the surgery notes of all family members with the date and details of the bereavement, so that the loss is not forgotten as a possible complicating factor when patients present with other problems.

Anniversaries can be a particularly poignant time, and the wise GP will be proactive. During the first year after bereavement, the three dates which the surviving spouse usually finds most difficult are the deceased's birthday, the wedding anniversary and, of course, the first anniversary of the death. These anniversaries can be marked in the practice diary or house call book for the coming year, and the GP can contact or visit the spouse or family before that date to see how they are doing. Small touches like this are often greatly appreciated.

SECTION CONTENTS

CHAPTER 57
Patient support organisations and cancer relief charities

There are many organisations working to support people with cancer, as well as their families and friends. Some are large, well-known national charities, such as Macmillan and CancerBACUP, many more are small but nonetheless equally important local groups. The type of help given varies greatly. Some provide financial assistance if required to help offset the unexpected costs of coping with cancer, for example, travelling expenses. Others aim to improve quality of life by providing holiday accommodation or "extras". Some provide health care personnel to work for the benefit of patients both in the hospital setting and in their own homes.

A generation ago most patients with cancer suffered in silence and ignorance, but today's patient is well informed and enquiring. This is thanks partly to those charitable bodies which provide a large amount of very high-quality information about cancer and its treatment, and seek to empower the patient to be an equal partner in the therapeutic relationship; and partly to the way in which the "information superhighway" has made access to information from so many different sources available so easily to many.

GENERAL ORGANISATIONS LISTED IN THIS CHAPTER

- The National Cancer Alliance
- CancerBACUP
- Cancerlink
- Bristol Cancer Help Centre
- Cancer Care Society
- The Hospice Information Service
- Ian Rennie Hospice at Home
- Macmillan Cancer Relief
- Marie Curie Cancer Care
- Richard Dimbleby Cancer Information and Support Service
- Royal London Homoeopathic Hospital
- The Sue Ryder Foundation
- Tak Tent Cancer Support
- Tenovus Cancer Information Centre (TCIC)

This chapter is designed to act as a guide to those organisations providing generic information and practical support. Those bodies, which exist to serve only the interests of patients with a specific tumour type, for example,

breast cancer, are listed in Chapter 58. Unfortunately, no list of this sort can be completely comprehensive. It concentrates on the principal national and regional organisations, though a few with a more limited geographical remit are mentioned as examples. This chapter should be read in conjunction with Chapter 60, which includes other information sources that patients, as well as their doctors, might find informative.

ORGANISATIONS LISTED IN THIS CHAPTER FOR PATIENT GROUPS WITH SPECIAL NEEDS

- Cancer Black Care
- Cancer You Are Not Alone – Newham
- Chai Lifeline Cancer Care
- Coping With Cancer – Leicestershire
- GaysCan

ORGANISATIONS LISTED IN THIS CHAPTER FOR CHILDREN WITH CANCER

- Association for Children with Life-threatening or Terminal Conditions and their Families (ACT)
- Cancer and Leukaemia in Childhood (CLIC)
- Children's Hospice Association Scotland (CHAS)
- Christian Lewis Trust
- Make-a-wish Foundation UK
- Rapid Effective Assistance for Children with Potentially Terminal Illness (REACT)
- Sargent Cancer Care for Children
- Starlight Children's Foundation

GENERAL ORGANISATIONS

The National Cancer Alliance
PO Box 579, Oxford OX4 1LP
Tel.: 01865 793566
Fax: 01865 251050
E-mail: nationalcanceralliance@btinternet.com
Website: www.nationalcanceralliance.co.uk

The NCA represents the interests and concerns of all people affected by cancer. Its aims are: to increase public and professional awareness about cancer diagnosis, treatment and care; to represent the interests, concerns and views of patients and their carers; to encourage those involved in all aspects of cancer care to work cooperatively to provide the most effective care; and to promote and monitor high-quality national standards for cancer care and treatment throughout the UK. Towards meeting its aims, the NCA has published a directory of cancer specialists, and networks with kindred organisations.

CancerBACUP

3 Bath Place, Rivington Street, London EC2A 3JR
Tel.: 020 7696 9003
Fax: 020 7696 9002
Helpline: 0808 800 1234 and 020 7613 2121 (Monday to Friday 9 am to 7 pm)
Website: www.cancerbacup.org.uk

The British Association of Cancer United Patients and their families and friends, now known as CancerBACUP was founded in 1986 by a doctor, Vicky Clement-Jones, who, facing treatment for ovarian cancer, found herself looking for information and help which was not easily available. From its early beginnings, CancerBACUP has grown into one of the pre-eminent cancer information organisations. CancerBACUP publishes a wide range of booklets and information leaflets covering almost every aspect of cancer. There are ones on specific tumour types, ones on different treatments both established and experimental, and others on coping with the physical and psychological difficulties, which often come hand in hand with a diagnosis of cancer, and also booklets on difficult areas in communication, such as "what do I tell the children?" The complete range of leaflets and booklets can be seen on the website in full text format. They can be ordered directly from the website, or by phone. CancerBACUP has a team of trained specialist nurses, backed up with a library of information, who are well equipped to try to answer almost any question. They can be accessed by a telephone helpline, or contacted by letter. CancerBACUP information centres staffed by nurses and with the full range of literature are situated in a number of cancer centres, including several locations in London, and in Nottingham, Manchester, Kendal, Coventry and Jersey. At some locations, London, Glasgow and Jersey, CancerBACUP offers a free one-to-one confidential counselling service.

Cancerlink

Freephone: 0808 808 0000 (10 am to 6 pm Monday, Wednesday and Friday)
E-mail: cancerlink@cancerlink.org.uk
Website: www.cancerlink.org

Formerly an independent organisation, Cancerlink is now part of Macmillan Cancer Relief (see below). It offers free consultancy, training and resources to over 700 UK cancer self-help and support groups and organisations. Through the website or the helpline, anyone can find if there is a specific local or national support group relating to a particular tumour type or other special factor, such

as ethnic group. CancerVOICES, part of Cancerlink, is a national network of cancer service users including cancer self-help and support groups, users, carers and professionals linked on a regional basis.

Bristol Cancer Help Centre

Grove House, Cornwallis Grove, Clifton, Bristol BS8 4PG
Tel.: 0117 980 9500
Fax: 0117 923 9184
E-mail: info@bristolcancerhelp.org
Website: www.bristolcancerhelp.org

The Bristol Cancer Help Centre aims to be a centre of excellence offering healing and positive health care to people affected by cancer, and to their supporters. Its aim is to practise, teach, research and develop the holistic approach as an integral part of cancer care. This pioneering institution, founded in 1980, is regarded as the gold standard of holistic complementary therapy. It offers cancer patients and their families healing programmes, which give them the opportunity to mobilise inner strength through the whole range of complementary therapies.

Cancer Care Society

11 The Corn Market, Romsey, Hampshire SO51 8GE
Tel.: 01794 830300 (Monday to Friday, 9 am to 5 pm)
Fax: 01794 518 133
E-mail: info@cancercaresociety.org
Website: www.cancercaresociety.org

The Cancer Care Society offers help for anyone whose life has been touched by cancer. Their services include emotional and practical support, counselling, a telephone link and groups around the country for patients, family and friends before, during and after treatment. There are local groups in Norfolk, Hampshire, Bedfordshire and South Wales.

The Hospice Information Service

Saint Christopher's Hospice, 51–59 Lawrie Park Road, Sydenham, London SE26 6DZ
Tel.: 010 8778 9252
Fax: 020 8776 9345
E-mail: info@his2.freeserve.co.uk
Website: www.hospiceinformation.info

Provides a comprehensive listing of all hospices, palliative care services and home care teams in the UK and abroad.

Ian Rennie Hospice at Home

52a Western Road, Tring, Hertfordshire HP23 4BB
Tel.: 01442 890222
Fax: 01442 891276
E-mail: info@irhh.org
Website: www.irhh.org

Ian Rennie Hospice at Home is an organisation dedicated to the care of terminally ill patients in their own homes in the Chilterns region of Hertfordshire and Buckinghamshire.

Macmillan Cancer Relief

89 Albert Embankment, London SE1 7UQ
Macmillan Cancerline: 0808 8082020
Tel.: 020 7840 7840
Fax: 020 7840 7841
E-mail: cancerline@macmillan.org.uk
Website: www.macmillan.org.uk

Now known as Macmillan Cancer Relief, the Society for the Prevention and Relief of Cancer was founded in 1911 by Douglas Macmillan following the death from cancer of his father. MCR is now one of Britain's oldest, largest and best known cancer charities. With the NHS and others, it funds and promotes the development of cancer care and support at many levels, in order to meet the physical, emotional psychological, practical and financial needs of people with cancer. It works from a network of regional offices throughout the UK (contact details available on the website). Macmillan is a major employer of health care professionals, funding over 2000 specialist nurses working in hospitals and the community and about 200 doctors in both academic and service posts as GPs, hospital trainees and consultants. In addition, it contributes to the physical infrastructure with building projects for cancer care, and has an information service. Macmillan also offers grants to patients in financial need, to cover, for example, the costs of installing a telephone line, fuel bills and short breaks and holidays.

Marie Curie Cancer Care

89 Albert Embankment, London SE1 7TP
Freephone: 0800 716146
Tel.: 020 7599 7777
Fax: 020 7599 7708
E-mail: info@mariecurie.org.uk
Website: www.mariecurie.org.uk

Founded in 1948, Marie Curie Cancer Care is the UK's most comprehensive cancer charity, providing community-based palliative care nurses, hospices day care centres and undertaking research. The 11 Marie Curie Centres, although receiving some NHS funding, constitute the largest provider of hospice beds outside the NHS.

Richard Dimbleby Cancer Information and Support Service

Saint Thomas' Hospital, Lambeth Palace Road, London SE1 7EH
Helpline: 020 7960 5682
Tel.: 020 7960 5689
Fax: 020 7960 5687
E-mail: richarddimblebycentre@gstt.sthames.nhs.uk
Website: www.richarddimbleby.org

A library and information service for health care professionals as well as patients and their families, also offering complementary therapies.

Royal London Homoeopathic Hospital

Greenwell Street, London W1W 5BP
Tel.: 020 7391 8833
Fax: 020 7391 8829
Website: www.uclh.org/services/rlhh

An NHS hospital, which accepts referrals from general practitioners (GPs) and hospital doctors for its complementary cancer care service that runs alongside and supports conventional medical therapy for cancer. Treatments available include homoeopathy, Shiatsu massage, iscador therapy, relaxation therapy, aromatherapy and psychological support. All these are delivered by health care professionals under the leadership of an NHS consultant, and are aimed to improve the quality of life of the patient, with no claims or expectation that the treatments will affect the progress of the cancer.

The Sue Ryder Foundation

Second Floor, 114–118 Southampton Row, London WC1B 5AA
Tel.: 020 7400 0440
Fax: 020 7400 0441
E-mail: info@sueryder.com
Website: www.sueryder.com

The Sue Ryder Foundation, established in 1953 by Lady Ryder of Warsaw, has 20 homes in the UK to care for people with all manner of disabilities and life-shortening illnesses including cancer.

Tak Tent Cancer Support

Flat 5, 30 Shelley Court, Gartnavel Complex, Glasgow G12 0YN
Tel.: 0141 211 0122
Fax: 0141 211 3988
E-mail: tak.tent@care4free.net
Website: www.taktent.org.uk

Tak Tent's logo is a four-pointed knot, signifying the four main methods of cancer treatment: surgery, radiotherapy, chemotherapy and hormone therapy. It also signifies the four main needs of the cancer patient: the physical, psychological, the emotional and spiritual. The knot is bound together by an "O" to represent oncology – the study and treatment of tumours. Tak Tent offers counselling and complementary therapies, and there is a network of support groups across Scotland. The Tak Tent Youth Project aims to encourage and assist young people affected by cancer to continue with normal family, social, student, and working life by providing communication, support and recreation. In every aspect of the project the young people are in control.

Tenovus Cancer Information Centre

43 The Parade, Cardiff CF24 3AB
Helpline: 0808 808 1010
Tel.: 02920 482000

Handbook of Community Cancer Care

E-mail: tcic@velindre-tr.wales.nhs.uk

Website: www.tenovus.com

The TCIC although based in Cardiff has a nationwide function. TCIC has oncology nurse specialists, social workers, welfare rights officers and counsellors located at several hospitals in England and Wales. There are now over 28 such staff acting as a full-time support network.

ORGANISATIONS FOR PATIENT GROUPS WITH SPECIAL NEEDS

Cancer Black Care
16 Dalston Lane, London E8 3AZ

Tel.: 020 7249 1097

E-mail: info@cancerblackcare.org

Website: www.cancerblackcare.org

Cancer Black Care provides information and support for black people affected by cancer. There are three branches in London, and ones in Birmingham and Manchester. Counselling, advocacy, grants and benefits advice are among the services provided. There is a monthly support and massage therapy group.

Cancer You Are Not Alone (CYANA) – Newham
31 Church Road, Manor park, Newham, London E12 6AD

Tel.: 020 8553 5366

CYANA is a general cancer support and self-help group. It holds monthly meetings with invited speakers, and has an information library of books and tapes. There is an Asian link worker with language skills working to offer specific services for people from Asian communities, and an Asian drop-in group.

Chai Cancer Care
Shield House, Harmony Way, off Victoria Road, London NW4 2BZ

Helpline: 0808 808 4567

Tel.: 020 8202 2111

Fax: 020 8202 2111

E-mail: info@chaicancercare.org.uk

Website: www.chaicancercare.org

Chai Cancer Care is a comprehensive cancer support organisation for members of the Jewish community. It offers a telephone helpline, financial, legal and religious surgeries in addition to genetic counselling, psychological counselling and complementary therapies. There is also a home care service and well-man and well-woman screening clinics.

Coping With Cancer – Leicestershire
Helen Webb House, 35 Westleigh Road, Fosse Road South, Leicester LE3 0HH

Language line: 0116 223 0020

Tel.: 0116 223 0055

This is a group giving emotional support and practical help to people with cancer. Services include information, visiting, transport, social and complementary therapy meetings, drop-in, providing support within ethnic communities and a quarterly newsletter. The language line offers information and advice in Gujarati and Hindi.

GaysCan
7 Baron Close, Friern Barnet, London N11

Tel.: 0208368 9027 (10 am to 8 pm)

E-mail: gayscan@blotholm.dircon.co.uk

A national organisation offering confidential help and support to gay men living with cancer.

ORGANISATIONS FOR CHILDREN WITH CANCER

Association for Children with Life-threatening or Terminal Conditions and their Families (ACT)
Orchard House, Orchard Lane, Bristol BS1 5DT

Helpline: 0117 922 1556

Administration tel./Fax: 0117 930 4707

E-mail: info@act.org.uk

Website: www.act.org.uk

The principal group working for the provision of palliative care for children with fatal or potentially fatal conditions including cancer in the UK. It does not directly provide palliative care services, but functions as an advocate for terminally ill children and acts as an umbrella organisation bringing together many local charities and providers, and giving support and information to health workers, other professionals and families.

Cancer and Leukaemia in Childhood (CLIC)
Abbey Wood, Bristol BS34 7JU

Tel.: 0117 311 2600

Fax: 0117 311 2649

E-mail: clic@clic-charity.demom.co.uk

Website: www.clic.uk.com

Originating in the West Country, CLIC is now a national organisation, which funds paediatric oncology outreach nurses, play specialists and homes from home. It funds transport and provides crisis breaks for children and their families. It recognises the separate needs of teenagers as being different from, yet equally important to, those of children. CLIC also funds education, training and research.

Children's Hospice Association Scotland (CHAS)
18 Hanover Street, Edinburgh EH2 2EN

Tel.: 0131 226 4933

Fax.: 0131 220 1626

E-mail: info@chas.org.uk

Website: www.chas.org.uk

The CHAS was founded in 1992 when Scotland had no children's hospice, forcing families to make long journeys south of the border. It now runs Rachel House, Scotland's first children's hospice, which provides specialist palliative support through respite care and emergency care for children with life-limiting, life-threatening and terminal conditions; regular short-term breaks for children and their families; terminal care and bereavement counselling and support; friendship, information, advice and practical support for families, with help available in their own homes at times of particular stress.

Christian Lewis Trust
62 Walters Road, Swansea, West Glamorgan SA1 4PT
Tel.: 01792 480 500
Fax: 01792 480 700
E-mail: clt@aol.com

The Christian Lewis Trust provides care for children with cancer and their families, including respite care, nurses, social workers and play specialists. There is an information service, and a number of local support groups.

Make-a-Wish Foundation UK
Make-A-Wish House, Minster Court, Tuscam Way, Camberley, Surrey GUIS 3YY
Tel.: 01276 24127
Fax: 01276 683727
Website: www.make-a-wish.org.uk

The Make-a-Wish Foundation is an international organisation with the sole aim of granting special things to children suffering from life-threatening illnesses including cancer, aged between 3 and 18 years.

Rapid Effective Assistance for Children with Potentially Terminal Illness (REACT)
Saint Luke's House, 270 Sandycombe Road, Kew, Richmond, Surrey TW9 3NP
Tel.: 020 8940 2575
Fax: 020 8940 2050

E-mail: react@reactcharity.org
Website: www.reactcharity.org

REACT works to give children with life-limiting illnesses including cancer comfort, dignity and where possible, greater independence. REACT responds quickly to deal with emergencies, and provides practical support to families by way of grants for equipment, holidays and funerals. It also supports research and education projects to improve the quality of life of severely ill children.

Sargent Cancer Care for Children
Griffin House, 161 Hammersmith Road, London W6 8SG
Tel.: 020 8752 2800
Fax: 020 8752 2806
E-mail: care@sargent.org
Website: www.sargent.org

This organisation funds over 100 health care professionals, principally social workers, whose responsibility is to provide social care and practical support for children and young people up to the age of 20 years with cancer and their families at this difficult time. Grants are available to cover additional expenses, such as clothing, travel and fuel bills for those in need. In addition, they have a number of residential centres, which act as home from home for holidays and respite care.

Starlight Children's Foundation
Macmillan House, Paddington Station, London W2 1HD
Tel.: 020 7262 2881
Fax.: 020 7402 7403
E-mail: info@starlight.org.uk

Starlight is an international children's charity, which aims to improve the happiness and quality of life of children with serious, life-threatening and terminal illnesses through the provision of entertainment in hospital, fun centres in hospitals and hospices and wish-granting.

Guide to tumour-specific groups and organisations

LIST OF ORGANISATIONS MENTIONED IN THIS CHAPTER BY TUMOUR TYPE

Breast and gynaecological cancers
- Breast Cancer Care
- The Haven Trust
- Breast Care Campaign
- Hysterectomy Support Network
- Lymphoedema Support Network
- Ovacome

Lung cancer
- The Roy Castle Lung Cancer Foundation
- The June Hancock Mesothelioma Research Fund

Upper and lower gastro-intestinal tract cancers
- British Colostomy Association
- The British Liver Trust
- Colon Cancer Concern
- Oesophageal Patients' Association

Central nervous system cancers
- British Brain and Spine Foundation
- The Brain Tumour Foundation
- British Brain Tumour Association
- Glaxo Neurological Centre

Head and neck cancers
- Changing Faces
- National Association of Laryngectomee Clubs
- Let's Face It

Leukaemia and lymphoma
- Anthony Nolan Bone Marrow Trust
- Leukaemia Care
- The Lymphoma Association
- International Myeloma Foundation (UK)

Urological cancers
- The Urostomy Association
- Kidney Cancer UK
- The Prostate Cancer Charity
- Testicular Cancer Group
- Testicular Cancer Support

Children's cancers
- The Joshua Gilbert Rhabdomyosarcoma Appeal
- The Neuroblastoma Society
- The Retinoblastoma Society

This chapter is designed to help the general practitioner point patients with specific cancer types and their relatives and friends in the direction of relevant patient support groups and kindred organisations. Generic psychological support groups for patients with any type of cancer, and organisations that provide practical help with the financial burden of cancer, have been covered in Chapter 57. Many of the organisations listed here double up as cancer research charities in their limited field, and so also receive mention in Chapter 59. No list such as this can be completely comprehensive, and in addition to the major national groups listed, many district general hospitals and cancer centres will have their own groups to support local patients. Some of these more local groups are mentioned as examples of what may be available.

BREAST AND GYNAECOLOGICAL CANCERS

Breast Cancer Care
Kiln House, 210 New Kings Road, London SW6 4NZ
Tel.: 020 7384 2984
Fax: 020 7384 3387
Freephone (10 am to 5 pm, Monday to Friday): 0808 800 6000
E-mail: info@breastcancercare.org.uk
Website: www.breastcancercare.org.uk

This organisation provides advice on many of the practical aspects of life following surgery for breast cancer, for example with prosthesis fitting and by supplying information about retailers of bras and swimming costumes. In addition, it supplies information leaflets and booklets, and co-ordinates face-to-face support for women with breast cancer from volunteers, who have experienced it for themselves.

The Haven Trust
Effie Road, London SW6 1TB
The Haven Helpline: 08707 272 273
Services information tel.: 020 7384 0099
Administration tel.: 020 7384 0000
Fax: 020 7384 0002
E-mail: info@thehaventrust.org.uk
Website: www.thehaventrust.org.uk

This organisation is a national charity providing a network of support centres for people affected with breast cancer. Havens offer information, advice, counselling and complementary therapies free of charge to complement medical treatment. The first Haven in Fulham, London, was opened in 2000; the second in Hereford is due to open in 2003.

Breast Care Campaign
Blythe Hall, 100 Blythe Road, London W14 0HB
Tel.: 020 7371 1510
Fax: 020 7371 4598
E-mail: uk@breastcare.co.uk
Website: www.breastcare.co.uk

While cancer is the foremost concern for readers of this book, many more women, especially younger ones, suffer from benign breast disease. The Breast Care Campaign is uniquely dedicated to raising awareness about benign breast disease. An important focus is to reassure women that the detection of a breast problem need not signal the worst, by putting risk factors into perspective.

Hysterectomy Support Network
3 Lynne Close, Green Street Green, Orpington, Kent BR6 6BS.

This organisation co-ordinates a number of local groups and publishes literature. It facilitates patients who have recently had, or are about to have, a hysterectomy meeting with others who have been through this experience, whether for cancer or benign disease, to share the experience and receive emotional and practical support.

Lymphoedema Support Network
Saint Luke's Crypt, Sydney Street, London SW3 6NH
Tel.: 020 7351 4480
Fax: 020 7349 9809
E-mail: adminlsn@lymphoedema.freeserve.co.uk
Website: www.lymphoedema.org

The network provides information, practical advice and emotional support for patients suffering from lymphoedema as a consequence of breast cancer or its treatment.

Ovacome
Saint Bartholomew's Hospital, West Smithfield, London EC1A 7BE
Tel.: 020 7600 5141
E-mail: internetfriends@ovacome.org.uk
Website: www.ovacome.org.uk

This organisation is a national support group for women with ovarian cancer. It provides information on diagnosis, treatment and research and has a network of telephone contacts for patients to speak to others for emotional support and practical advice.

LUNG CANCER

The Roy Castle Lung Cancer Foundation
200 London Road, Liverpool L3 9TA
Helpline tel.: 0800 358 7200
Tel.: 0151 794 8800
Fax: 0151 794 8888
Website: www.roycastle.org

In addition to funding research on lung cancer treatment, the Roy Castle Foundation provides information, help and advice about lung cancer and smoking cessation. The Roy Castle Patient Support and Information Network comprise, at present, 13 local groups, where patients and their families can meet and exchange experiences.

The June Hancock Mesothelioma Research Fund
Saint Peter's House, Hartshead, Sheffield S1 2EL
Helpline tel.: 0113 206 6466
E-mail: mavisro@ulth.northy.nhs.uk
Website: www.leeds.ac.uk/meso

June Hancock was the first person never to have worked with asbestos, who was awarded damages following the diagnosis of mesothelioma: as a child she grew up in the shadow of an asbestos factory and had regularly inhaled the deadly pollutant. The Mesothelioma Information Service, supported by the June Hancock fund, offers information, advice and support to patients, carers and health care professionals, and provides access to a nationwide network of specialist nurses.

UPPER AND LOWER GASTRO-INTESTINAL TRACT CANCERS

British Colostomy Association
15 Station Road, Reading, Berkshire RG1 1LG
Tel.: 0118 939 1537
Fax: 0118 956 9095
Helpline tel.: 0800 328 4257
E-mail: sue@bcass.org.uk
Website: www.bcass.org.uk

This association is the national registered charity, which represents the interests of people with a colostomy and provides support, reassurance and practical information to anyone with, or about to have an "ostomy". It does not dispense prescriptions, stock stoma care supplies or do home deliveries. It does not sponsor stoma care or colorectal nurses.

The British Liver Trust
Ransomes Europark, Ipswich IP3 9QG
Tel.: 01473 276326
Fax: 01473 276327
E-mail: info@britishlivertrust.org.uk
Website: www.britishlivertrust.org.uk

The work of this trust relates both to cancer affecting the liver, and to other forms of liver disease. Its aims are to publish up to date information for patients, to support individuals with liver disease and those who care for them, and to fund research within the charity's resources.

Colon Cancer Concern
9 Rickett Street, London SW6 1RU
Infoline: 08708 506050 (10 am–4 pm Monday to Friday)
Tel.: 020 7381 9711
E-mail: queries@coloncancer.org.uk
Website: www.coloncancer.org.uk

This organisation is the UK's first national charity devoted solely to colorectal cancer. The aims are to disseminate information to the public and health care professionals, fund pioneering research and campaign for improved quality and accessibility of services for patients with cancer of the large bowel. Other aims are to improve early diagnosis, increase the cure rate, and prolong and improve the quality of life of those with colorectal cancer. Information is provided through leaflets, the website and a telephone information service manned by a nurse specialist.

Oesophageal Patients' Association
16 Whitefields Crescent, Solihull, West Midlands B91 3NU
Tel.: 0121 704 9860
Website: www.opa.org.uk

Members of this association provide information and support to others with oesophageal cancer.

CENTRAL NERVOUS SYSTEM CANCERS

British Brain and Spine Foundation
7 Winchester House, Cranmer Road, Kennington Park, London SW9 6EJ
Helpline: 0808 808 1000
Tel.: 020 7793 5900
Fax: 020 7793 5939
E-mail: info@brainandspine.org.uk
Website: www.brainandspine.org.uk

Since its inception in 1992, the Foundation has worked towards achieving four objectives: increased levels of research into neurological disorders, greater access to quality information and support for patients and carers, improved medical skills and delivery of service to the public, and greater awareness of neurological disorders and disability.

The Brain Tumour Foundation
PO Box 162, New Malden, Surrey KT3 4HW
Tel. and Fax: 020 8336 2020
E-mail: btf.uk@virgin.net

This organisation provides information and support for patients with brain tumours in the UK.

British Brain Tumour Association
2 Oakfield Road, Hightown, Merseyside L38 9GQ
Tel.: 0151 929 3229

This association provides information for patients suffering from the effects of brain and spinal tumours. It promotes public awareness, develops support groups and promotes research.

Glaxo Neurological Centre
Norton Street, Liverpool L3 8LR
Tel.: 0151 298 2999
Fax: 0151 298 2333
Website: www.glaxocentre.merseyside.org

This organisation is a unique non-medical advice and information centre for people with neurological conditions and their carers.

HEAD AND NECK CANCERS

Changing Faces
1–2 Junction Mews, London W2 1PN
Tel.: 020 7706 4232
Fax: 020 7706 4234
E-mail: info@changingfaces.co.uk
Website: www.changingfaces.co.uk

This group, not specifically for patients with head and neck cancer, aims to provide support for individuals with facial disfigurement from any cause, congenital or acquired, and their families. This may be by personal contact, booklets and videos, and workshops. It also provides help for health care professionals, teachers and employers. The goal is to permit full social re-integration of the disfigured individual.

National Association of Laryngectomee Clubs
Ground Floor, 6 Rickett Street, Fulham, London SW6 1RU
Tel.: 020 7381 9993
Fax: 7381 0025
E-mail: rtunnard@ntlworld.com
Website: www.laryngectomees.inuk.com

This is the umbrella organisation for over 90 clubs nationwide, which are devoted to the rehabilitation of patients who have undergone laryngectomy. It offers literature and other information including a training video on resuscitation of the patient with a tracheostomy. The association promotes and supports the development of new local clubs.

Let's Face It
Christine Piff, 14 Fallowfield, Yately, Hampshire GU17 7LW
Tel.: 01252 879630
Fax: 01252 872633
Website: www.letsfaceit.force9.co.uk

This organisation was founded by Christine Piff who underwent major, disfiguring surgery for a facial cancer. It is a support network, which brings together others with similar problems and allows them to share experiences and pass on advice.

LEUKAEMIA AND LYMPHOMA

Anthony Nolan Bone Marrow Trust
The Royal Free Hospital, London NW3 2QG
Website: www.anthonynolan.com
The principal aim of this trust is to provide a register of potential bone marrow donors, so that all those who may require an unrelated donor bone marrow transplant may find one. In addition, the organisation also provides information for patients and their families through their website and publications.

Leukaemia Care
2 Shrubbery Avenue, Worcester WR1 1QH
Tel.: 01905 330003 or 0845 7673203
Fax: 01905 330090
E-mail: enquiries@leukaemiacare.org
Website: www.leukaemiacare.org
This is an organisation for patients with Hodgkin's disease, non-Hodgkin's lymphoma, myelodysplasia and aplastic anaemia, as well as all types of leukaemia. Its website provides basic information for patients, without going into all the treatment details or giving individual medical advice. The Leukaemia Care Society network of volunteers provides local support through a co-ordinated national network.

The Lymphoma Association
PO Box 386, Aylesbury, Buckinghamshire HP20 2GA
Helpline tel.: 0808 808 5555
Administration tel.: 01296 619400
Website: www.lymphoma.org.uk
This association offers information and support to people with Hodgkin's disease and non-Hodgkin's lymphoma. The association works closely with the British National Lymphoma Investigation (BNLI), one of the largest organisations co-ordinating research into the diagnosis and treatment of lymphomas.

International Myeloma Foundation (UK)
2nd Floor, 31 York Place, Edinburgh, EHI 3HP
Helpline tel.: 0800 980 3332
Tel.: 0131 557 3332
Fax: 0131 556 9720
E-mail: theimf@myeloma.org.uk
Website: www.myeloma.org.uk
This organisation offers information through a freephone helpline, its website and literature. It co-ordinates a patient and family support network.

UROLOGICAL CANCERS

The Urostomy Association
18 Foxglove Avenue, Uttoxeter Staffordshire ST14 8UN
Tel.: 0870 770 7931
Fax: 0870 770 7932
E-mail: ua@centraloffice.fsnet.co.uk
Website: www.uagbi.org
This organisation provides advice and support for all those living with urostomies whether necessitated by cancer or by some other disease. There is information on different appliances, and advice regarding work and home life.

Kidney Cancer UK
Tel.: 024 7647 0584
Website: www.kcuk.org
Founded in 2000, Kidney Cancer UK is the country's first support organisation specifically for patients with kidney cancer and their families. It aims to provide reliable and up to date information, raise public awareness and bring patients together to share experiences and discuss common problems.

The Prostate Cancer Charity
Du Cane Road, London W12 0NN
Helpline: 0845 300 8383
Tel.: 020 8383 8124
Fax: 020 8383 8126
E-mail: info@prostate-cancer.org.uk
Website: www.prostate-cancer.org.uk
This organisation offers support and information to patients, their families and friends through their telephone helpline, internet website and range of literature. In addition, they have a nationwide network of patients and their families who are willing to talk to people about their experiences. This organisation is also committed to both research into, and raising public and political awareness of, prostate cancer.

Testicular Cancer Group
312 Parkgate, Upper College Street, Nottingham NG1 5AQ
Tel.: 0115 912 6761
E-mail: tcgroupeastmids@aol.com
This group was set up by men who all have had testicular cancer, and is a local group based in the East Midlands. It exists to provide support and help to men with testicular cancer and their families, but it does not provide medical advice.

Testicular Cancer Support
14 Blighmont Crescent, Millbrook, Southampton SO15 8RH
Tel.: 023 8077 5611
This is another local voluntary group of men, who have been treated for testicular cancer offering self-help.

CHILDREN'S CANCERS

The Joshua Gilbert Rhabdomyosarcoma Appeal
1 Ransworth Gardens, Potters Bar, Hertfordshire EN6 3PD
Tel. and Fax: 01707 662227
E-mail: info@jg-rabdo.com
Website: www.jg-rabdo.com

This organisation's principal aim is to fund research into rhabdomyosarcoma, but the website offers some information and support.

The Neuroblastoma Society
Alderwood, 9 Dominic Court, Beaulieu Drive, Waltham Abbey, Essex EN9 1JT
Tel.: 01992 719696
E-mail: nsoc@ukonline.co.uk
Website: web.ukonline.co.uk/nsoc/

This small charity provides information and support for families of children with neuroblastoma, and offers grants for neuroblastoma research.

The Retinoblastoma Society
Saint Bartholomew's Hospital, West Smithfield, London EC1A 7BE
Tel.: 020 7600 3309
Fax: 020 7600 8579
E-mail: rbinfo@rbsociety.org.uk
Website: www.rbsociety.org.uk

This group aims to support families of children with eye cancer throughout diagnosis, treatment and follow-up, by providing information, contact with other families, national and local meetings and a newsletter.

CHAPTER 50

CHAPTER 59

The cancer research charities

Much progress has been made in cancer treatment over recent decades. Some improvements are attributable to organisational changes, some to a recognition of the importance of psycho-social aspects of care. However, the greatest advances have been through a combination of scientific and clinical research. Collectively, there has been an enormous international research effort, made up of a largely unco-ordinated mosaic of activity comprising government, through the NHS and the MRC, the universities and professional associations, and industry together with a large number of charities. These various bodies sometimes work independently, but often together. For example, a university clinical department based in a teaching hospital may have income streams from the NHS, the MRC, the cancer charities and the pharmaceutical industry. Many clinical studies will be done on a multicentre basis, and involve different cancer centres nationally or internationally. Recently, there have been attempts to bring a sense of order and planning into cancer research, by joining these stakeholders together to work for their common aims. The UK Coordinating Committee on Cancer Research (the UKCCCR) has now been superseded by the National Cancer Research Institute and the National Cancer Research Network.

Patients with a question often turn first to their general practitioner (GP), and so it is useful for the GP to know a little about the structure and funding of cancer research. Patients become aware of cancer research in different ways, and this in turn influences the questions they may ask. They may have been asked to take part in a clinical trial, and seek further information. They may have been told that nothing more can be done in their case, and wonder if there is a new approach, which can be tried. Patients often talk to one another in the hospital setting, in the context of support groups or independently. As a result they hear of new or experimental treatments, which they think might be worthwhile. The broadcast and printed news media often sensationalise modest advances, promoting the discovery of a "cure for cancer". In addition, many patients and their families are altruistic and genuinely seek to promote the cause of cancer research and ask for advice as to where their charitable efforts should be directed.

There are many charities, which are involved in the field of cancer research. Some, such as Cancer Research UK (CRUK) are very large organisations whose entire efforts are directed towards this end. Others, such as Marie Curie and Tenovus, are equally committed to the support and care of cancer patients, and to research. There are many organisations, large and small, which are concerned only with one type of cancer, for example, Breakthrough Breast Cancer and the Neuroblastoma Society. Some of these organisations are multipurpose, funding both research and providing information and support. Other cancer research charities are geographically based, and exist to support research in one hospital or cancer centre.

In a book of this type it is neither possible nor appropriate to provide a comprehensive directory of organisations involved in cancer research, but it may be helpful to give contact details and briefly describe the work of a few selected bodies. Disease specific organisations which also support research are listed in Chapter 58.

Cancer Research UK

P.O. Box 123, Lincoln's Inn Fields, London, WC2A 3PX
Tel.: 020 7242 0200
Fax: 020 7269 3100
Website: www.cancerresearch.uk.org

Cancer Research UK (CRUK) appeared in 2002 as a result of the merger of The Cancer Research Campaign (CRC) and The Imperial Cancer Research Fund (ICRF). CRUK is the world's largest voluntary sector cancer research organisation. It employs over 3,000 scientists, and its annual research budget is more than £176 million. It runs several large basic science research institutes across the country, as well as funding some university clinical departments. It runs the patient orientated website Cancer Help UK.

Marie Curie Cancer Care

89 Albert Embankment, London SE1 7TP
Tel.: 020 7599 7777
Fax: 020 7599 7708
E-mail: info@mariecurie.org.uk
Website: www.mariecurie.org.uk

Marie Curie Cancer Care is perhaps best known for its community-based palliative care nurses and hospices. In addition to this, Marie Curie has an important research role with its own laboratories.

Medical Research Council

20 Park Crescent, London W1B 1AL
Tel.: 020 7636 5422
Fax: 020 7436 6179
Website: www.mrc.ac.uk

The MRC is not a charity, but a government funded body. It funds cancer research as well as other types of medical research. It is a partner with the CRC and the ICRF in the new National Cancer Research Institute. It employs full-time scientists to work on important research topics in its own research establishments; it supports university researchers through a range of grant schemes designed to meet scientific needs, and gives personal awards for research training and career development.

Tenovus

43 The Parade, Cardiff CF24 3AB
Tel.: 029 2048 2000
Website: www.tenovus.com

The Tenovus cancer charity was set up in 1943 by 10 businessmen (the "ten-of-us") and now invests around £2 million each year on cancer research, patient care, counselling and education. Its research efforts are based at the Tenovus Institute for Cancer Research at the University Hospital of Wales in Cardiff, and other scientists and clinicians are employed in Southampton, Liverpool and Bournemouth.

United Kingdom Children's Cancer Study Group

University of Leicester, 3rd Floor, Hearts of Oak House, 9 Princess Road West, Leicester LE1 6TH
Tel.: 0116 249 4460
Fax: 0116 254 9504
E-mail: ukccsg@le.ac.uk
Website: www.ukccsg.org

The United Kingdom Children's Cancer Study Group (UKCCSG) aims to improve the management of children with cancer and to advance the knowledge and study of childhood malignancy. The Group has over 400 members, including all disciplines involved in the treatment of children with cancer, working in 22 specialised paediatric oncology centres throughout the British Isles.

Guide to further reading

It is the authors' aspiration that this small book will prove to be a valuable source of reference for general practitioners (GPs) seeking the answer to a question about cancer. Nonetheless, it is inevitable that the need for more information on a particular topic will arise from time to time. The final chapter in this book will guide the reader to other, more substantial, general works of reference; to monographs on specific subjects, and to some of the increasing number of online oncology information services. Several books are also listed, which the GP may recommend to enquiring patients. Such a listing cannot be comprehensive, and so what follows is an eclectic, rather personal choice.

MAJOR TEXTBOOKS ON CANCER

The Oxford Textbook of Oncology, second edition, R. Souhami, I. Tannock, P. Hohenberger and J.-C. Horiot (Editors), 2001, 2 volumes, 2,956 pages, £295, Oxford University Press.

Nowadays, oncologists wonder how they ever managed without this pre-eminent cancer text before publication of the first edition in 1995. Written by a very distinguished international panel of authors from all branches of cancer medicine and surgery, it covers every aspect of cancer from pathology and epidemiology through to diagnosis and treatment. It is as up to date as any book of this sort can be, but each edition will age rapidly in such a fast moving field.

Cancer – The Principles and Practice of Oncology, sixth edition, V.T. De Vita Jr, S. Hellmann and S.A. Rosenberg, 2001, 2 volumes, 3,125 pages, Lippincott Williams & Wilkins.

This textbook with a largely US authorship is just about as comprehensive as any such work can be. It will offer an answer to almost any question, but treatment philosophy and policy is offered from a North American viewpoint, which is not always accepted as standard practice in the UK.

Treatment of Cancer, fourth edition, P. Price and K. Sikora (Editors), 2002, 1,137 pages, £129, Arnold.

This is a valuable British textbook covering the underlying principles of cancer treatment and practical management of every tumour type. Many chapters are co-authored by a team comprising a surgeon, a medical and a radiation oncologist with special experience in malignancies of a particular organ or system to reflect the best multidisciplinary practice.

Oncology – A Multidisciplinary Textbook, A. Horwich (Editor), 1995, £95, Arnold.

This large book covers the whole practice of cancer management. It is written from a modern multidisciplinary standpoint, reflecting the fact that the skill of effective cancer treatment, nowadays, lies not in the talents of an individual, but in effective teamworking.

SMALLER BOOKS ON CANCER MANAGEMENT

Clinical Oncology, second edition, A.J. Neal and P.J. Hoskin, 1997, £18.99, Arnold.

This small book written principally with medical students in mind gives a balanced account of cancer and its management with enough detail to make it worthwhile to a broader readership.

Cancer and Its Management, fourth edition, R.L. Souhami and J.S. Tobias, 2002, 480 pages, £34.95, Blackwell Science.

This excellent book, written by a medical oncologist and a clinical oncologist who have the gift of explaining difficult issues well, is a very valuable mid-range cancer book. It goes well beyond the most basic concepts and addresses issues of complexity and controversy.

Concise Notes in Oncology, second edition, K. Mokbel, 1999, 131 pages, £12.95, Petroc Press.

This brief book, as it name suggests, is a set of lists and telegraphic notes, probably more suited to the junior doctor or nurse preparing for an examination than for the practising doctor when faced with a clinical problem. Nonetheless, it contains an amazing array of facts relating to both common and rarer cancers, and is a useful *aide memoire*.

Cancer Care in the Community, B. Hancock (Editor), 1996, 198 pages, Radcliffe Medical Press.

A short book whose value lies in useful chapters covering such diverse aspects as communication and psychosocial aspects of cancer treatment, needs assessment, economics, and purchasing and provision of cancer care. The chapters relating to cancer treatment and management of individual cancer types are probably too brief to be of much value.

BOOKS ON PARTICULAR ASPECTS OF CANCER

American Cancer Society's Guide to Complementary and Alternative Cancer Methods, 2000, American Cancer Society.

This is a clear and understandable guide to the many different types of alternative and complementary therapies, which are on offer today. There are hundreds of entries relating to all the various therapeutic strategies, which document, wherever possible, the evidence base for their use. It attempts to distinguish between methods, which may be valuable adjuncts to conventional treatment, those which are merely harmless distractions and approaches that are, in one way or another, potentially dangerous.

TNM Classification of Malignant Tumours, fifth edition, L.H. Sobin and C. Wattekind (Editors), 1997, 227 pages, Wiley Liss.

The TNM Classification of Malignant Tumours is only a small volume, yet it is the recognised compendium of cancer staging. Published on behalf of the UICC, the International Union Against Cancer, it carries full details of the staging of individual cancer types referred to in brief throughout this book.

Symptom Management in Advanced Cancer, third edition, R. Twycross and A. Wilcock, 2001, 415 pages, Radcliffe Medical Press.

This very valuable book offers a symptom-based approach to difficult situations in patients with advanced cancer, and will be of use to hospital specialists and GPs as well as to key medical and nursing palliative care personnel.

Directory of Cancer Specialists, 1995 (being updated) £5.70 including post and packing, National Cancer Alliance.

This book is aimed at helping patients, and GPs acting as their advocates, select appropriate specialists.

BOOKS FOR THE LAY READER

Living with Cancer: Symptoms – Diagnosis – Treatment, J. Tobias and K. Eaton, 2001, £14.99, 224 pages, Bloomsbury.

This book, written to compliment the BBC television series "Living with Cancer" is written with the informed and educated lay person in mind. Nonetheless, it gives a significant amount of detail about treatment and prognosis, even about rarer tumour types. While the general tenor is one of optimism about what can be done for patients with cancer, it does not paint an inappropriate picture when discussing areas in which a successful outcome is uncommon.

Cancer – The Evolutionary Legacy, M. Greaves, 2001, £9.99, Oxford University Press.

This somewhat philosophical and speculative book, written by an eminent cancer scientist, explores how the study of the evolutionary biology may help to unravel some of the mysteries of cancer. Darwinian selection may go some way to explaining why women seem to have a raw deal from this dread disease, and why some malignancies, such as prostate cancer, seem to be on the increase.

Cancer – What Every Patient Needs to Know, revised edition, J.S. Tobias, 1997, £7.99.

This small paperback is written in characteristically readable style. It covers all types of cancer and all modalities of cancer treatment. It is illustrated with short case histories giving a personal touch, allowing the reader, who may have cancer to identify with a similar patient.

ONLINE INFORMATION

The American Cancer Society Website, www.cancer.org

This website provides its own information about the many types of cancer and the various treatments available for patients. In addition, it provides a guide to books and journals stratified for both a lay and a professional audience, and links to other helpful sites.

CancerHelp UK, www.cancerhelp.org.uk

CancerHelp UK is a free online information service about cancer and cancer care for people with cancer and their families. It is a service of Cancer Research UK.

Cancernet, www.cancernet.nci.nih.gov

This excellent website, which describes itself as credible, current and comprehensive, is produced by the National Cancer Institute of the US. It has sections describing all types of cancer, treatment options and clinical trials. There is a choice for information to be presented for the patient or for the health care professional. There are links to over 100 other websites, although these are mainly American ones.

CancerBACUP, www.cancerbacup.org.uk

This is the UK's leading cancer information service. The full text of all CancerBACUP information booklets is available, as well as the answers to over 500 frequently asked questions. There is a resources database, and professionals' section, with links to authoritative UK guidelines. Literature searches using Medline, for example, and other bibliographic databases can be performed through this site.

Department of Health, www.doh.gov.uk/cancer

Most government publications relevant to cancer, for example the *National Cancer Plan* and *The Nursing*

Contribution to Cancer Care can be accessed and downloaded from this website. Other important documents to be found on this website are the *Improving Outcomes* series related to cancers of different sites. For each site, there are paired publications: the *Manual* and the *Research Evidence*. Cancers covered so far in this series are breast cancer, colorectal cancer, lung cancer, gynaecological cancers and upper gastro-intestinal cancers. More will be published in due course.

Palliative Care Formulary, www.palliativedrugs.com

This website provides essential, comprehensive and independent information for health professionals about the use of drugs in palliative care. It highlights drugs given for unlicensed indications or by unlicensed routes and the administration of multiple drugs by continuous subcutaneous infusion.

Index

Note: Drugs are listed by their generic name.

chronic lymphocytic leukaemia
   (CLL) 194–5
chronic myeloid leukaemia (CML) 195–6
cigarette smoking 4–5
   preventive health interventions
      10–11, 125–6
CIN grades for cervical dysplasia 43
cisplatin 73
   auditory impairment from 98
   renal toxicity 99
citalopram 254
cladribine 73
Clark's classification, for malignant
      melanoma 172–3
clinical trials 95–6
   breast cancer 39, 78–9
CNS lymphoma, and AIDS 206
CNS metastases, palliative treatment
      238–40
CNS tumours
   in children 31, 224–7
   classification 190–1
   corticosteroid therapy 81
   investigations 189–90
   presentation 29, 189
   support organisations 286
co-analgesics 248
codeine 245–6
Colon Cancer Concern 286
colorectal cancer
   aetiology 118
   and diet 5–6
   geographical incidence 13
   histopathology reporting 45
   inherited susceptibility 8, 17–18, 19
   investigations 119–20
   presentation 26, 119
   screening 39–40, 118–19
   staging 120–1
   treatment
      adjuvant chemotherapy 121–2
      adjuvant radiotherapy 122
      follow-up 122–3
      locally advanced disease 123
      metastatic disease 123–4
      palliative radiotherapy 124
      surgery 120
Committee on Safety of Medicines 96
communication
   with children 271–2
   and domiciliary terminal care 266
community services
   and domiciliary terminal care 265–6
   and hospice care 268–9
   and shared care 54–5
co-morbidity
   diabetes mellitus 263
   heart disease 262
   liver disease 263
   renal failure 263–4
   respiratory disease 262–3
   and treatment options 261–2
complementary therapies 90–1
computed tomographic
      colonography 40

computed tomography (CT),
      lung cancer screening 41
confusion 254–5
connective tissue tumours see sarcomas
constipation, treatment 251
contraceptive pill, and breast cancer 9,
      116
Coping with Cancer (support
      organisation) 282
corticosteroids 81–2
   for anorexia 249
   as antiemetics 250
   for pain 248
   visual impairment from 97–8
cosmic radiation, and breast cancer 7
cough 255–6
counselling 89
   genetic counselling 18
craniopharyngioma 191
   in children 226
   radionuclide therapy 63–4
crocidolite (blue asbestos)
   and mesothelioma 216
   occupational cancers 4
cutaneous cancers see skin cancer
cyclizine 250
cyclophosphamide 73
   and second malignancies 102
cyproterone acetate 79–80
cytarabine 73
cytology 42–3
cytotoxic drugs see chemotherapy

dacarbazine 73
dactinomycin 73
daunorubicin 73
death
   bereavement care 275
   in childhood 272
   at home 273–4
   hospice care 268–9
dental problems 99, 255
depression 254
dexamethasone 81–2
   for anorexia 249
   as antiemetic 93–4, 250
   for pain 248
dextromoramide 248
dextropropoxyphene 245–6
diabetes mellitus, and treatment
      options 263
diagnosis
   early detection 11–12
   genetic testing 18–19
   presentation see presentation
   staging 47–9
   tissue diagnosis 42
      cytology 42–3
      histology 43–6
   see also screening
diamorphine 247–8
diarrhoea
   from chemotherapy 70
   treatment 251–2

diazepam 250, 254
   as muscle relaxant 248
diclofenac 246
dietary factors
   and cancer aetiology 5–6
   and chemotherapy 94
   complementary therapy 90
   preventive health interventions 11
dietetics 88
differentiating agents 83–4
diffuse large B-cell lymphoma 202
dihydrocodeine 245–6
dipipanone 248
disodium pamidronate 84–5
DNA intercalating agents 73, 75
DNA repair mechanisms, and cancer
      susceptibility 8
docetaxel 74
domiciliary terminal care 265–7
domperidone 93–4, 250
doxorubicin 74
   cardiotoxicity 100
drugs, cytotoxic see chemotherapy
dry mouth 99, 255
ductal carcinoma in situ (DCIS)
   pathology 106–7
   treatment 108
Dukes' staging, for colorectal
      cancer 120–1
dysphagia 252–3
dysplasia, cervical
   cytology 42–3
   screening 36–7
   treatment 159
dyspnoea 256–8

ear, tumours of 155
elderly patients
   breast cancer therapy 115–16
   treatment options 233–4
electron beam therapy 62
endocrine system
   and cancer aetiology 8–9
   late effects of therapy 99, 229
endocrine therapy see hormone
      therapy
endometrial cancer 166–7
   brachytherapy 62–3
   geographical incidence 14
   hormonal influences 9
   hormonal therapy 80
   presentation 26–7
ependymomas 190–1, 226
epidemiology 13–15
epirubicin 74
Eptstein–Barr virus (EBV) 6–7
estramustine 74
etoposide 74
   and second malignancies 102
evidence-based oncology, clinical
      trials 95–6
Ewing's sarcoma 30, 212
exemestane 78–9
exfoliative cytology 42–3

lymphoma (*continued*)
    support organisations 287
    and viral infection 6–7
Lymphoma Association 287

Macmillan Cancer Relief 281
Make-a-wish Foundation UK 283
male breast cancer 117
malignant fibrous histiocytoma
    of bone 213
malignant melanoma
    aetiology 169
    diagnosis 170–1
    incidence 14, 169
    presentation 29–30
    time trends 15
    treatment 172–3
malnutrition, and dysphagia 252–3
mammography 19, 38–9
mantle cell lymphoma 201
marginal zone lymphoma 201
Marie Curie Cancer Care 281, 289
massage 91
mastectomy 109–10
    and familial cancer syndromes 19
medical physicists 88
Medical Research Council 289
medroxyprogesterone acetate 79
megestrol acetate 79
melaena 258–9
melphalan 74
meningiomas 191
menopause, induction of, breast cancer
    therapy 76–7
mercaptopurine 74
Merkel cell carcinoma 173–4
mesothelioma 4, 216
    June Hancock Mesothelioma
        Research Fund 285
metal dust exposure, occupational
    cancers 4
metastases
    image-guided ablation 86
    neck lymph nodes 155–6
    palliative treatment
        bone marrow disease 242
        bone metastases 237–8
        brain metastases 238–40
        liver metastases 240–1
        pulmonary metastases 241–2
        spinal cord compression 240
        superior vena cava obstruction 242
    salvage surgery 59–60
    TNM classification 48–9
    and treatment choices 56–7
methadone 247
    for cough 256
methotrexate 68, 74–5
    renal toxicity 99
metoclopramide 93–4, 250
midazolam
    as antiemetic 250
    as muscle relaxant 248
mitomycin 75

mitoxantrone 75
molar pregnancies 168
monoclonal antibodies
    and histopathology 45
    therapeutic 82–3
morphine 246–7
mouth
    cancer *see* oral cavity cancer
    dry/sore 99, 255
mucosa associated lymphoid tissue
    (MALT) lymphoma 201
mucositis, from chemotherapy 70
multidisciplinary cancer teams 53–4
    see also shared care
multiple myeloma 202
muscle relaxants 248
muscle weakness 259–60
musculoskeletal effects of therapy
    100, 229
mustine (chlormethine) 73
mycosis fungoides 174, 201–2
myeloma 202
    International Myeloma
        Foundation (UK) 287
    presentation 28
myelosuppression 69–70, 92–3
myopathy 260

naproxen 246
nasal cancer 154
    and occupational exposure 4
    presentation 28–9
nasopharyngeal cancer
    age variations 14
    geographical variations 13
    inherited susceptibility 8
    presentation 28–9
National Association of Laryngectomee
    Clubs 286
National Cancer Alliance 279–80
National Cancer Research Institute 289
National Cancer Research Network 289
National Health Service (NHS)
    breast cancer screening programme
        38–9
    cervical cancer screening programme
        37
nausea 70
    antiemetic therapy 93–4, 249–50,
        271
neck cancer *see* head and neck cancer
neoadjuvant chemotherapy 66
nephrotoxicity, from therapy 70,
    99, 230
    tumour lysis syndrome 94
nerve root compression 260
neuroblastoma
    in children 31–2, 227
    differentiating agents 83–4
    monoclonal antibody therapy 83
    screening 41
Neuroblastoma Society 288
neuroectodermal tumours, intracranial
    191

neuroendocrine tumours
    carcinoid tumours 214–15
    radionuclide therapy 63–4
    somatostatin analogue therapy 82
neuropathy, from therapy 98, 111
neuropsychological effects of therapy,
    late effects 98–9, 229
neurotoxicity, from chemotherapy 71
neutropenia 69, 92–3
nicotine-replacement therapy 10
non-Hodgkin's lymphoma (NHL)
    and AIDS 205–6
    in children 31, 223–4
    classification 200–3
    corticosteroid therapy 81
    monoclonal antibody therapy 82–3
    presentation 28, 199–200
non-seminomatous germ cell tumours
    see testicular cancer
non-small cell lung cancer (NSCLC)
    see lung cancer
nonsteroidal anti-inflammatory drugs
    (NSAIDs) 246
norethisterone 79
nurse specialists 87
    and domiciliary terminal care 265–7
    and hospice care 268–9
nutritional factors
    and cancer aetiology 5–6
    and chemotherapy 94
    complementary therapy 90
    dietetics 88
    and dysphagia 252–3

occult blood testing 19, 40
occupational cancers 4
occupational therapy 89
octreotide 82
oesophageal cancer
    geographical incidence 13
    investigations 136–7
    outcomes 138
    palliative treatment 137–8
    presentation 25–6, 136
    risk factors 4–5, 136
    treatment 137
Oesophageal Patients' Association 286
oestrogen deprivation therapy 76–7
oestrogen receptor antagonists
    for breast cancer 77–8
    for endometrial cancer 80
oestrogens
    and breast cancer 9, 116–17
    for prostate cancer 79
oligodendrogliomas 190–1
oncology pharmacists 88
ondansetron 93, 250
'one stop clinics', and early
    detection 11–12
oophorectomy 19, 76–7
opioids
    analgesics 245–8, 271
    for cough 256
    for dyspnoea 257